CHEST AND CARDIAC RADIOLOGY

Chest and Cardiac Radiology

NICER Series on Diagnostic Imaging

Edited by

Charles B. Higgins, MD
Professor of Radiology
University of California
School of Medicine
San Francisco, USA

Holger Pettersson, MD
Professor and Chairman
Department of Radiology
University of Lund, Lund, Sweden

Merit Communications

ISBN 1 873413 25 4

Published by
Merit Communications
7 Salisbury Place
Langton Road
London SW9 6UW
England

Printed by
Butler & Tanner Ltd
Frome and London

NYCOMED

Reprinted papers
are available from
Merit Communications

Contents

Contributors

Sylvia Heywang, MD
Radiology Clinic and Polyclinic
in Grosshadern Clinic of
Ludwig-Maximilians-University
Munich, Germany

Chisato Kondo, MD
Department of Radiology
University of California
School of Medicine
San Francisco, California, USA

David Naidich, MD
Department of Radiology
Bellevue Hospital
New York, New York, USA

Stuart S. Sagel, MD
Mallinckrodt Institute of
Radiology
Washington University School of
Medicine
St Louis, Missouri, USA

Lynn Steinbach, MD
Department of Radiology
University of California
School of Medicine
San Francisco, California, USA

Richard D. White, MD
Section of Cardiovascular Imaging
Division of Radiology
Cleveland Clinic Foundation
Cleveland, Ohio, USA

Charles B. Higgins, MD
Department of Radiology
University of California
School of Medicine
San Francisco, California, USA

Nestor Müller, MD
Department of Radiology
Vancouver General Hospital
Vancouver, British Columbia
Canada

Rainer Reinmüller, MD
Radiology Clinic and Polyclinic
in Grosshadern Clinic of
Ludwig-Maximilians-University
Munich, Germany

Udo Sechtem, MD
Clinic for Inner Medicine
University of Cologne
Cologne, Germany

Peter Vock, MD
Department of Diagnostic
Radiology
University of Berne Hospital
Berne, Switzerland

Elias A. Zerhouni, MD
Department of Radiology
The Johns Hopkins Hospital
Baltimore, Maryland, USA

Carl J. Zylak, MD
Breast Screening Program for
Ontario
McMaster University Medical
Center
Hamilton, Ontario, Canada

Preface

Progress in diagnostic imaging has proceeded at a staggering rate during the past decade. The increment in new knowledge resulting from new diagnostic procedures have eclipsed even the most optimistic predictions. Consequently the need to disperse this new knowledge and to promulgate the proper and efficient use of new diagnostic imaging techniques has considerably taxed the traditional modes for dissemination of this information. A timely synthesis of such information as it relates to specific organ systems is important for the worldwide implementation of these technologic and diagnostic innovations. Such worldwide dissemination of evolving concepts is provided by the NICER program of educational courses, books and newsletters. This volume represents the first of a series of books which provide a synthesis of updated information pertaining to Radiology of the Chest and Heart.

The thirteen chapters for this volume were carefully chosen in order to provide information on topics about which considerable new information has appeared in the past few years. Plain radiography and computed tomography remain the most frequently utilized techniques for imaging of the chest. A chapter demonstrates the use of plain radiography and CT for solving a recurring diagnostic dilemma, the differentiation between lung abscess and empyema. The most frequent uses of CT for chest diagnosis are reviewed in separate chapters focussed on: the staging of lung carcinoma; evaluation of mediastinal masses; and the assessment of parenchymal lung diseases. The role of MRI in thoracic disease is explored in chapters dealing with mediastinal masses and disorders of the chest wall. It is now becoming evident that MRI is the most effective technique for assessing abnormalities of the brachial plexus. This new application of MRI is discussed in one of the chapters.

The potential of MRI for the evaluation of cardiovascular disease is now recognized. Accordingly, separate chapters explore its application to: thoracic vascular disease, acquired heart disease and congenital heart disease. Speculative applications of MRI are also described in chapters on the use of MRI for quantifying blood flow in the central circulation and for the diagnosis of diseases of the breast.

We recognize the invigorating intellectual challenge required to keep these volumes relevant to the rapidly advancing wave of knowledge in diagnostic imaging. We feel that this volume is current for 1991–1992; moreover, the task of timely updating this knowledge is enthusiastically accepted.

San Francisco and Lund, Oct. 1991
Charles B. Higgins, M.D.
Holger Pettersson, M.D.

Computed tomography of parenchymal lung disease

Elias A. Zerhouni
Johns Hopkins University School of Medicine, Baltimore, USA

Introduction

Since the 1980s, computed tomography (CT) has played an increasingly important role in the evaluation of pulmonary parenchymal disease. With the advent of scanners permitting studies during suspended respiration and the development of high resolution software, both focal and diffuse pulmonary parenchymal processes can now be reliably evaluated. The increasing availability of CT scanners has led to a dramatic increase in the use of CT in assessing diffuse pulmonary parenchymal pathology. In this chapter we address the state of the art in the investigation of focal and diffuse parenchymal lung disease.

Focal Lung Disease

Good technique is essential for interpreting focal lung pathology with CT. The plain chest radiograph should be available whenever possible as a guide to the CT study. As a general rule, a non-contrast examination with contiguous 8 - 10 mm thick sections should be performed first. Thick sections are advantageous because they demonstrate blood vessels as branching structures, allowing easy recognition. On thinner sections, vessels may simulate small parenchymal nodules, and are more difficult to recognize (Fig. 1). Once a focal abnormality is localized with the thick sections, thin sections may then be used for accurate densitometry or to better define the features of the focal process. In most cases, intravenous contrast enhancement is not needed except to differentiate vascularized parenchyma from non-vascularized collections or necrotic parenchymal regions. Administration of contrast should preferably be done with a fast bolus injection with rapid acquisition of scans over a 30 - 60 second period. For vascular lesions such as arteriovenous malformations, a dynamic CT

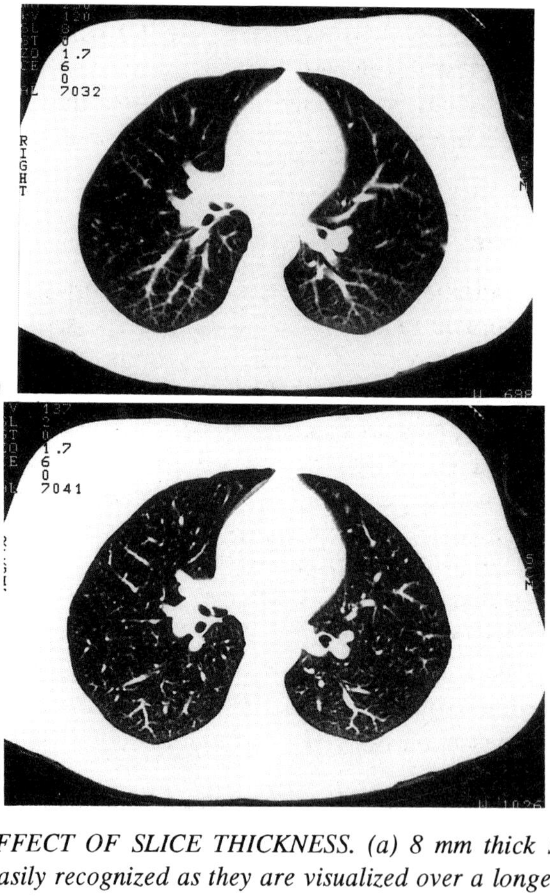

(a)

(b)

Figure 1. *EFFECT OF SLICE THICKNESS. (a) 8 mm thick scan. Blood vessels are easily recognized as they are visualized over a longer portion of their course as branching structures. (b) 2 mm section at the same anatomical level. Except for those within the thin slice, vessels are seen in cross section as small dots. Differentiation of small focal abnormalities from blood vessels is easier on thick section scans.*

angiographic technique should be used. For more complex parenchymal processes, bolus injection followed by rapid infusion is preferable. Contrast medium should never be used when attempting densitometry of lung nodules because it may increase the attenuation values and falsely simulate a benign calcified nodule. Proper window settings for hard copies are essential. Display of thoracic CT images requires at least two window settings. Window levels should be selected at the mid-point between the average density of the structure or abnormality one wants to demonstrate and the average density of the surrounding medium. In the lung parenchyma, most focal lesions measure between 20 and 80 Hounsfield Units (HU), and the lung measures about -750 to -850 HU. Therefore, for parenchymal studies, appropriate window levels are between -350 and -450 HU. The window width should be selected to encompass the entire range of densities present in the thorax which ranges between 1400 and 2000 HU.

Nodular Lesions

Evaluation of pulmonary nodules is one of the most common clinical problems in thoracic imaging. CT is helpful in cases where a questionable nodule is suspected on plain radiographs. By overcoming the problem of summation of structures in complex anatomic areas, such as the apices, the paraspinal, perihilar, pericardiac and peridiaphragmatic regions, CT is of value in confirming or excluding the presence of a suspected nodule. Often, confusing shadows due to osseous or vascular structures can be easily clarified with CT. CT has the intrinsic advantage of providing a high contrast image in which nodular lesions appear white against a black background, thus enhancing recognition. The real challenge, however, is to determine the benign or malignant nature of the detected lung nodule. Indeed, the majority of solitary pulmonary nodules represent benign granulomas. Systematic biopsy or resection of all pulmonary nodules would be clinically impractical. Diagnostic radiologists have long searched for effective methods of differentiating benign from malignant nodules. A major diagnostic clue to the granulomatous nature of a nodule is the presence of calcific deposits in typical patterns such as in a central nidus, or in a laminated or diffuse pattern. The presence of such calcific deposits is a widely accepted non-histological criterion for certifying nodules as benign. CT, with thin sections to reduce partial volume effects, can demonstrate small amounts of calcification not detectable by conventional radiography or tomography. Furthermore, CT permits objective and quantifiable assessments of nodule density.

In an early study by Siegelman et al, 30% of benign nodules in a group of 91 lesions demonstrated unsuspected calcification by thin section CT [1]. Initially, CT densitometry of lung nodules could not be reproduced on all scanners owing to lack of standardization and limited understanding of the technical issues involved in accurately measuring CT numbers in the lung environment [2]. With the advent of modern and more reliable scanners and standardization of CT measurements with either reference phantoms or special calibration, accurate detection of the calcified nodule has become possible and effective on any scanner [3]. In 1986, a co-operative study involving ten centers in the United States demonstrated the usefulness of CT in the management of lung nodules [4]. This study demonstrated that thin-section CT can detect unsuspected calcification in about one-half of benign nodules. Although a reference phantom was the most sensitive and reliable way of performing CT densitometry for pulmonary nodules, obvious calcification can often be seen with the simple use of thin-section scans (Fig. 2). At the present time, thin-section CT scanning has replaced conventional tomography in most centres for the evaluation of the lung nodule. CT densitometry is helpful in the management of lung nodules, not only by detecting calcification but also by reliably demonstrating absence of calcification. Indeed, with optimal CT densitometry, the lack of calcification has become a strong indicator of malignant disease. In our experience, more than 80% of lesions less than 2 cm in diameter, with no evidence of calcification on thin-section CT, turn out to be malignant. Thus, CT provides a means of effectively segregating small nodules that can be conservatively followed by repeat radiographs from those in which a high probability of malignancy can be inferred by reliable demonstration of the absence of any calcification. Such non-calcified nodules are, justifiably, aggressively managed by needle biopsy and surgery.

Today, CT has become an integral part of the diagnostic approach to the pulmonary nodule. There are, however, important caveats. First, CT has proven effective only in nodules less than 3 cm in diameter and in those with discrete, smooth or slightly lobulated margins. CT rarely yields a confident diagnosis of benign disease in

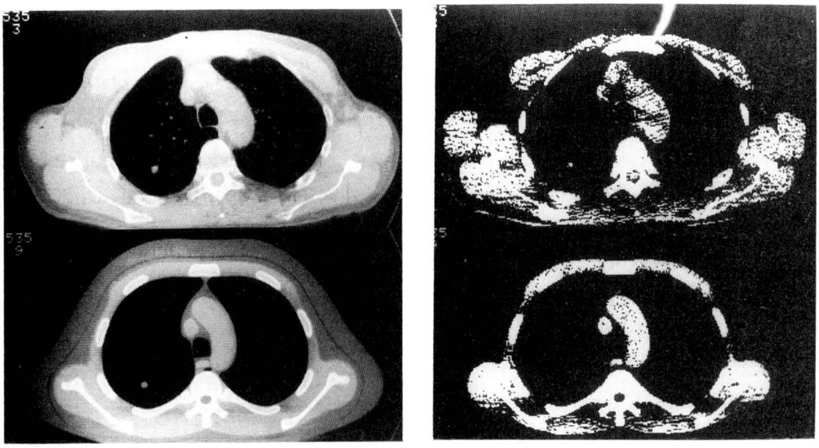

(a) (b)

Figure 2. *LUNG NODULE DENSITOMETRY. An 8 mm nodule was discovered on a plain film in a 42-year-old smoker. (a) The patient was scanned with thin sections and the nodule can be seen in the right upper lobe (top half image). One or two pixels of slightly higher attenuation can be recognized on this thin-section scan. To achieve more precise quantification of calcification a reference phantom test was performed consisting of scanning a standard phantom that simulates the patient's anatomy as well as size and position of the nodule (bottom half of a) (b) Same image as (a) but using a minimum window width. With the phantom method, the presence of calcification is determined by comparing a scan of the patient to that of the reference phantom. In this case at a level of 54 HU, several pixels of high value can be seen in the patient's nodule (top half) whereas the reference nodule (bottom half) is no longer seen. Extensive calcification is present in this nodule, which is thus most likely benign.*

larger nodules or in those with irregular or spiculated borders [4]. In such cases, proceeding directly to tissue sampling with either needle biopsy, bronchoscopy, or surgery is more appropriate. Areas of calcification can be routinely demonstrated in a small percentage of carcinomas. Calcified carcinomas occur near pre-existing scars, when engulfing nearby granulomas or when demonstrating intrinsic dystrophic calcifications. With CT, up to 10% of carcinomas may demonstrate calcifications. In carcinomas, the calcifications are generally eccentric with a stippled pattern. The great majority of calcified carcinomas are lesions larger than 3 cm in diameter. However, a few cases less than 3 cm in diameter have been reported. Thus, one should exercise caution and certify a nodule benign only when the typical patterns of benign calcification are seen.

In addition, extreme caution should be used when scanning patients with a higher likelihood of calcified malignant nodules such as patients with known history of tumours (mucinous adenocarcinomas or sarcomas) with a high propensity for calcification. In addition, any nodule diagnosed as benign by CT should be followed for at least 2 years by repeat radiographs.

Besides increased accuracy in assessing nodular calcification, CT has the unique capability of demonstrating fat in solitary nodules, certifying the diagnosis of pulmonary hamartoma. The pulmonary hamartoma is the third most common cause of resected pulmonary nodules, accounting for 6 - 8% of lesions. Typically, it is indistinguishable from other nodules unless the distinctive 'popcorn-like' calcification is present. The fatty tissue component of hamartoma can be uniquely recognized with CT (Fig. 3). In a series of 47 cases of hamartomas, fat alone was detected in 18 and fat plus calcification in 10 [5]. Except for lipoid pneumonias, no other focal parenchymal pathology harbors fat in significant amounts, making this CT sign a strong aetiological indicator of the hamartomatous nature of a nodule. Thin section scans of excellent quality are mandatory to avoid the risk of misinterpreting air cavities within nodules as low-density fat.

Metastatic Nodules

CT is clearly the most sensitive means of detecting metastatic lung disease. However, the increased sensitivity of CT also leads to the discovery of many incidental focal pulmonary densities. Detection of such abnormalities in the oncologic patient, who is generally prone to pulmonary infections, increases the need to ensure that these lesions truly represent metastatic disease.

This problem is one of the most commonly encountered in the management of oncological patients. Even though no single criterion or combination of criteria permit a specific diagnosis, some features are typical of metastatic disease such as multiplicity of lesions, predominantly distributed in the outer one-third of the lower lobes within 3 cm of the pleural surfaces is characteristic. Metastatic lesions are more likely to be spherical or ovoid, whereas linear triangular, irregularly shaped, or multiple ill-defined lesions, especially centrally located, are less likely to represent metastasis. In a study of multiple

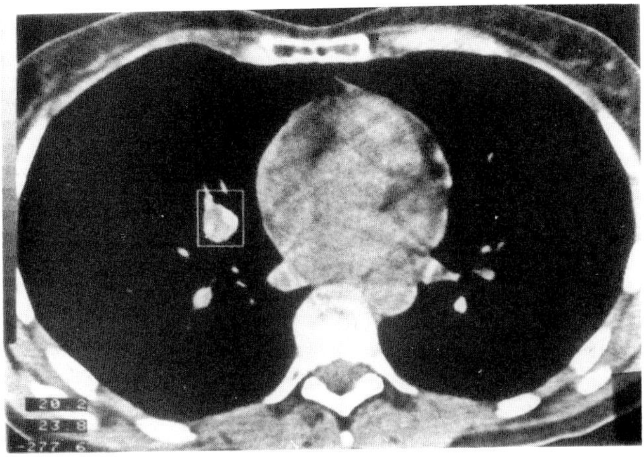

Figure 3. *PULMONARY HAMARTOMA. A 2.5 cm lesion is seen on the right side. This lesion demonstrates peripheral calcification. In addition, areas of low attenuation in the range of fat were detected in the centre of the lesion. Finding of fat with or without calcification on a thin section scan of a smooth or slightly lobulated nodule is pathognomonic of pulmonary hamartoma.*

pulmonary nodules detected by CT, non-calcified round lesions larger than 2.5 cm or numbering more than 10 were always metastatic [6]. In such cases, biopsy of the lesions is recommended if a diagnosis of metastasis would significantly alter therapy. In other instances, an increasingly used alternative is to assess the growth rate of lesions by comparing changes in size on sequential examinations In addition, helpful morphological signs, such as the demonstration of a vascular connection between the pulmonary arterial bed and a peripheral lung lesion, can be extremely helpful. Typically, metastatic nodules appear connected to a pulmonary artery branch when the vessel runs parallel to the scanned plane (Fig. 4). Although not specific, the finding of such a sign should strongly suggest the diagnosis of haematogenous metastasis [7,8]. CT has also proven helpful in evaluating the patient who presents with an apparently solitary pulmonary nodule after detection and treatment of an extrathoracic malignancy. In such cases the critical question is to determine whether this new nodule represents a primary cancer of the lung or a solitary metastasis from the previously diagnosed malignancy. Statistically, the likelihood of a new primary lesion is high for epidermoid carcinomas (65%) and

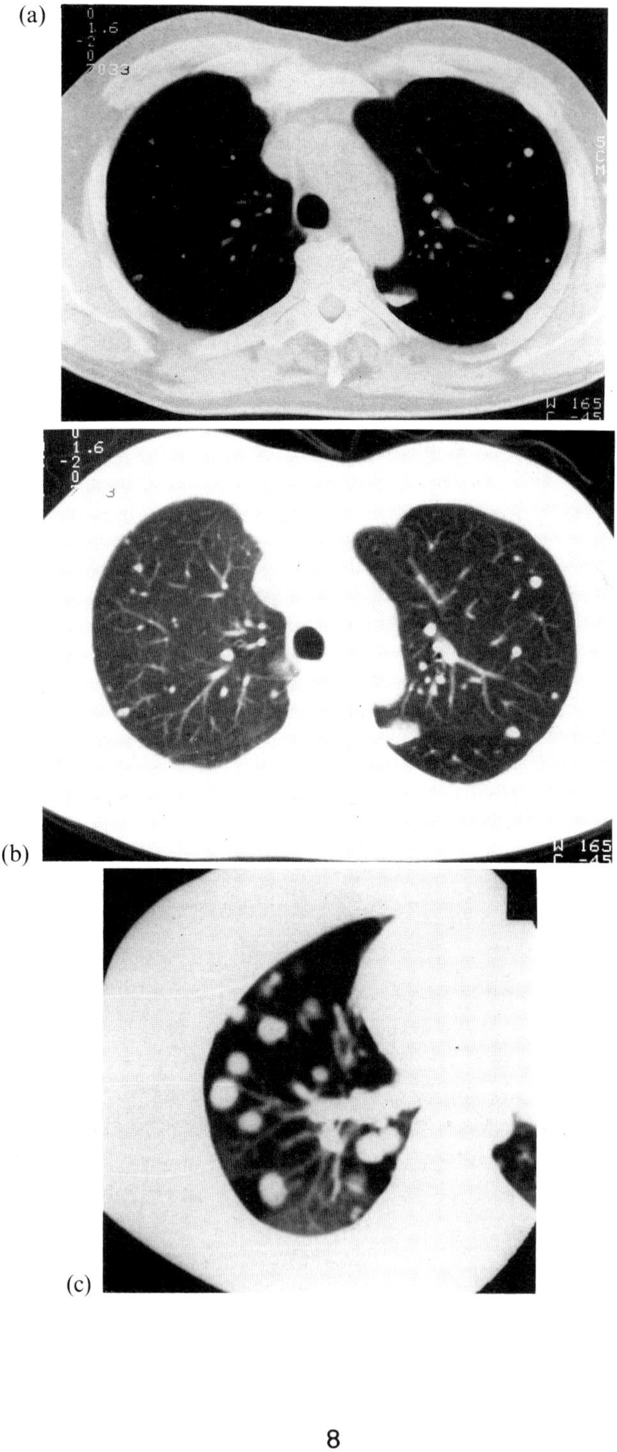
(a)
0
1.6
-20
0
7033
5CM
W 165
(b)
0
1.6
-20
0
W 165
(c)

adenocarcinomas (50%). With extrathoracic sarcomas, a solitary nodule is much more likely to represent a metastatic lesion. Thus, CT examination of the remainder of the lung is mandatory to ensure that the visualized nodule is truly solitary. If additional lesions are found, the diagnosis of metastatic disease is much more likely. If no other lesion is found with CT, the newly discovered nodule should be considered a new primary lung cancer until proven otherwise.

Bronchial Carcinoid

The bronchial carcinoid tumor is another focal lesion that can often be recognized by its morphologic features and anatomic relationships. Carcinoids are most commonly found at bifurcations of lobar or segmental bronchi, an anatomical association that is very suggestive of the diagnosis. Characteristically, these lesions demonstrate smooth borders with splaying but without destruction of the nearby bronchi. In a third of the lesions, coarse calcification can be seen due to areas of cartilaginous or bony transformation [9]. Classically, atelectasis of the lobe or segment can be seen. Today, however, early detection afforded by CT leads to the frequent discovery of such lesions before the development of atelectasis. These lesions should be considered low grade malignancies and managed as such [10]. The long term prognosis when these lesions are removed is excellent, with a 95% survival rate at 5 years.

Arteriovenous Malformations

Most arteriovenous malformations (AVMs) are easily recognizable

---

Figure 4. *METASTATIC LUNG DISEASE. (a and b) Patient with known osteosarcoma presenting with multiple calcified nodules. Scan at lung window settings demonstrates scattered tiny nodules which appear connected to adjacent pulmonary vessels on this 2 mm thin section scan. (c) More advanced case of metastatic disease. Note again vascular connection with vessels leading to the metastatic lesions which are predominantly distributed in the outer third of the lung parenchyma. This appearance and distribution is characteristic. Note also the presence of a zone of low attenuation between the metastatic nodule and the pleural surface, presumably due to hypoperfusion of the parenchyma secondary to embolization of the pulmonary artery by the metastatic process.*

with CT through the demonstration of their vascular connections. Typically, an enlarged feeding artery and an enlarged draining vein can be demonstrated. With dynamic CT scanning and intravenous contrast enhancement, a vascular pattern can be seen and a firm diagnosis established.

Pulmonary Embolus and Infarction

CT has not been useful in the demonstration of peripheral pulmonary emboli in the lung parenchyma, although large central pulmonary emboli can be demonstrated using contrast enhancement. CT, however, is helpful in recognizing pulmonary infarcts and septic embolic processes. As for haematogenous metastasis, a vascular correction is often recognized when septic emboli or pulmonary infarcts are present. Typically, septic emboli or lung infarcts can be recognized by a subpleural location, a triangular shape with the apex of the lesion directed toward the pulmonary hilum, and thickening of the adjacent pleura (Fig. 5) [11]. Cavitation of such lesions is a common finding [12]. In addition, following intravenous contrast injection, the periphery of the lesion enhances in a rim-like fashion without enhancement of the centre.

Focal Inflammatory Disease

A focal infiltrate that persists despite presumably effective therapy is one of the most vexing problems in clinical practice. In such cases, the possibility of a proximal obstructive lesion should be excluded. CT is well-suited to such a task as an adjunct to bronchoscopy. Often, bronchoscopy is hampered by the presence of associated inflammation due to postobstructive pneumonia. Such inflammation may obscure underlying lesions. In this context, CT is most valuable by providing a map of the bronchial tree and an accurate guide for the bronchoscopist. CT is helpful in demonstrating the absence of significant obstruction in many cases. Of critical importance in these cases is a perfect technique using thin 4 - 5 mm contiguous sections throughout the area of interest with the liberal use of intravenous contrast enhancement. Bronchiectasis is frequently the cause of a focal persistent infiltrate. This entity can be accurately depicted and staged with CT, and even minor degrees of the disease can be identified using thin-section scanning. One should remember that bronchiectasis can be reactive to the presence of infection in the lung and the possibility of a central obstructing lesion as the cause of underlying bronchiectasis should be excluded.

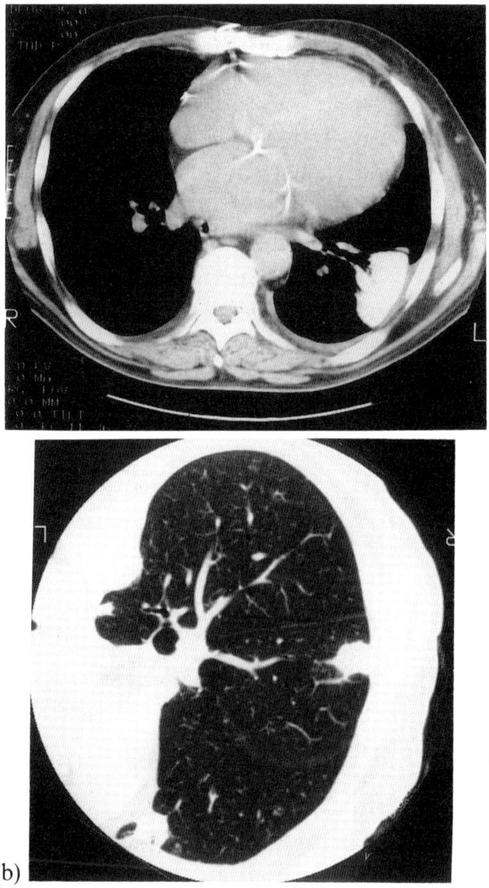

(a) (b)

Figure 5. *PULMONARY INFARCTS. (a) Embolic infarct in a patient with renal failure. Note the triangular shape of the infarct with its apex directed towards the hilum. Note adjacent pleural thickening. Note that vessels are seen connected to the apex of the lesion. In this case, the lesion exhibits high attenuation values due to diffuse calcification, a common phenomenon-in patients with chronic renal failure and pulmonary infarction. (b) Septic infarcts in an intravenous drug abuser. Note several subpleural lesions with vessels leading to apex of each lesion.*

Focal Lesions in the Immunocompromised Patient

With the increasing incidence of immune deficiency and the increasing risk of opportunistic infection in the patient population, CT is used more often in the monitoring and early detection of these potentially lethal complications. In our experience, aggressive use of CT as early as possible in the course of the disease is of critical importance in the management of these patients. In some cases, a specific aetiology such as invasive aspergillosis is suggested (Fig. 6) [13]. CT helps direct tissue sampling by demonstrating the areas of the lung that are most involved.

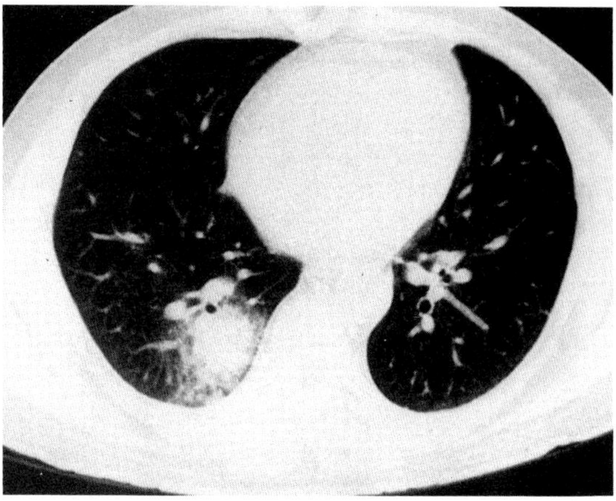

Figure 6. *EARLY INVASIVE PULMONARY ASPERGILLOSIS. 29-year-old patient after bone marrow transplant. Focal lesion is seen in right lower lobe with a halo of intermediate density. This halo sign is typical in the early phase of invasive aspergillosis. Case courtesy of Dr J. Kuhlman.*

Complex Pleural Parenchymal Pathology

CT has become a powerful tool for the management of patients with complex combined pleural and parenchymal pathology. In such patients, radiographs are difficult to interpret. CT is a helpful guide to therapy and helps distinguish pleural loculated fluid components that should be drained from parenchymal components that do not require intervention. This task is made easier by using adequate intravenous contrast enhancement. Normal vascularized parenchyma will demonstrate enhancement, whereas abscesses, areas of necrosis, and pleural collections will not.

CT of Diffuse Pulmonary Parenchymal Disease

CT is playing an increasingly important role in the investigation of diffuse lung disease. Plain radiography remains the standard technique for detection and characterization of diffuse pulmonary processes. However, one of the main limitations of plain radiography for the evaluation of such processes is the superimposition of structures due to the projectional format of that imaging method. With the advent of high resolution CT (HRCT), detailed analyses of the lung parenchyma have become possible. A body of work now exists establishing the basis for the interpretation and clinical application of HRCT.

Technical Considerations

Detailed analysis of parenchymal structure requires the use of HRCT techniques. HRCT consists of the combination of three essential elements: (1) The use of thin, 1 - 2 mm sections; (2) targeted reconstructions with fields-of-view (FOVs) restricted to each lung field individually; and (3) the use of high spatial resolution algorithm of reconstruction. On modern scanners, HRCT images can be acquired in a short scan time of less than 2 seconds with a 512 × 512 matrix and a mA factor typically varying between 140 and 170, depending upon the size of the patient. The exact scanning protocol may vary depending upon the expected pathology. When diffuse disease is known to be present and HRCT is used for further characterization, our recommendation is to use a limited number of scans encompassing the upper, middle and lower thorax. For example, in asbestosis, a widely used protocol includes scanning the entire thorax with 7 - 8 scans distributed at 3-cm intervals in the upper lungs and 2-cm intervals in the lower lungs. Others recommend scanning the entire thorax with 1 - 2 mm sections every 10 - 15 mm. In cases where diffuse disease is not known to be present, a standard CT scan may first be performed. Thin section scans can then be prescribed at levels where a suspicion of pathology is found on the conventional thick section scans. In the great majority of cases, conventional thick section scans will demonstrate some ill-defined abnormality which can then be characterized further by HRCT scans at the appropriate anatomic levels.

The display of lung structure requires the use of appropriate electronic window settings. Precise settings are often a matter of subjective preference. However, there are guidelines that should be followed to ensure that pathology is not over or underestimated. Indeed, the appearance of lung structures can be drastically affected by the inappropriate use of window settings (see above).

Patient-related factors can also affect image quality in HRCT. Most important is the need to acquire images at full inspiration. Full inspiration promotes separation of parenchymal structures and aids analysis. A common patient-related artefact that can simulate pathology is the presence of dependent densities in the subpleural regions. These dependent densities have been shown to relate to areas of micro-atelectasis due to the effect of gravity on the dependent lung in supine patients. With HRCT, these areas can simulate pulmonary fibrosis. In such cases. it is critical to also examine the patient in the prone position. Pulmonary fibrosis will persist in the prone position whereas physiologically dependent densities will disappear (Fig. 7). Additionally, chest wall abnormalities that protrude in the lung parenchyma can also mimic pathology, presumably by compressing the adjacent lung parenchyma and creating areas of local atelectasis.

Normal Lung Structure by HRCT

The HRCT appearance of the normal lung is essentially determined by the limits of resolution of current scanners. This limit is about 300 μm. This resolution limit determines what structures and pathological processes will or will not be visualized by HRCT. At inspiration, the normal lung is composed of 80% air, 10% blood and 10% tissue. As the small mass of lung tissue is distributed over an enormous surface about the size of a tennis court, lung tissue is extremely delicate. The thickness of alveolar walls is about 20 - 30 μm and is an order of magnitude below the resolution of HRCT. Consequently, most of the lung tissue appears as homogeneous and featureless on HRCT. As the primary function of the lung is gas exchange, maintaining an extremely thin barrier between alveolar air and interstitial capillaries is essential. The lung is maintained in a stable position within the chest by its hilar connections to which the central or 'core' structures are

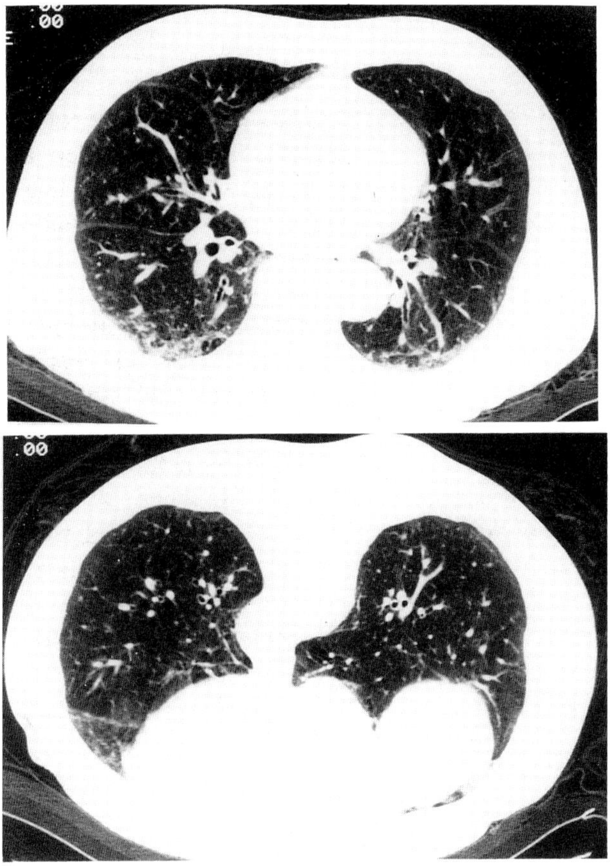

(a)

(b)

Figure 7. *DEPENDENT DENSITIES SIMULATING PULMONARY FIBROSIS. (a) Thin section scan in the supine position. Increased dependent densities are seen in the posterior aspect of the lower lobes bilaterally with apparent reticulation which closely resembles pulmonary fibrosis. (b) Same patient in the prone position. Almost complete clearing of the abnormalities seen in (a) is noted. Note increasing density now in the anterior aspects of the pulmonary parenchyma.*

attached. These core structures are represented essentially by the bronchovascular tree which forms the stem upon which the functional parenchyma distributes itself. At the periphery of the lung is the visceral pleura from which emanate connective tissue septa which support the pulmonary parenchyma. A well-organized fibre network extending from the central bronchovascular structures to the visceral pleura supports all the delicate alveolar wall structures, keeping capillaries and alveoli open for functional exchange. Bronchi and pulmonary arteries divide by dichotomous branching. There are about 23 generations of dichotomous branching in airways from the trachea to the alveolar sacs. Bronchi with wall thicknesses of less than 300 μm cannot be visualized. This corresponds to seventh to ninth generation bronchi. Thus, only centrally located bronchi can be seen on normal HRCT.

By contrast, there are 28 pulmonary arterial branchings; 300 μm pulmonary arteries represent the sixteenth to seventeenth generation branching, corresponding to arteries at the level of the terminal bronchioles and the most proximal respiratory bronchioles. Vascular structures, therefore, can be visualized to within a few millimeters of the pleural surfaces (see Fig. 1). Clearly, the vascular tree is a better landmark for defining the lung architecture by HRCT, since it can be followed to the level of the secondary lobule, which includes parenchyma supplied by about five terminal bronchioles. Characteristically, pulmonary arteries run parallel to the bronchi, whereas pulmonary veins course within the secondary lobule septa and are not accompanied by bronchi.

Basic Signs of Diffuse Lung Disease by HRCT

The alveolar interstitium is a complex structure of cells and extracellular matrix bounded by the alveolar epithelium on one side and the endothelium of the capillaries on the other. The most important constituent of the interstitium is connective tissue which help keep the alveoli open and regulate the movement of water, proteins, and cells within the alveolar walls. A large variety of agents can injure the lung. Remarkably, the response of the lung to such injuries appears stereotyped and relatively independent of the type of injury. Thus, there are a limited number of basic HRCT signs which express this lung response to injury [14]. HRCT signs are best approached by understanding the effects of this response on the CT appearance of the lung parenchyma.

Acute and Subacute Phase

Capillary endothelial cells and type I alveolar cells are most vulnerable to injury. Damage alters the permeability of these cells, leading to swelling and fragmentation. Leaks in the cellular lining of capillaries and/or alveoli promote the development of interstitial and alveolar oedema. Depending upon the type and severity of injury, this process can be self-limited. If massive, the epithelial lining becomes completely destroyed over vast areas. The denuded underlying tissue is then covered by a thick layer of fibrin and cell debris, leading to partial or complete filling of the alveolar air spaces. Consequently, in the acute phase, there is a relative reduction in the amount of air in the affected areas of the lungs. In addition, an increase in the alveolar wall thickness and the presence of debris, interstitial and alveolar oedema all lead to an increase in the background density of the lung parenchyma. This sign has been termed 'ground glass' opacification and is the most basic sign of acute pulmonary injury (Fig. 8). Muller et al have shown a correlation between the presence of ground glass opacities and activity of disease in patients with idiopathic pulmonary fibrosis [15]. They found that biopsies performed in areas of ground glass opacity most often corresponded to acute or subacute phases of the disease process and that tracking the extent and density of these opacities was useful in assessing response. Often, prominence of septal structures and thickening of the peribronchial soft tissues can

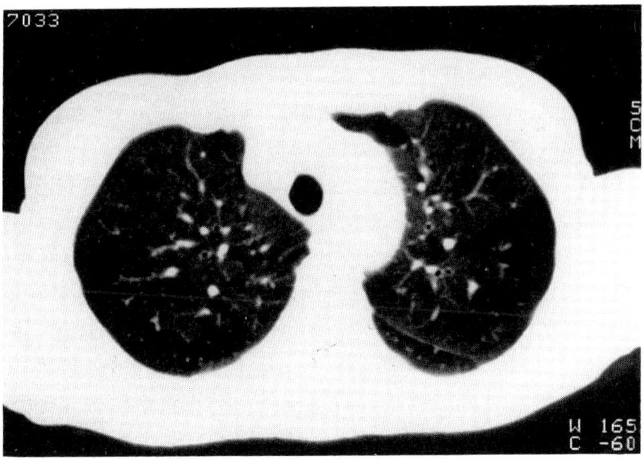

Figure 8. *ACUTE PHASE: GROUND GLASS OPACIFICATION. Note slightly increased background densities distributed in a geographic-like fashion. This is the most common sign of early acute diffuse alveolar damage by HRCT. At this stage, the plain film is often normal. This patient was diagnosed as having Pneumocystis carinii pneumonia.*

also be noted in these stages [16,17]. This is most probably due to lymphatic engorgement related to the removal of necrotic debris through airways or by macrophagic action and clearance through the lymphatic system.

With more severe stages of injury, complete filling of air spaces can precede the demonstration of air space nodules, eventually leading to the more typical alveolar infiltrate with air bronchograms [18].

Chronic Phase

In the chronic phase, various types of cells migrate into the interstitium. This recruitment of new cell types expands and thickens the interstitium. The type and proportion of these cells vary depending upon the injury but the physical result is similar and is characterized by thickening of the interstitium. On HRCT, this stage is manifested by thickening of the visceral pleural surfaces which appear finely irregular. Interlobular septa become more visible, forming reticular patterns which can be classified by the size of the reticular element. The most commonly recognizable reticular pattern is that of a network of polyhedral lines measuring 15 - 25 mm in diameter with, at their centre, a core pulmonary artery. This reticular pattern is characteristic of the secondary lobule architecture and can be seen in interstitial pulmonary oedema and in cases of lymphangitic carcinomatosis. Other reticular patterns can be recognized by HRCT. A medium reticulation with elements measuring 5 - 10 mm can be seen in many cases representing various degrees of severity in interstitial thickening. A very fine pattern with elements measuring 2 - 3 mm can often be seen in severe diffuse involvement of the interstitium such as that seen in miliary tuberculosis for example. During the evolution of a chronic interstitial process with reticulation, nodularity may appear. Typically, these nodules are localized at the junction points of the lines forming the reticular patterns. These nodules appear sharply marginated as opposed to air space nodules which typically have a very ill-defined border (Fig. 9).

End Stage Lung

In the later stages of the lung response to injury, alveolar structures are destroyed and the interstitium is no longer recognizable as a distinct entity. Local fusion of alveolar walls and destruction of

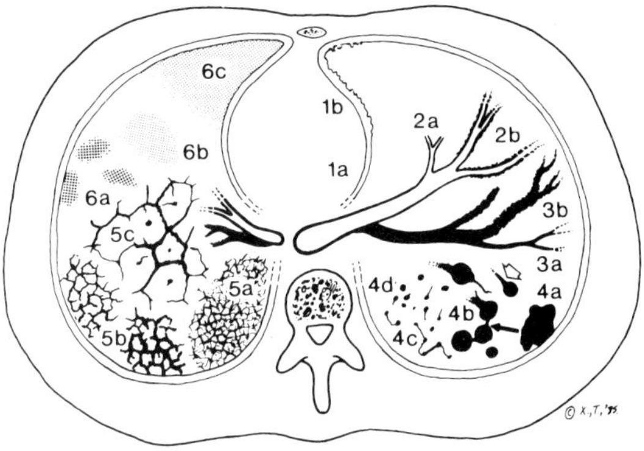

Figure 9. *HRCT SIGNS OF DIFFUSE PULMONARY PARENCHYMAL DISEASE. (1a) Normal appearance of visceral pleura. (1b) Slightly irregular serrated appearance of visceral pleura is typical of early interstitial disease. (2a) Normal bronchus. Normal bronchi are only visible to the mid lung field. (2b) When interstitial disease is present, bronchi are seen more distally as their wall thickens. The interface of bronchi with the surrounding pulmonary parenchyma also appears irregular and serrated due to the thickening of the interstitium. (3a) Normal pulmonary arteries. (3b) With interstitial disease the interface between vessels and lungs appears irregular. (4a - b) Examples of interstitial nodules. Note the sharp margination as well as the association with linear abnormalities in some cases. (5a) Fine reticulation. (5b) Medium reticulation. (5c) Large reticulation with a central pulmonary artery typical of secondary lobular architecture. (6a - c) Ground glass opacification typical of acute phase. (Reprinted from ref. 16).*

neighbouring acini is noted. Healing by fibrosis leads to the formation of dense areas of collagen interspersed with regions of parenchymal destruction and cystic formation. In such areas, bronchi appear dilated and 'tethered' by the destructive process. Large cystic and bullous areas rimmed with remnants of alveoli can be seen leading to the typical 'honeycombed' lung (Fig. 10). This ultimate destruction of lung tissue, the final act in the pulmonary defence process, is the surest sign on HRCT of end stage lung disease. This stage can be recognized very early even when cysts are less than 2 - 3 mm in size.

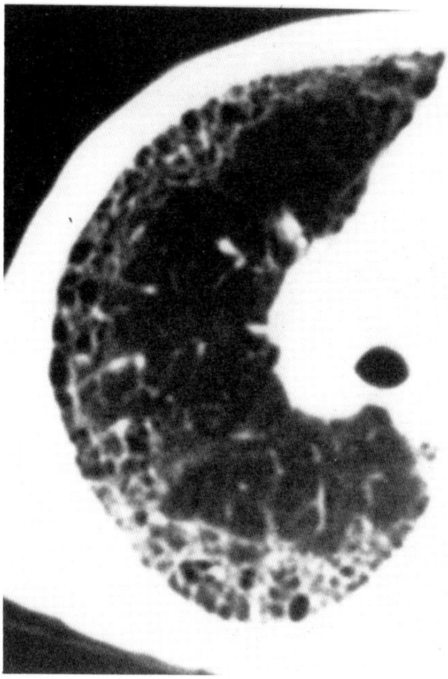

Figure 10. *'HONEYCOMB' LUNG IN END STAGE PULMONARY FIBROSIS. Note that the peripheral distribution of the honeycombing which consists of a combination of reticular changes interspersed with cystic spaces corresponding to destroyed alveolar structures.*

Characteristically, open lung biopsies performed in areas of honeycombing have a low diagnostic yield, since it represents a very late stage of response at which time the causative agent may no longer be recognizable. Thus, HRCT can provide preoperative guidance to the surgeon performing lung biopsy by steering him away from areas of honeycombing toward areas of ground glass opacities which are more likely to represent an early phase of the process.

Specific Disease Entities

A few specific entities will be presented here to familiarize the reader with the use of HRCT.

Lymphangitic Carcinomatosis

Pulmonary lymphangitic carcinomatosis refers to the spread of tumor within pulmonary lymphatics. This entity was one of the earliest to be specifically recognizable by HRCT [19]. Thickening and infiltration of interlobular septa and bronchovascular sheath is typical, with a large network of polyhedral reticular elements with a beaded appearance [20]. Pathologically, areas of beaded septal change have been found to correspond to non-uniform expansion of the septa by irregular tumour infiltration (Fig. 11).

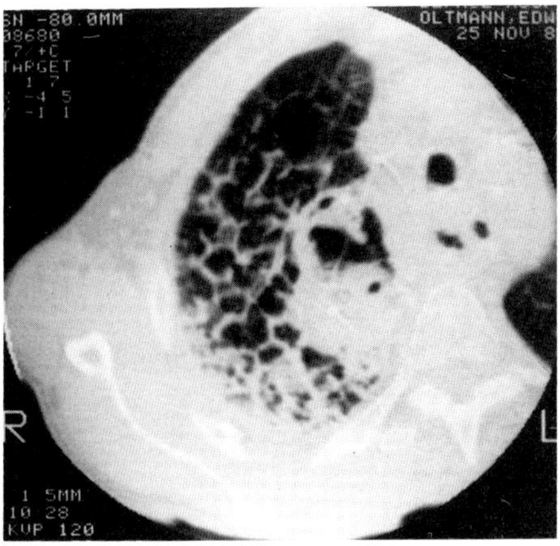

Figure 11. *LYMPHANGITIC CARCINOMATOSIS. Note polyhedral pattern of reticulation with elements corresponding to secondary lobule septa. Note beaded appearance of the thickened septa. Large central tumour seen near the mediastinum from which lymphangitic spread occurred.*

Miliary disease

The radiographic appearance of miliary processes is well known. HRCT appears capable of detecting the process before it becomes visible on plain radiography. Typically, a very fine diffuse reticular network of 2 - 3 mm basic elements is apparent throughout the interstitium (Fig. 12). As the process evolves, tiny nodules can be seen at the junction points of the reticular network. In addition to tuberculosis, numerous other diseases have been associated with a miliary pattern including pulmonary alveolar microatiasis, histoplasmosis, and reactions to methotrexate therapy.

Idiopathic Pulmonary Fibrosis (IPF)

IPF is a specific disorder defined by a combination of clinical, morphological, and radiological features. It is characterized by diffuse inflammation confined largely to the pulmonary interstitium. That in

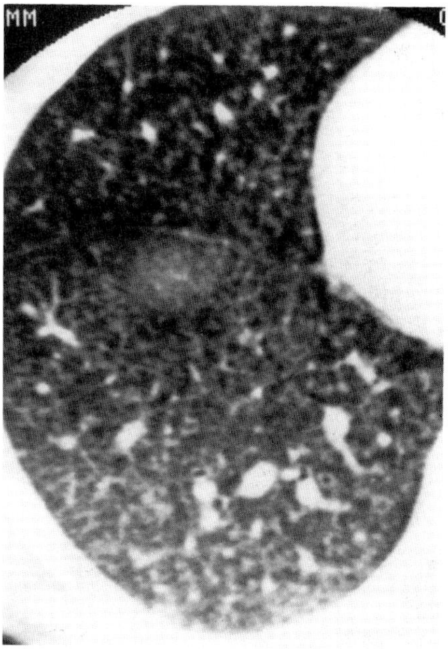

Figure 12. *MILIARY DISEASE. Example of early miliary tuberculosis. Note diffuse tine reticulation throughout the pulmonary parenchyma. Note also early micronodularity.*

itself is not specific and may be the result of numerous and diverse processes such as collagen vascular disease, pulmonary infections, and exposure to industrial agents, as well as a wide variety of genetic, metabolic, or inflammatory disorders. HRCT findings in patients with IPF have been extensively reported [16,21]. Patchy areas of ground glass opacification corresponding to areas of active inflammation are often seen [15]. IPF is characterized by a distinctive pattern of reticulation with medium-sized elements distributed preferentially at the periphery of the lungs in the subpleural regions (Fig. 13). Initially, linear subpleural lines with irregular visceral pleural surfaces can be seen with a progression towards reticulation and eventual cystic destruction with a characteristic pattern of honeycombing (Fig. 10). Not surprisingly, HRCT better delineates the full extent of IPF and in many cases can establish the presence or absence of the disease with a higher degree of diagnostic confidence.

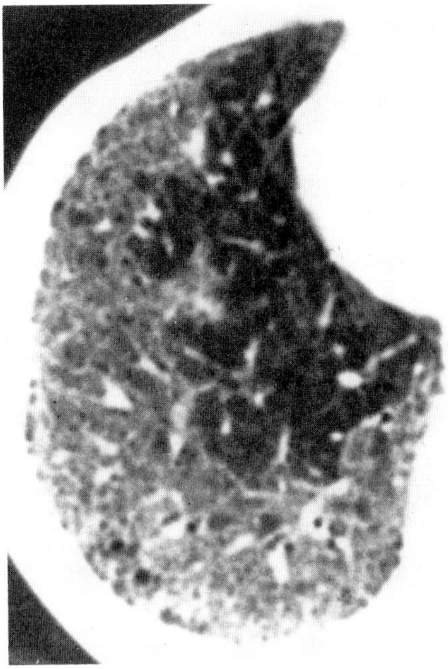

Figure 13. *IDIOPATHIC PULMONARY FIBROSIS. Note predominant involvement of the periphery of the lung. Note irregular appearance of the visceral pleural surfaces with formation of 'arcades' due to septal fibrosis. Note the presence of a ground glass opacity corresponding to a component of acute and subacute alveolitis. Note the presence of underlying reticulation of small to medium size with multiple tiny consist with early cystic destruction. (see also Fig. 10).*

Asbestosis

Asbestosis is defined as diffuse lung fibrosis due to asbestos exposure. It is one of the major occupationally-related causes of lung damage. The role of HRCT in evaluating patients with documented exposure to asbestos is becoming increasingly important. As shown by Aberle et al [22], characteristic findings in patients with asbestosis are: (1) subpleural lines; (2) thickened subpleural septa identified as single or branching lines; (3) parenchymal bands defined as coarse linear opacities extending through the lung; (4) increased non-dependent subpleural densities; and (5) honeycombing (Fig. 14).

Changes due to asbestosis are predominant in the subpleural regions of the lower lobes. As documented by Friedman et al, in an analysis of chest radiographs and HRCT in 60 patients, the positive predictive value of HRCT is much greater than that of chest radiography (100% vs. 79%, respectively) [23]. HRCT appears to be of great value in both excluding as well as confirming the presence or absence of this disease in its early stages.

(a) (b) (c)

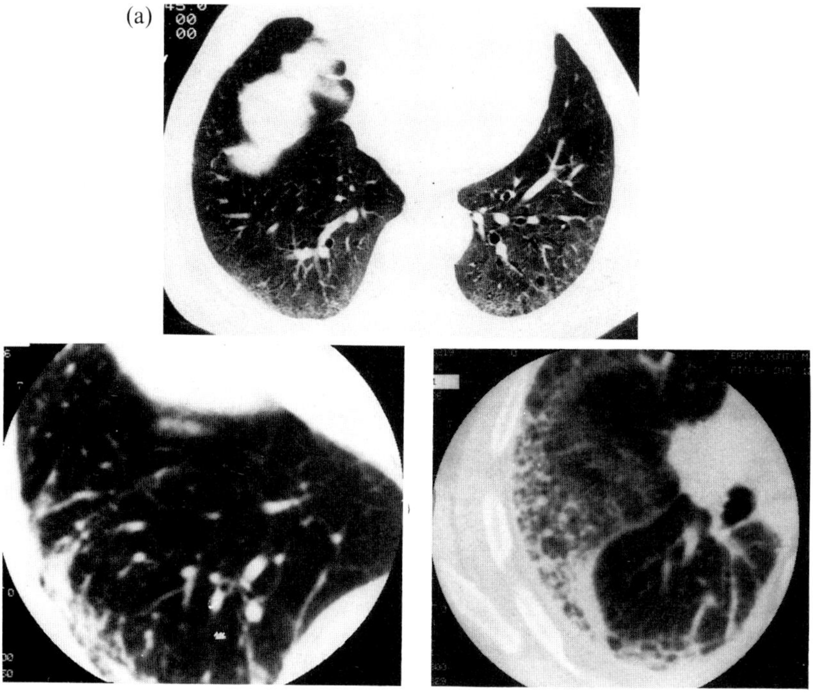

Figure 14. *EXAMPLES OF ASBESTOSIS. (a) Early changes of asbestosis found in a patient with negative chest radiographs. Note the irregular interface between pulmonary arteries and surrounding pulmonary parenchyma. The pulmonary arteries appear tethered. Note the fine reticulation which is predominantly distributed in the subpleural regions of the lower lobes. Very early cystic formation can also be seen consistent with early honeycombing. (b) More advance case. This case demonstrates reticulation in the subpleural regions with evidence of transparenchymal bands throughout the parenchyma of the lower lobe. (c) More severe case of proven asbestosis. Note irregular surfaces of the visceral pleura including the major fissure. Note subpleural reticulation. This appearance is indistinguishable from idiopathic pulmonary fibrosis.*

Sarcoidosis

The pulmonary manifestations of sarcoidosis are protean. HRCT findings typically include nodules and thickening located predominantly along bronchovascular sheaths in the central regions of the lungs bilaterally (Fig. 15). In addition, micronodules corresponding to non-caseating granulomas can be seen throughout the parenchyma and are extremely well-demonstrated by thin section CT [24,25]. In addition, ground glass opacities which can lead to alveolar infiltration may be seen throughout the lungs. The association of such changes with hilar and mediastinal lymphadenopathy is pathognomonic of sarcoidosis. As the disease evolves, typical findings of pulmonary fibrosis can also be seen with honeycombing and central retraction with crowding of vessels and bronchi.

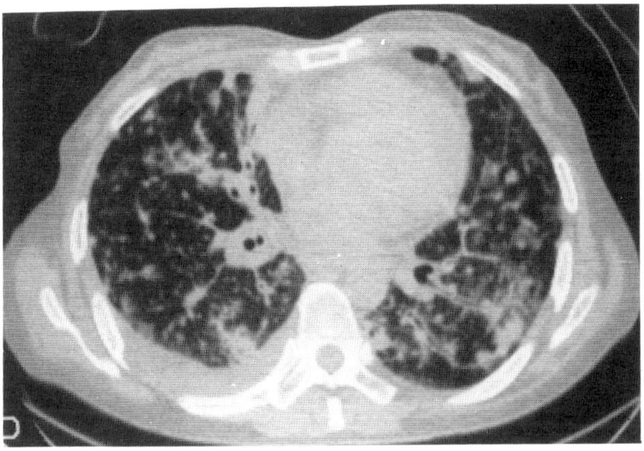

Figure 15. *SARCOIDOSIS. Note marked thickening of the bronchovascular sheaths associated with nodularity and prominent septa. The central predominance of this disease is characteristic.*

Pulmonary Histiocytosis X

Also known as eosinophilic granuloma of the lung, pulmonary histiocytosis X is a disorder of unknown aetiology that typically affects young or middle-aged adults. In the majority of cases, a history of smoking is also present. Pathologically, pulmonary histiocytosis X is characterized by nodules and cysts, most often located near bronchovascular structures in the central regions of the lungs.

This distribution is not unlike that of sarcoidosis. However, the main differentiating feature is the frequent presence of cysts of various sizes which appear connected or adjacent to bronchi. As shown by Moore et al, the predominant HRCT finding is the presence of cystic spaces [26]. These cystic spaces are differentiable from emphysematous blebs due to the presence of identifiable walls. Reticulation is not a prominent feature in histiocytosis X even though plain films may suggest reticulation. Presumably, superimposition of the multiple cystic walls is responsible for the pseudo-appearance of reticulation on pain radiographs.

Pulmonary Lymphangioleiomyomatosis (LAM)

Lam is a rare disease characterized by disorderly proliferation of smooth muscle within the pulmonary interstitium. The disease affects only women of childbearing age. Patients present typically with progressive dyspnoea and/or haemotysis, either with recurrent pneumothoraces due to rupture of peripheral dilated air spaces or with chylous effusions. The disease is often confused with asthma in its early stages. Plain film findings are not pathognomonic. However, the HRCT appearance of LAM has been described as one of the most characteristic [27]. Innumerable, thin-walled cysts can be identified throughout the lungs without evidence of intervening abnormal lung densities (Fig. 16). These cysts are the results of air space ectasia secondary to progressive airway obstruction. These cysts typically vary in size from a few millimeters to up to 5 centimeters. Nodularity, thickened interlobular septal lines and vascular destruction are significant in their absence. Superficially, LAM may be difficult to differentiate from pulmonary emphysema. However the uniform distribution throughout both lungs strongly favours LAM.

Emphysema

HRCT is capable of detecting emphysematous changes of the lung before pulmonary function test become abnormal. Correlation of pathological specimens and HRCT have been uniformly excellent. In high risk populations such as those with suspected alpha I antitrypsin deficiency, HRCT van be of great value. Cystic spaces with no definable walls are the hallmark of pulmonary emphysema. Predominant distribution to the upper lobes is helpful in differentiating the disease from LAM.

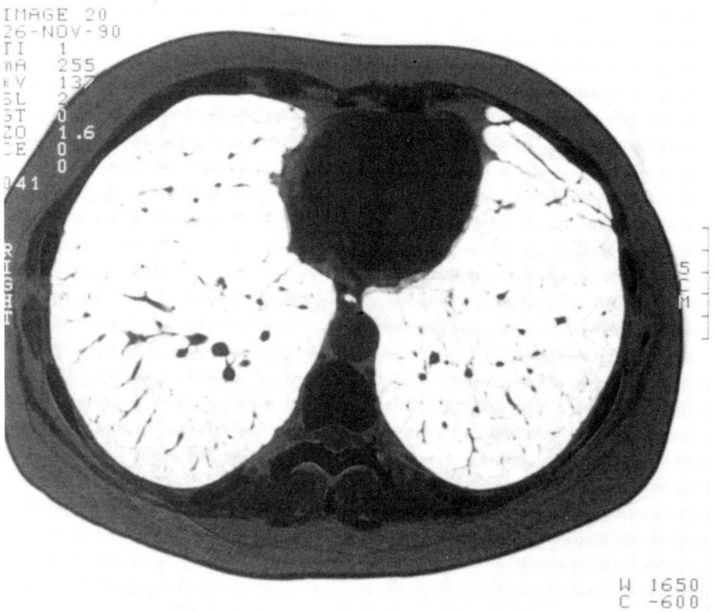

Figure 16. *LYMPHANGIOLEIOMYOMATOSIS. Characteristic appearance of LAM with numerous cysts of various sizes distributed uniformly throughout the lung to involve upper and lower lobes equally. Although this superficially resembles emphysema, the clinical context and the global involvement of the lungs allows easy differentiation.*

Conclusion

As shown by these specific examples, HRCT is very effective in visualizing the disordered architecture of the lung parenchyma in the presence of diffuse lung disease. HRCT has become the premier technique of investigation and evaluation of the lung parenchyma. In addition to its ability to specifically recognize several entities, one of the most important aspects of HRCT is its sensitivity. Indeed, compared to pulmonary radiographs, HRCT appears capable of detecting disease processes much earlier in their evolution. Clinically, a perhaps more important role has been the impact of HRCT on the management of immunocompromised patients. In such patients, HRCT often permits detection of infectious complications such as Pneumocystis carinii infection or cytomegalovirus infection days before it would become apparent on pain chest radiographs. In bone marrow transplants, HRCT has been found to be valuable in the early detection of invasive aspergillosis. Clearly, with the increasing availability of CT scanners, HRCT is becoming a very important tool in the clinical management of diffuse lung processes.

References

1. Siegelman SS, Khouri NF, Leo FP, Fishman EK, Braverman RM, Zerhouni EA. Solitary pulmonary nodules: CT assessment. *Radiology* 1986;**160:**307-312.
2. Zerhouni EA, Spivey JF, Morgan RH, Leo FP, Stitik FP, Siegelman SS. Factors influencing quantitave CT measurements of solitary pulmonary nodules. *J Comput Assist Tomogr* 1982;**6:**1075-1087.
3. Zerhouni EA, Boukadoum M, Siddiky MA, Newbold JM, et al. A standard phantom for quantitative CT analysis of pulmonary nodules. *Radiology* 1983;**149:**767-773.
4. Zerhouni EA, Stitik FP, Siegelman SS, Naidich DP, et al. CT of the pulmonary nodule: A cooperative study. *Radiology* 1986;**160:**319-327.
5. Siegelman SS, Khouri NF, Scott WW jr, Leo FP, Hamper U-M, Fishman EK, Zerhouni EA. Pulmonary hamartoma: CT findings. *Radiology* 1986;**160:**313-317.
6. Gross BH, Glaser GM, Buchsein FL. Multiple pulmonary nodules detected by computed tomography: Diagnostic implications. *JCAT* 1985;**9:**880-885.
7. Meziane MA, Hrunab RH, Zerhouni EA, Wheeler PS, Khouri NF, et al. High resolution CT of the lung parenchyma with pathologic correlation. *Radiographics* 1988;**8:**27-54.
8. Milne ENC, Zerhouni EA. Blood supply of pulmonary metastases. *J Thorac Imag* 1987;**2:**15-23.
9. Magid D, Siegelman SS, Eggleston JC, Fishman Ek, Zerhouni EA. Pulmonary carcinoid tumors: CT assessment. *J Comput Assist Tomogr* 1989:**13:**244-247.
10. McCaughan BC, Martini N, Bains MS. Bronchial Carcinoids: A review of 124 cases. *J Thorac Cardiovasc Surg* 1985;**89:**8-17.
11. Huang RM, Naidich DP, Lubat E, Schinella R, Garay SM, McCauley DI. Septic pulmonary emboli: CT radiographic correlation. *AJR* 1989;**153:**41-45.
12. Kuhlman JE, Fishman EK, Teigen C. Pulmonary septic emboli: Diagnosis with CT. *Radiology* 1990;**174:**211-213.
13. Kuhkman JE, Fishman EK, Siegelman SS. Invasive pulmonary aspergillosis in acute leukemia: Characteristic findings on CT, the CT halo sign and the role of CT in early diagnosis. *Radiology* 1985;**157:**611-614.
14. Zerhouni EA, Naidich DP, Stitik FP, Khouri NF, Siegleman SS. Computed tomography of the pulmonary parenchyma. 2. Interstitial disease. *J Thorac Imaging* 1985;**1:**54-64.
15. Muller NL, Staples CA, Miller RR, Vedal S, Thurlbeck WM, Ostrow DN. Disease activity in idiopathic pulmonary fibrosis: CT and Pathologic correelation. *Radiology* 1987;**165:**731-734.
16. Meziane MA, Hruban RH, Zerhouni EA, Wheeler PS, Khouri NG, Fishman EK, Hutchins GM, Siegelman SS. High resolution CT of the lung parenchyma with pathologic correlation. *Radiographics* 1988;**8:**27-54.

17. Webb WR, Stein MG, Finkbeiner WE, Im JG, Lynch D, Gamsu G. Normal and diseased isolated lungs: High-resolution CT. *Radiology* 1988;**166:**81-87.
18. Naidich DP, Zerhouni EA, Hutchins GM, Genieser NB, McCauley DI, Siegelman SS. Computed tomogtraphy of the pulmonary parenchyma. Part 1. Distal airspace disease. *J Thorac Imag* 1985;**1:**39-53.
19. Munk PI, Muller NL, Miller RR, Ostrow DN. Pulmonary lymphangitic carcinomatosis: CT and pathologic findings. *Radiology* 1988;**166:**705-709.
20. Ren H, Hruban RH, Kuhlman JE, Fishman EK, Wheeler PS, Zerhouni EA, Hutchins GM. Comuted tomography of inflation-fixed lungs: the beated septum sign of pulmonary metastases. *J Comput Assist Tomogr* 1989;**13:**411-416.
21. Muller NL, Miller RR, Webb WR, Evans KG, Ostrow DN. Fibrosing alveolitis: CT-pathologic correlation. *Radiology* 1986;**160:**585-588.
22. Aberle DR, Gamsu G, Ray CS, Feuerstein IM. Asbestos-related pleural and parenchymal fibrosis: detection with high-resolution CT. *Radiology* 1988;**166:**729-734.
23. Friedman AC, Fiel SB, Fisher MS, Radecki PD, Lev-Toaff AS, Caroline DF. Asbestos-related pleural disease and asbestosis: a comperison of CT and chest radiography. *AJR* 1988;**150:**269-275.
24. Hamper UM, Fishman EK, Khouri NF, Johns CJ, Wang KP, Siegelman SS. Typical and atypical CT manifestations of pulmonary sacroidosis. *J Comput Assist Tomogr* 1986;**10:**928-936.
25. Muller NL, Kullnig P, Miller RR. The CT findings of pulmonary sarcoidosis: analysis of 25 patients. *AJR* 1989;**152:**1179-1182.
26. Moore ADA, Godwin JD, Muller NL, Naidich DP, Hammar SP, Buschman DL, et al. Pulmonary histiocytosis X: comparison of radiographic and CT findings. *Radiology* 1989;**172:**249-254.
27. Rappaport DC, Weisbrod GL, Herman SJ, Chamberlain DW. Pulmonary lymphangioleimyomatosis: high-resolution CT findings in four cases. *AJR* 1989;**152:**961-964.

Computed tomography of pleural infection and lung abscess

Carl J. Zylak
McMaster University Medical Center, Hamilton, Ontario, Canada

Introduction

Differentiation of empyema from lung abscess, and empyema from subphrenic abscess are important diagnostic challenges. Accurate diagnosis facilitates the appropriate therapeutic intervention. Lung abscess generally responds to appropriate antibiotic therapy; empyema almost always requires tube drainage [1,2]. This classic approach to therapy, however, is being modified, particularly in conjunction with treatment of lung abscess. A lung abscess may be treated with an indwelling transbronchial catheter [3] or with percutaneous chest tube drainage in situations where the abscess abutts adjacent involved pleura [4,5]. These alternative approaches may seemingly make accurate differentiation less important, however, the majority of pulmonary abscesses are treated in the traditional manner.

Accurate differentiation of an empyema from a subphrenic abscess clearly has more important therapeutic implications. Successful therapy is related to prompt drainage requiring placement of the drainage tube in the appropriate anatomic compartment, that is, above or below the respective hemidiaphragm.

The radiological features which enable accurate diagnosis and differentiation of empyema, pulmonary abscess and subphrenic abscess form the essence of this section.

Pleural versus Parenchymal Processes

Morphology [6]

The pleura consists of two serous membranes arranged in the form of a closed invaginal sac which invests each lung. The visceral pleura forms the inner layer of the pleural surface. It is intimately adherent to the surface of the lung and its fissures between lobes. The parietal pleura forms the outer margin of the pleural space. It is in intimate contact with the inner surface of the chest wall, covering a large part of the diaphragm and the mediastinum. The pulmonary and parietal pleura are continuous with one another and join at the hila. Ordinarily the two surfaces are in contact during all phases of respiration. The potential space or pleural cavity becomes apparent when air or fluid collects between the visceral and parietal pleura. The right and left pleural sacs have no connection between them. They frequently come into immediate contact behind the body of the sternum to form the well known anterior junction line; less frequently they come in contact posterior to the oesophagus to form the posterior junction line.

The parietal pleura has names which reflect its relationship to various regions within the thoracic cavity: the costal pleura, the diaphragmatic pleura, the cervical pleura and the mediastinal pleura.

The costal pleura lines the internal aspect of the ribs and transversus thoracis in addition to the sternum and sides of the bodies of the vertebrae. Outside the costal pleura is a thin layer of loose areolar tissue called the endothoracic fascia which corresponds to the transversalis fascia of the abdominal wall. On each side the costal pleura extends laterally over the inner surface of the costal cartilages, ribs and the constituent parts of the transversus thoracis. In the posterior portion of the thorax, it passes over the sympathetic trunk and its branches, then onto the sides of the bodies of the vertebrae where it becomes continuous with the mediastinal pleura. In the cephalad direction the costal pleura is continuous with the cervical pleura at the inner margin of the first rib. Inferiorly, or caudad, it is continuous with the diaphragmatic pleura. This costodiaphragmatic line of reflection of the pleura begins behind the xiphoid process and passes posteriorly and inferiorly behind the seventh costal cartilage, reaching the mid axillary line at the level of the tenth rib. The line then ascends slightly crossing the twelfth rib to reach the level of the upper border of the spine of the twelfth thoracic vertebra. The line on the left side is similar except that initially it follows the ascending part of the sixth costal cartilage.

The diaphragmatic pleura is continuous with the costal pleura as just described and immediately is continuous with the mediastinal pleura along the line of attachment of the pericardium to the diaphragm. The diaphragmatic pleura covers part of the upper surface of the corresponding side of the diaphragm.

The mediastinal pleura forms the lateral boundary of the mediastinum. Cephalad to the root of the lung it is a continuous sheet between the sternum and the vertebral column. At the root of the lung the mediastinal pleura extends laterally as a tube of serous membrane which encloses the structures of the lung root, and passes into continuity with the visceral pleura. Below the hila it extends as a double layer from the lateral edge of the esophagus to the medial surface of the lung where it is continuous with the pulmonary pleura. The double layer is the pulmonary ligament. The ligament is continuous above with the tube investing the hila: below it ends in a free falciform border (Fig. 1).

One should note that the inferior limit of the pleura is on a considerably lower level than the corresponding border of the lung. Also it does not extend to the attachment of the diaphragm, so that below the line of reflection of the pleura from the chest wall to the diaphragm, the latter is in direct contact with the rib cartilages and the muscles in the intercostal spaces. The most inferior part of the pleural space is that situated adjacent to the twelfth thoracic vertebra in intimate contact with the crura of the diaphragm [7].

When interpreting contrast enhanced computed tomograms knowledge of the vascular supply of the two layers of the pleura becomes an important consideration. The pariel pleura derives its arterial supply from somatic or body wall arteries, that is intercostal, internal thoracic and musculophrenic. Its veins join the systemic veins in the neighbouring parts of the chest wall. The visceral pleura derives its vascular supply from the bronchiol vessels.

In terms of morphology of the lung, an important consideration in the differentiation of a pleural versus a parenchymal process is the effect on the pulmonary vessels and bronchi. The arborization of these channels will be displaced by an extrapulmonary process whereas with a pulmonary process such as an abscess the supplying arteries and bronchi are sometimes seen to 'enter' the abnormal area.

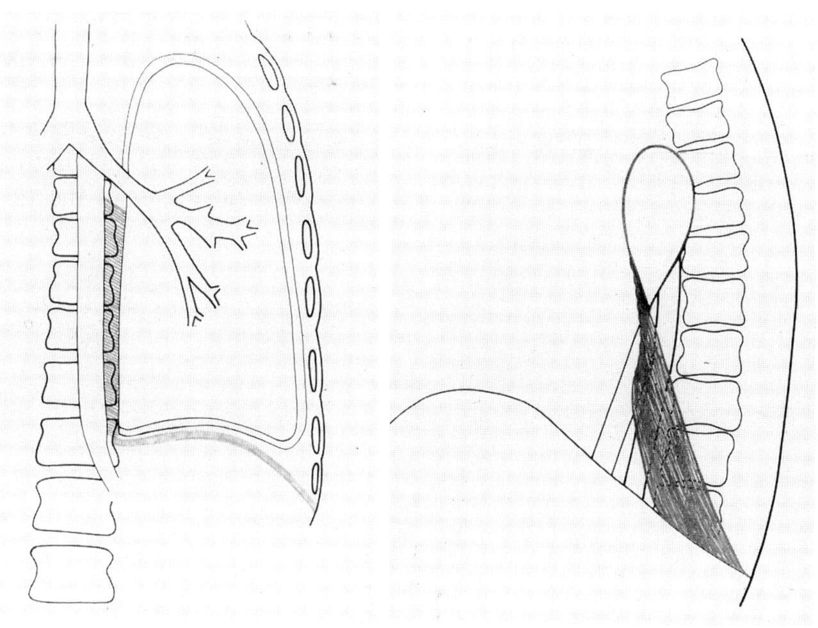

(a) (b)

(c)

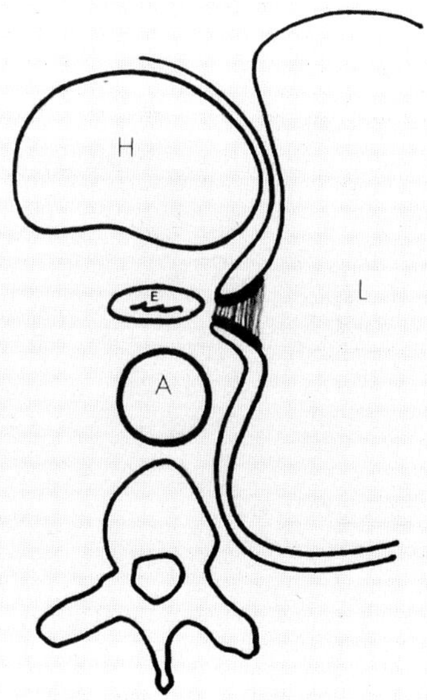

Figure 1. *SCHEMATICS OF THE PULMONARY LIGAMENT. (a) The pulmonary ligament (cross hatched) consists of a double pleural layer from the lateral edge of the oesophagus to the medial surface of the lung where it is continuous with the visceral pleura. (b) The pulmonary ligament sweeps laterally and posteriorly to project over the dorsal spine. (c) Axial schematic showing intimate relationship of oesophagus to pulmonary ligament.*

Clearly, depending on the size of the lesion some accompanying distortion and displacement occurs.

Pathology [8]

An abscess is a localized collection of pus caused by suppuration within a tissue, organ or confined space. The term pulmonary abscess describes a local suppurative process within the lung characterized by necrosis of lung tissue. Abscesses can occur anywhere in the lung, however, often they are close to or in contact with the pleura. Abscesses begin as a focus of hyperaemia followed in time by central necrosis. The enclosing wall initially may be poorly defined, however, with time and progressive fibrosis it becomes more discrete. If communication develops with a bronchus, air enters the cavity.

Causative organisms can be introduced into their sites of focal destruction by the following mechanisms: aspiration of infective material, antecedent primary bacterial infection, septic embolism, neoplasia and miscellaneous considerations including penetrating trauma and contiguous spread of infection from neighbouring organs or cavities.

An empyema is essentially a suppurative pleuritis consisting of a frank purulent exudate. Contamination of the pleural space most commonly occurs by contiguous spread of organisms from intrapulmonary infection, but occasionally it occurs by lymphatic or haematogenous dissemination from a more distant infection.

Radiologic Features

Conventional Radiography

Empyema

The shape of an empyema is influenced by the contour of the adjacent structures particularly the chest wall i.e. the shape may be lenticular, fusiform or somewhat triangular [9]. The appearance of the medial margin, formed by the visceral pleura, depends on the status of the adjacent lung. If the adjacent lung is not involved by an accompanying infection, the margin will be exquisitely sharp (Fig. 2). If there is an accompanying pneumonia, loss of sharpness of the interface will apply (silhouette sign) (Fig. 3). Another helpful feature is the shape of the angle formed at the cephalad and caudad interfaces of the pleural collection with the adjacent lung. The angle formed will generally be obtuse. The analogy can be made with the profile appearance of a loose-fitting laboratory coat which has been displaced away following insertion of a basketball underneath it. The laboratory coat will form an obtuse angle particularly at its superior or cephalad margin. If one now removes the basketball and places it in front of the lab coat the angle formed by the basketball and the lab coat will be acute as viewed in profile. This feature is very helpful in differentiating a pleural or extrapleural process from onc located in the pulmonary parenchyma. The effects of gravity can be examined by changing patient position, e.g. decubitus, upright vs. supine. If the fluid is relatively freely movable within the pleural space, one may appreciate a change in its distribution with change in patient position.

Pleural fluid collections may change their shape with varying levels of respiration - particularly as noted at fluoroscopy - however, their position will not alter.

With the development of a bronchopleural fistula, the introduction of air affords additional distinctive radiographic features (Fig. 3). The width of the air-liquid interface on orthogonal projections, as a rule, will be significantly different due to the lenticular shape of the pleural space. The width of the process will be much narrower (wider) on one view when compared to its depiction on the orthogonal projection [10]. The air-liquid interface may be seen to cross fissure lines, another indication that the abnormality is situated within the pleural compartment. The thickness of the wall can now be assessed. The visceral pleural side is usually thicker than the parietal component. This may well relate to accompanying compressive atelectasis and/or infection. The presence of air allows visualization of the inner margins of the empyema cavity. Generally, these are quite smooth.

Pulmonary Abscess

A pulmonary abscess is usually spherical or round. Distinctness of the margin depends on the stage of development. Early on, its margins may be obscured by adjacent areas of pneumonia. As the pneumonia clears the margin of the pulmonary abscess becomes quite well defined.

Gravity essentially has no effect. Respiration will not alter the shape of the abscess but it may move up and down on inspiration and expiration enabling correct placement of the lesion within the lung.

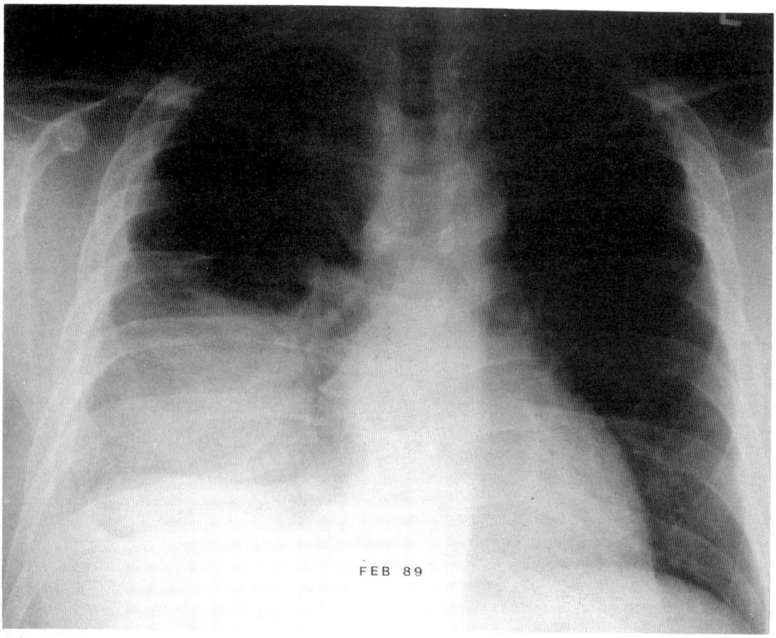

(a)

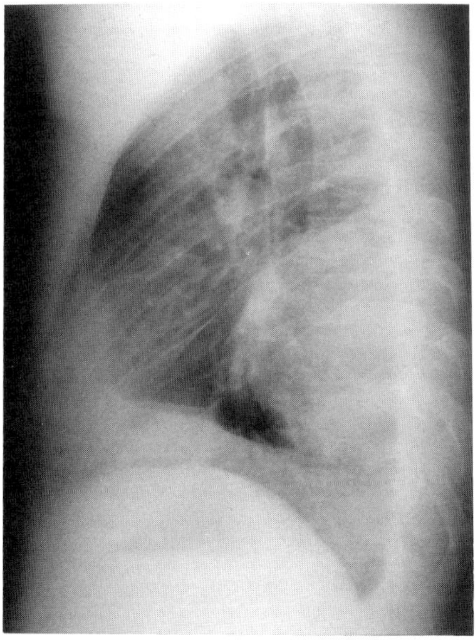

(b)

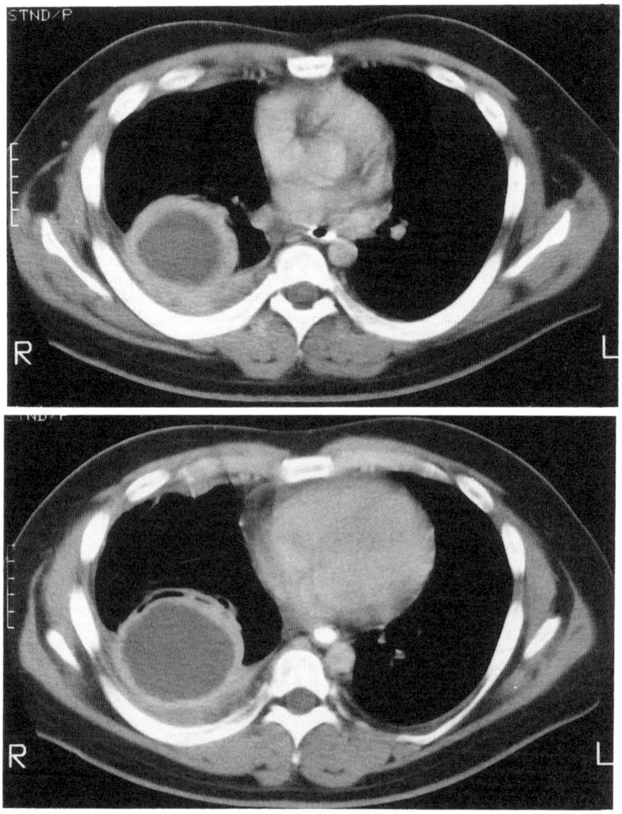

(c)

(d)

Figure 2. *FRONTAL (a) AND LATERAL (b) PROJECTIONS OF A 23-YEAR-OLD MALE WITH DOWN'S SYNDROME SHOW A POSTERIORLY PLACED QUITE WELL DEFINED LARGE DENSITY. Pleural thickening parallels the right lateral chest wall. The radiographic appearances are those of an empyema. (c) and (d) Enhanced axial CTs show a collection of fluid surrounded by thickened visceral pleura anteriorly and parietal pleura posteriorly (split pleura sign). The angle formed by the fluid collection with the lung at its lateral margin is somewhat obtuse. Medially, it merges with thickened pleura. There is compressed lung anterior to the empyema. There is also displacement of the vessels superiorly by the fluid collection.*

If communication with a bronchus is present an air-liquid interface will be evident on radiographs made tangent to the interface, e.g. upright, decubitus. Because of the spherical configuration of the abscess the width of the air-liquid interface will be approximately equal on orthogonal projections. The air liquid interface is generally

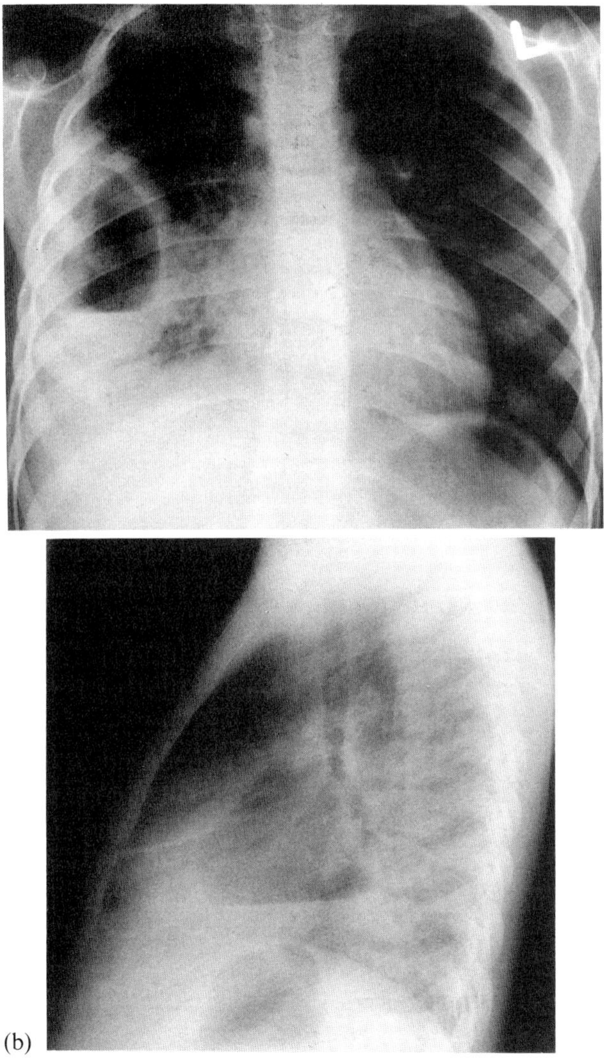
(a)
(b)

Figure 3. *5-YEAR-OLD PATIENT PRESENTING WITH FEVER AND RIGHT CHEST PAIN. Frontal (a) and lateral (b) projections demonstrate a smooth-walled cavity with air and liquid. Note the discrepancy in the width of the air-fluid level on orthogonal projections in keeping with location in the pleural space. There is evidence of air space disease in the surrounding middle and lower lobes effacing part of the medial border of the empyema.*

uniformly level; however, the presence of accompanying debris may result in an undulating appearance. The wall of a pulmonary abscess is generally thicker than that of an empyema and less uniform in its thickness. Its inner margin is, in contrast to empyemas, shaggy.

Computed Tomography

Computed tomography (CT) offers several advantages over conventional radiography. Serial sections afford a unique opportunity for studying images in the third dimension. Reconstruction techniques allow formation of coronal and sagittal images at any desired plane. Density and sensitivity differences enable distinction of many more tissue and liquid interfaces. Detail is, of course, enhanced due to the absence of over- or underlying structures. Intravenous contrast enhancement allows identification of hyperaemic regions within the lesion, facilitating more precise location of the abnormality (Fig. 2). Bolus contrast medium enhancement, in addition to usual contrast enhancement, may be helpful in distinguishing pleural from parenchymal disease [11].

Empyema and Pulmonary Abscess

CT features closely parallel those found on conventional radiography. However, because of the advantages discussed above several additional features are found only on CT.

The CT features which help in the differentiation of lung abscess from empyema include shape, attenuation values, angle at the interface between the lung and chest wall at its cephalad and/or caudad margins, interface with and effect on adjacent lung, and characteristics of the wall [12-16].

The shape of an encapsulated empyema on axial images can be surprisingly round, particularly when the section is made through that part of the empyema protruding most medially into the adjacent lung. Evaluation of the pleural parenchymal interface on such a section can be misleading. The angle formed may appear to be acute, however, when one views the sections serially, the more cephalad and caudad regions of the empyema collection will have an obtuse angle in the majority of cases (Fig. 4). In a study of 63 patients with a total of 70 inflammatory lesions 70% of empyemas had an obtuse chest wall angle; an obtuse angle was found in none of the abscesses. An acute chest wall angle was shown in 83% of abscesses and 14% of empyemas. In terms of shape, 63% of empyemas were lenticular; none of

(a)

(b)

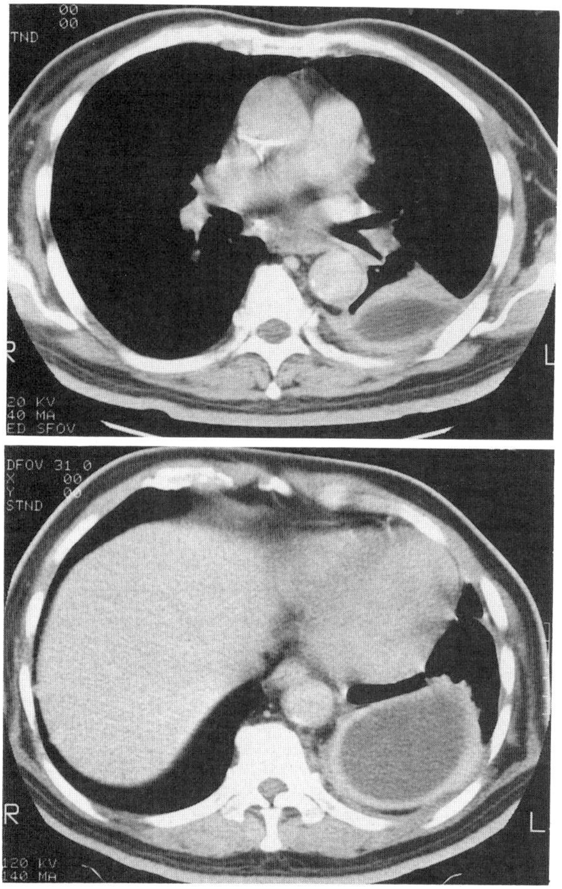

Figure 4. *TRANSAXIAL ENHANCED CT SCANS DEMONSTRATE A LENTICULAR SHAPE OF THIS EMPYEMA. In (a) the fluid collection forms an obtuse angle at its lateral lung interface; however, the more caudal cut through the largest part of the empyema demonstrates not surprisingly an acute angle with the chest wall. The pleura is split with the parietal layer being somewhat thinner than the visceral. The plain films were similar to those shown in Fig. 2.*

the abscesses had this shape. Abscesses were round in 67%; in empyemas, 11% [16].

Attenuation values of a lung abscess show a wide range of values because of a combination of consolidation and aerated lung. Attenuation values of empyemas are accordingly narrower due to the absence of lung (Fig. 5).

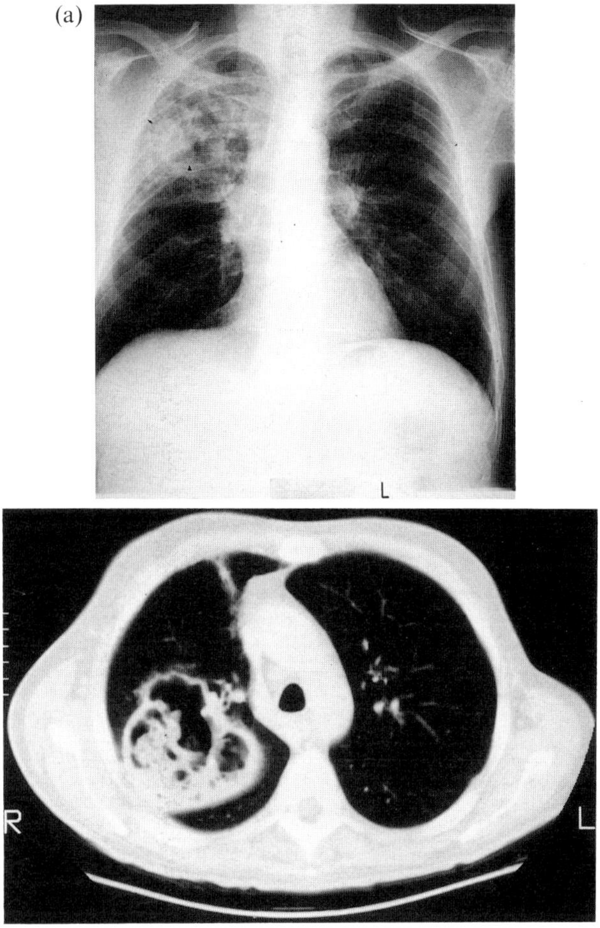

Figure 5. *PULMONARY ABSCESS. (a) Postero-anterior radiograph shows an air-fluid level (arrowhead) and necrotic material (arrow) in an abscess caused by aspergillosis in the right upper lobe. (b) Axial CT demonstrates varying thickness of the wall, irregularity of its inner margin, and a mixture of air and debris which accounts for the wide range of attenuation values as compared to the more uniform content of an empyema cavity. Note the acute angles at the interface of the abscess with the pleura/chest wall.*

Details of the interface with and the effect upon adjacent lung is enhanced with CT. This applies particularly to demonstration of the effect of the process on adjacent bronchi and pulmonary vessels. An empyema will compress the adjacent lung and displace adjacent vessels. With a pulmonary abscess the vessels can be seen to extend to or into the abscess with very little accompanying displacement (Fig. 6).

Details of the wall characteristics are enhanced on CT. If the adjacent lung is involved then its outer margin will be indistinct. The inner margin of an abscess, however, is always irregular in contrast to the smooth inner wall of an empyema.

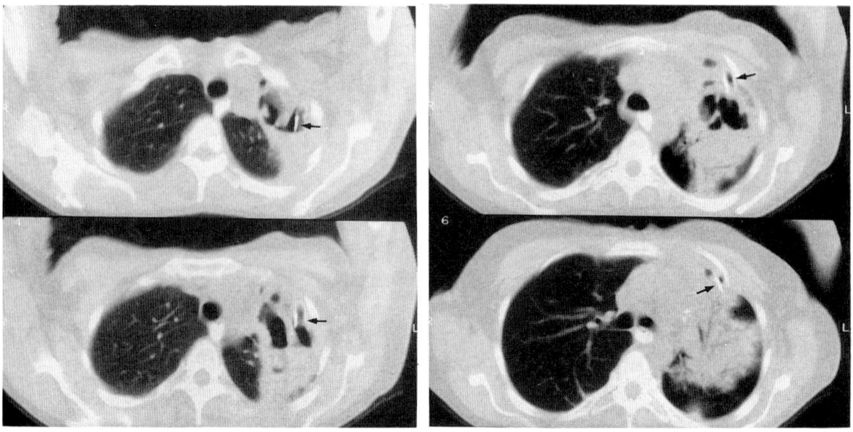

(a) (b)

Figure 6. *PULMONARY ABSCESS MASQUERADING AS AN EMPYEMA (a and b). Serial axial CTs show position of a drainage tube (arrow) thought to have been placed in an empyema. Note continuity of the space containing air and fluid, some unevenness of this interface, and merging of the adjacent pneumonia (air bronchograms) with the areas of lung necrosis that is the abscess. If this was an empyema, one would have expected to find fluid in the dependent region of the pleural space.*

The walls of the empyema are separated by the infective process. Due to the systemic vascular supply these surfaces will enhance with conventional contrast enhancement resulting in the splitting or separation of the visceral and parietal pleura. The visceral margin is often thicker as stated earlier because of a combination of compressive atelectasis and/or accompanying pneumonia (Fig. 7).

The presence of air within an empyema (bronchopleural fistula) enables enhancement of the features described as air becomes an added contrast agent (Fig. 8). Air within the pulmonary ligament may simulate a bronchopleural fistula (Fig. 9).

(a)

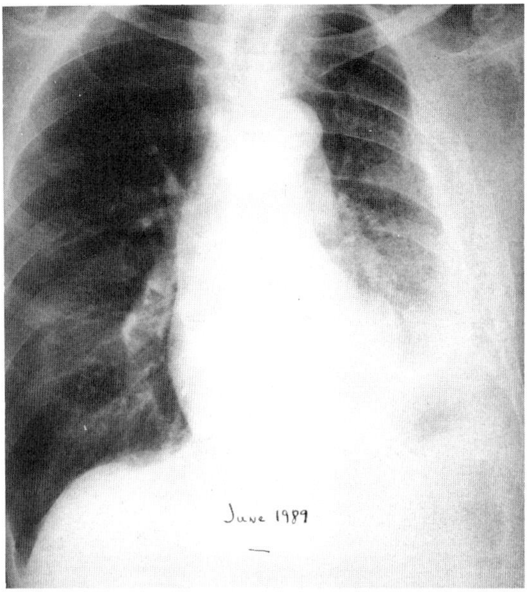

(b)

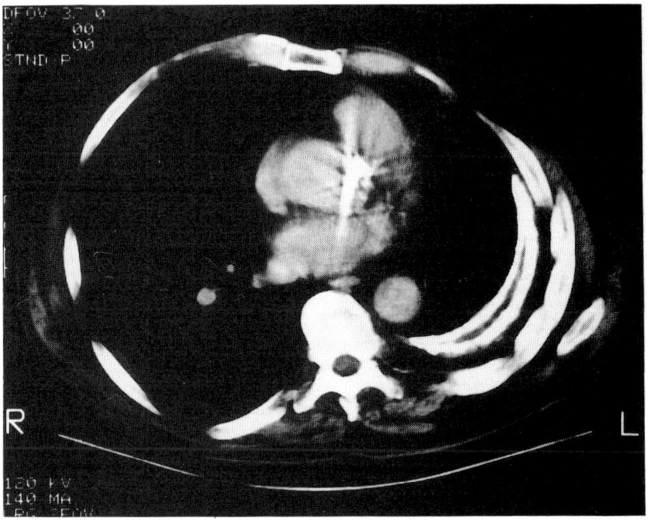

Figure 7. *78-YEAR-OLD MALE CALCIFIED TUBERCULOUS EMPYEMA DEMONSTRATING 'SPLIT PLEURA SIGN'. (a) PA view demonstrates extensive calcification of the visceral and parietal pleura plus thickening of the extrapleural soft tissues. (b) Axial CT demonstrates calcification of the visceral and parietal pleura - the split pleura sign as well as thickening of the extrapleural soft tissues. Extensive calcification is noted in the aortic valvular region.*

(a)

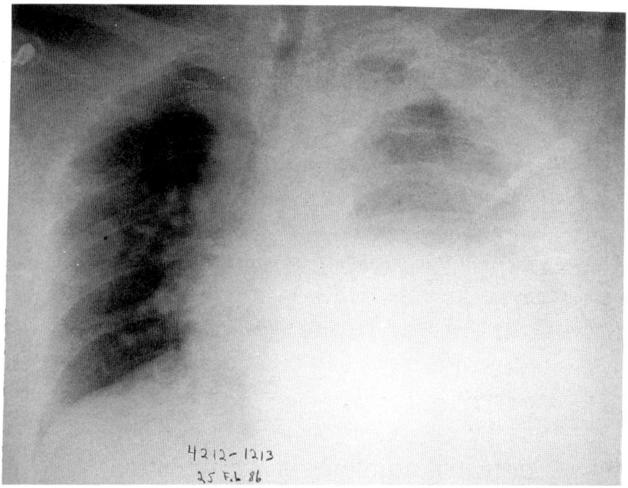

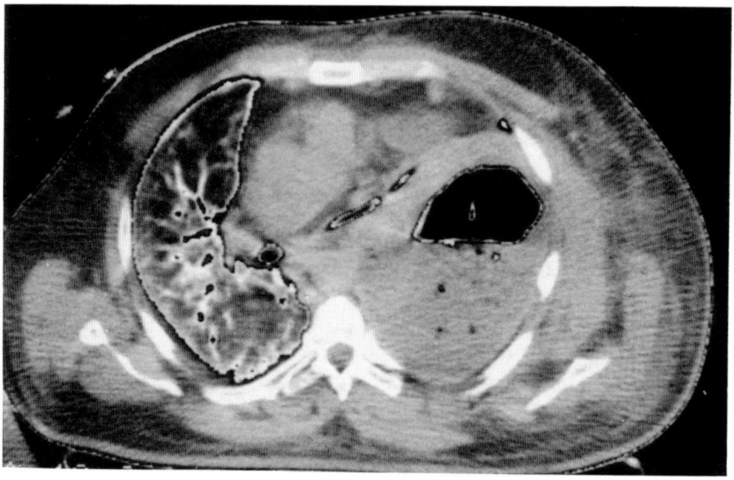

(b)

Figure 8. *44-YEAR-OLD DIABETIC WITH DEVELOPMENT OF A BRONCHOPLEURAL FISTULA. (a) Frontal projection demonstrates a large air fluid collection in the left pleural space. There is some shift of the mediastinum to the right. (b) An enhanced axial CT demonstrates air and fluid within the left pleural space with elevation of the airway as well as compressive atelectasis of the lung anteriorly. Note induration of soft tissues of the chest wall. This induration extended down to the flank in keeping with actinomycosis.*

Potential Pitfalls [17,18]

The presence of fluid in pre-existing pulmonary air spaces with or without accompanying bronchial communication can mimic the CT appearances of an empyema. These fluid filled air spaces have many of the same signs used both radiographically and in cross sectional imaging to characterize loculated pleural fluid collections. These include lenticular shape, air-fluid levels of different length on orthogonal projections, uniform smooth inner walls, mass effect on the adjacent lung and a pattern of enhancement resembling the appearance of split pleural surfaces, a pseudo split pleura sign.

Bullae tend to be located in the upper lobes with air-fluid levels limited by fissures assuming these can be identified. These fluid-filled cysts are rarely associated with accompanying pleural effusion. Clearly prior radiography or CT is invaluable in demonstrating the presence of pre-existing cavities or bullae. Nonetheless even when comparison films are available, fluid within pre existing air spaces may create significant problems in differentiating abscess from empyema.

Occasionally, large mediastinal masses, particularly those with smooth margins, may be confused with a large pleural effusion or empyema. An example of hydatid disease [19] of the pericardium is shown in Fig. 10.

In summary, lung abscess and empyema can frequently be distinguished with conventional radiography. However, it is clear that computed tomography has many advantages. Abscesses will be seen to be round whereas empyemas are lenticular. Separation of the pleural layers with an empyema is exquisitely demonstrated as is accompanying compression of the adjacent lung. Generally, the angles formed at the chest wall, particularly at the cephalad and caudad regions of the lesion will be obtuse with an empyema and acute with an abscess. An abscess will demonstrate a thick non uniform irregular wall whereas the empyema generally is thinner, more uniform and smooth. When all of these findings are taken into consideration, the distinction between empyema and pulmonary abscess is generally possible.

Pleural (Effusion/Empyema) versus Peritoneal (Ascites/Subphrenic Abscess)

Accurate differentiation of empyema from subphrenic abscess is of major clinical importance. Prompt tube drainage following insertion into the involved space facilitates a good outcome. Conventional

(a)
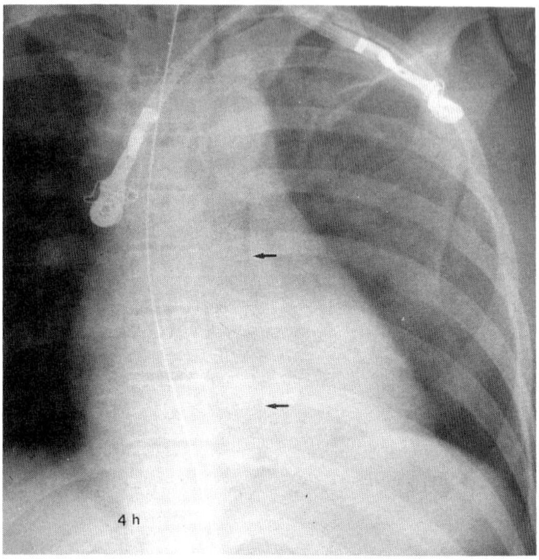

(b)
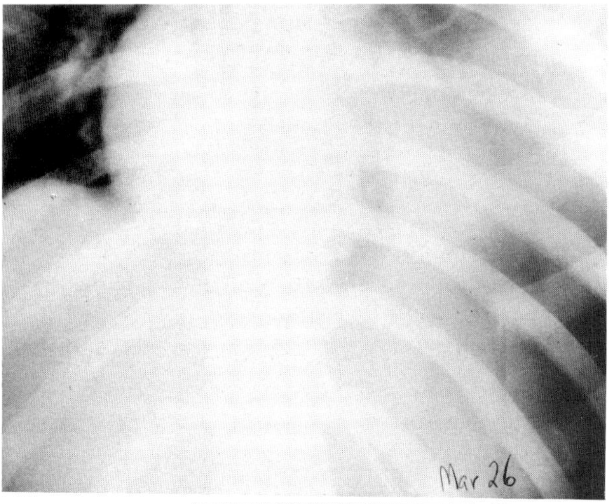

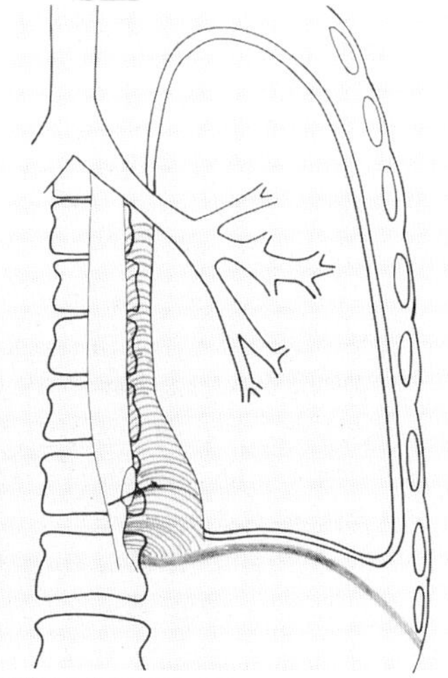

(d)
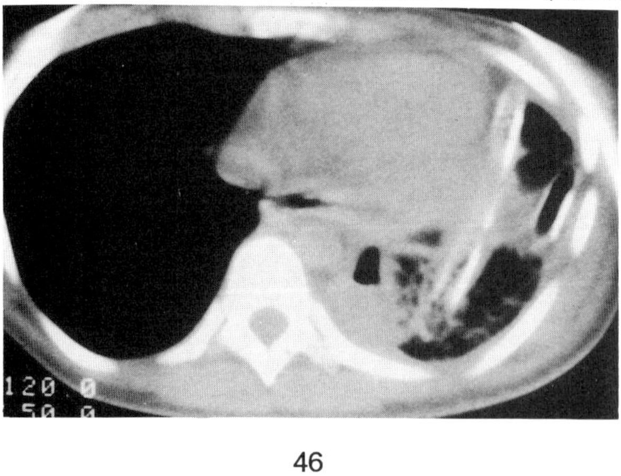

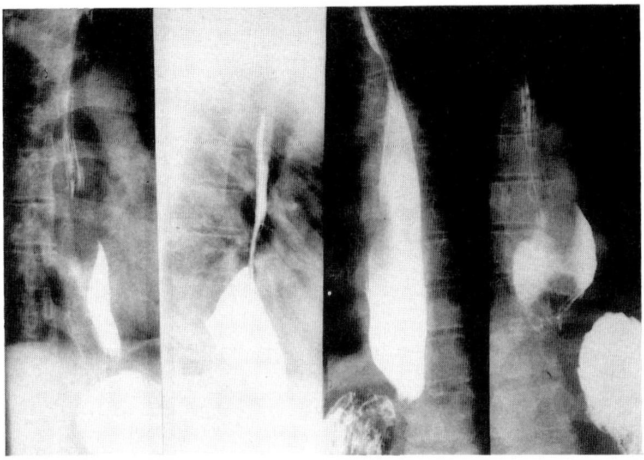

(e)

Figure 9. *24-YEAR-OLD FEMALE SUSTAINING BLUNT TRAUMA IN A MOTOR VEHICLE ACCIDENT. (a) A frontal projection made approximately four hours after the injury demonstrates a linear collection of air paralleling the aorta (arrows). Esophageal rupture was suspected. A study with Gastrografin failed to demonstrate adequately the lower esophagus (not shown). (b) A frontal projection made 24 hours later demonstrates a crescentric shaped left paravertebral air collection with an accompanying soft tissue density. (c) Schematic demonstrating communication (arrow) between the ruptured esophagus and the pulmonary ligament (crosshatched). The patient subsequently developed a large pleural effusion following rupture of the contents from the pulmonary ligament into the pleural space. (d) Axial CT scan made several weeks later. There is a medially positioned air fluid collection which may be within the pulmonary ligament. The patient was treated conservatively with tube drainage and survived. (e) Composite follow-up oesophagogram demonstrates aperistalsis of the lower third of the esophagus with an appearance of a myotomy representing the site of previous tear. The lower esophageal sphincter was incompetent with gross reflux.*

radiography can be helpful in making this differentiation, however, cross sectional imaging techniques offer a major advantage. Interpretation of these, however, requires an understanding of the anatomy of the diaphragm, the structure which separates the thoracic and peritoneal cavities. Ultrasound has an advantage due to its ability to image in the sagittal plane facilitating accurate identification of its position vis-a-vis peridiaphragmatic fluid collection.

Anatomy of the Diaphragm [20]

The diaphragm is a somewhat fan- or dome-shaped musculofibrinous sheet separating the thoracic and abdominal cavities. Its periphery consists of muscular fibres attached to the circumference of the thoracic outlet converging into a central tendon. The muscular fibres consist of three groups - sternal, costal and lumbar.

The sternal part arises by two fleshy slips from the back of the xiphoid process, the costal part from the internal surfaces of the cartilages and adjacent parts of the lower six ribs on each side, interdigitating with the transversus abdominis, the lumbar part from two aponeurotic arches, the medial and lateral lumbocostal arches, and from the lumbar vertebrae by two pillars or crura.

The lateral lumbocostal arch (lateral arcuate ligament) is a thickened band in the fascia covering the quadratus lumborum. It is attached medially to the front of the transverse process of the first lumbar vertebra and laterally to the lower margin of the twelfth rib. The medial lumbocostal arch (medial arcuate ligament) is a tendinous arch in the fascia covering the upper part of the psoas major. It is continuous with the lateral tendinous margin of the corresponding crus and is attached to the side of the body of the first or second lumbar vertebra. Laterally it is fixed to the front of the transverse process of the first lumbar vertebra.

The crura are tendinous in structure at their attachments and blend

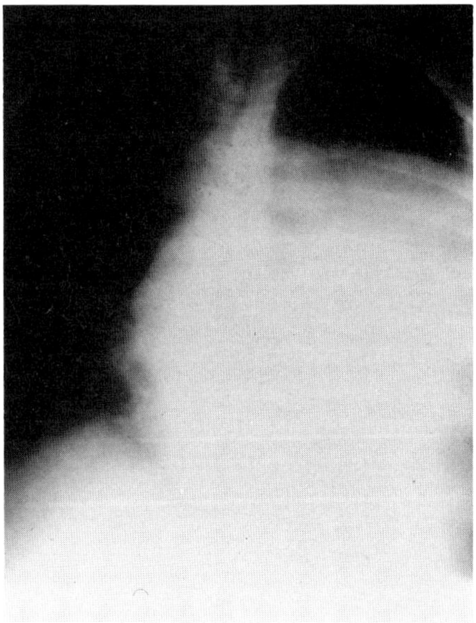

(a)

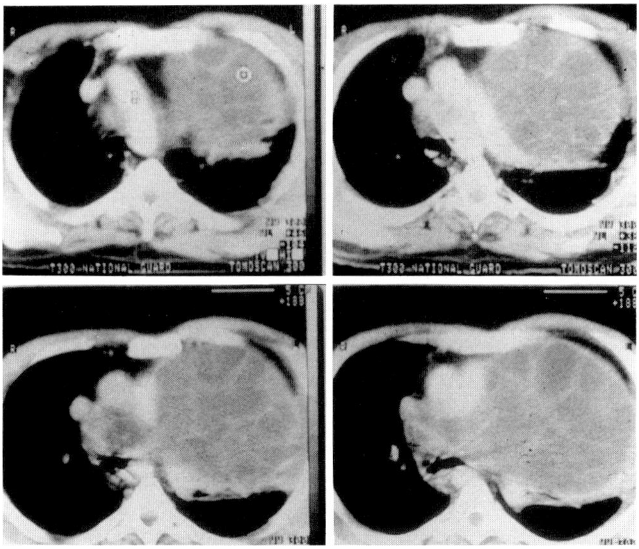

(b)

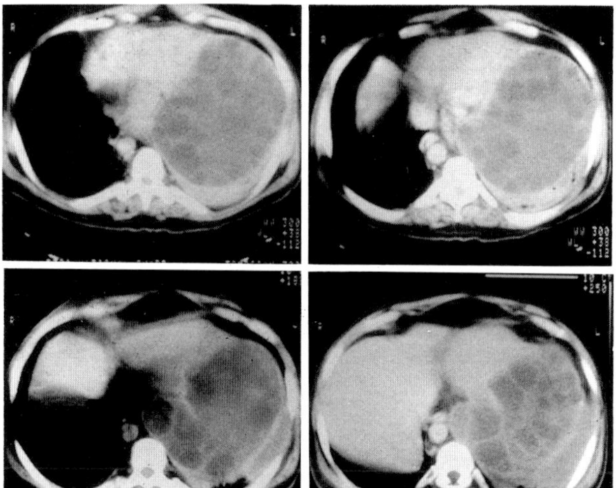

(c)

Figure 10. *26-YEAR-OLD MALE WITH PERICARDIAL ECHINOCOCCOSIS. (a) The frontal projection demonstrates a large opacity occupying most of the left hemithorax with displacement of the mediastinum to the right. (b and c) A series of axial CT's demonstrates the multi septated lesion entirely within the left side of the pericardial sac.*

with the anterior longitudinal ligament of the vertebral column. The right crus is broader and longer than the left. It arises from the anterolateral surface of the bodies and intervertebral discs of the upper three lumbar vertebrae. The left crus arises from the corresponding parts of the upper two. The medial tendinous margins of the crura meet in the median plane to form an arch across the front of the aorta.

From this circumferential attachment the fibres of the diaphragm converge into a central tendon. It is a thin but strong aponeurosis of closely interwoven fibres situated near the centre of the dome formed by the muscle, but closer to the front of the thorax, so that the posterior muscular fibres are longer. It is immediately below the pericardium with which it is partially blended.

The diaphragm is pierced for the passage of structures between the thorax and abdomen, the three large openings, i.e. the aortic, the oesophageal and the vena caval being of interest.

The aortic aperture is the lowest and most posterior of the large openings. It is situated at the level of the lower border of the twelfth thoracic vertebra. The aortic opening transmits the aorta and the thoracic duct and occasionally, the azygous vein.

The oesophageal aperture is in the muscular part of the diaphragm at the level of approximately the tenth dorsal vertebra, being formed by splitting of the medial fibres of the right crus. It is above, in front and somewhat to the left of the aortic opening and transmits the oesophagus, vagal trunks and oesophageal branches of the left gastric vessels.

The vena caval aperture, the highest of the three large openings, is at about the level of the eighth and ninth thoracic vertebrae. It is situated at the junction of the right leaf with the central area of the tendon. It is traversed by the inferior vena cava and some branches of the right phrenic nerve.

CT Signs

Four signs have been particularly helpful in the CT differentiation of pleural effusion/empyema from ascites/subphrenic abscess. These include the displaced crus sign [21,22], the interface sign [23], the diaphragm sign [24] and the bare area sign [25].

The Displaced Crus Sign

Kollins [21] made the initial observation of lateral displacement of the crus by a pleural effusion. Intraperitoneal fluid collections do not produce such displacement (Fig. 11). The crura appear as curvilinear slips extending from the aorta towards the posterior chest wall, maintaining a fairly close relationship to the vertebral column. The right crus is usually somewhat larger than the left. They are not to be confused with enlarged lymph nodes [26,27].

Interface Sign

This sign relates to the appearance of the interface between a fluid collection and the adjacent liver or spleen. When the collection is pleural, the interface is hazy and unsharp, whereas in the presence of ascitic fluid, the interface with these organs is sharp (Fig. 12). The absence of a sharp interface in the presence of a pleural effusion may well be related to the presence of the diaphragm between the fluid and the solid viscus and also partial volume averaging.

Diaphragm Sign

Due to its dome shape each hemidiaphragm on serial cross sections will he demonstrated as an oval or concentric circle, the circle becoming larger in the caudad direction. Structures within the circular or oval contour of the hemidiaphragm are intra-abdominal while those outside this contour are thoracic (Fig. 13a). The hemidiaphragm may appear as a stripe if there is sufficient subdiaphragmatic fat (Fig. 14), otherwise its location may be implied indirectly when the solid viscera are outlined by adjacent lung (Fig. 13a).

Bare Area Sign

The distribution of fluid in the right upper quadrant is influenced by the bare area of the liver. The superior and inferior coronary ligaments effectively preclude intraperitoneal fluid from extending posterior to the liver in the region of the bare area. There is nothing to stop the medial extension of fluid within the pleural space. Hence, fluid which is present behind the liver at the level of the bare area is pleural and not intraperitoneal.

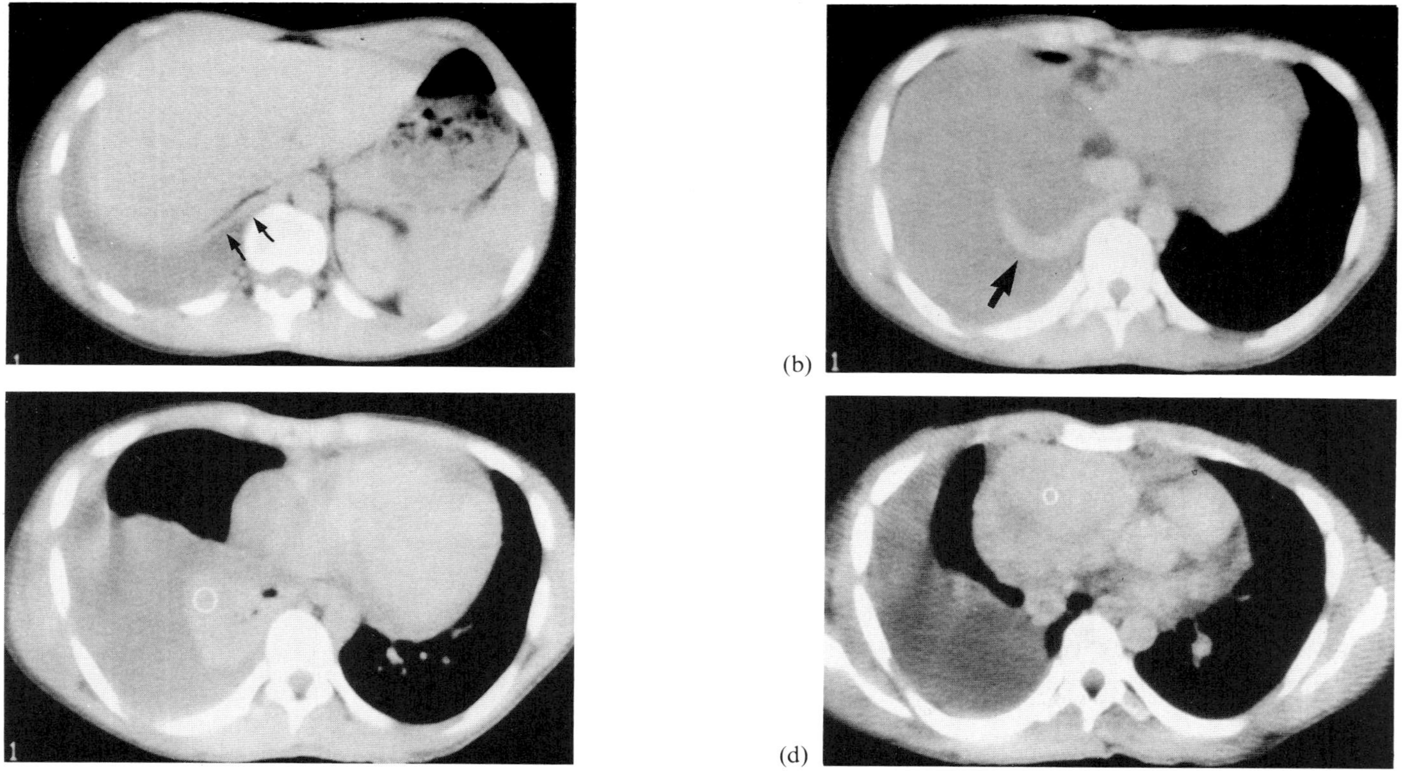

(a) (b) (c) (d)

Figure 11. *23-YEAR-OLD MALE WITH HODGKIN'S DISEASE. The enhanced serial axial CT images show: (a) Displacement of the right crus (arrows) and lack of definition of the lateral margin of the liver (interface sign) indicating presence of a pleural effusion. (b) The enlarged pleural effusion is noted. The curvilinear structure (arrow) does not represent displacement of the crus but a peripheral part of the collapsed right lower lobe. (c) Collapsed lower lobe (cursor) which is enhanced. (d) The large mediastinal mass in the prevascular space (cursor) demonstrates mixed attenuation in keeping with Hodgkin's disease.*

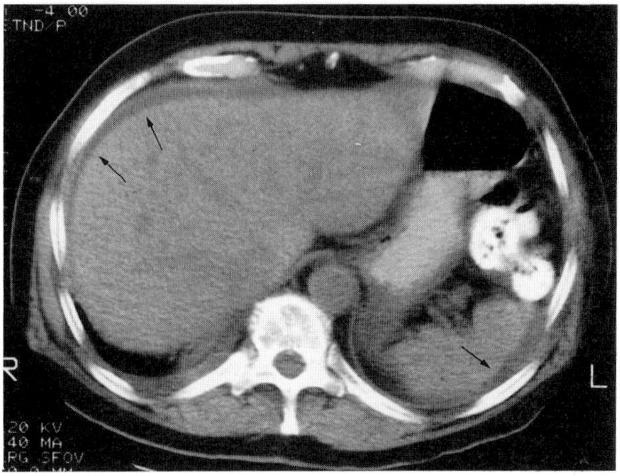

Figure 12. *AXIAL CT IMAGE IN A PATIENT WITH ASCITES AND PLEURAL EFFUSION. The interface between the liver, spleen and ascitic fluid is sharp (arrows). A small pleural effusion is present posteriorly on the right separated from the margin of liver and hemidiaphragm by intervening lung.*

The utility of these signs has been evaluated [28,29]. A study of 52 patients with ascites, right pleural effusion or both, showed that each of the individual criteria was reliable when only one abnormal fluid collection was present, that is, either a pleural effusion or ascites. When both a right pleural effusion and ascites were present, none of the four criteria individually reliably identified both fluid collections. However, the combined use of the four criteria did indeed lead to correct localization of all of the abnormal fluid collections.

Pitfalls

Atelectasis and Subpulmonary Fluid

The inferior surface of the lower lobe is concave. Intrusion of subpulmonary fluid into this concavity can create a spurious impression of a hemidiaphragm on cross sectional imaging. The peripheral portion of the atelectatic lobe may appear as a concentric band of increased density simulating the appearance of a hemidiaphragm. Should this be the case the fluid collection within this apparent hemidiaphragm would be incorrectly placed in the peritoneal cavity [30,31]. Differentiation is readily afforded by viewing contiguous

(a)

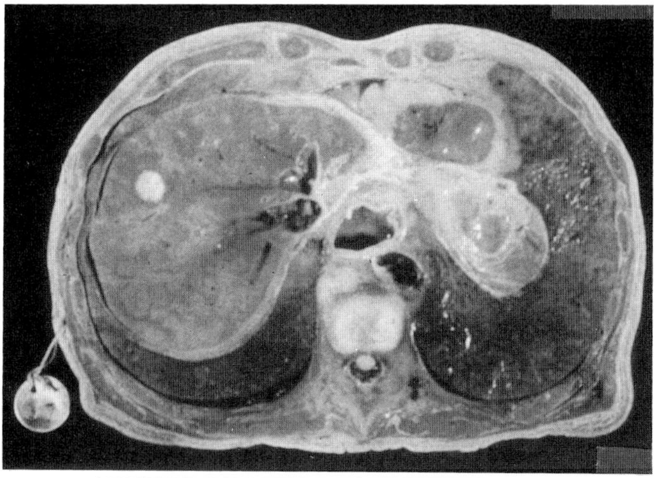

(b)

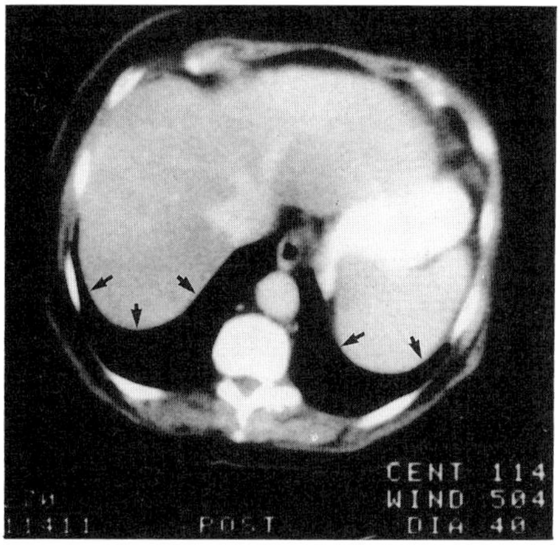

Figure 13. *ANATOMIC CROSS SECTION SHOWING RELATIONSHIP OF PERITONEAL AND THORACIC CAVITIES. (a) Structures inside the diaphragm are intraperitoneal, those outside are intrathoracic. (b) Normal anatomy. Indirect identification of hemidiaphragms by contour formed by juxtaposition of aerated lung and normal abdominal structures (arrows).*

axial images in the cephalad direction. By doing so it becomes obvious that the troublesome slice simply reflected the peripheral portions of a partially collapsed lobe. Conversely, when studying the images in a caudad direction, the true hemidiaphragm will become apparent.

It is unusual to produce a complete concentric false hemidia-

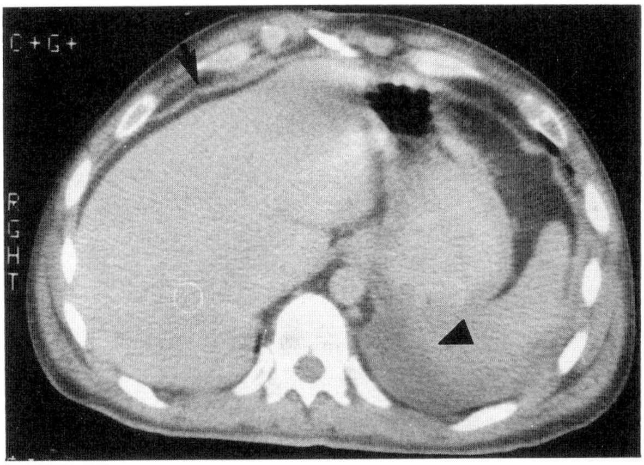

Figure 14. *AXIAL CT. Right hemidiaphragm appears as a stripe (arrow) because of availability of peridiaphragmatic fat. A pleural effusion on the left results in poor definition of the adjacent spleen (arrow-head) (interface sign).*

It is unusual to produce a complete concentric false hemidiaphragm. The more usual situation is to section a portion of the collapsed lobe producing a partial stripe, its lateral extent appearing to be suspended in the fluid (Fig. 11).

Thickening of the Parietal Pleura

Thickening of the pleura is most often the result of accompanying inflammation. In particular, with contrast enhancement the abnormal pleura will be demonstrated as a prominent soft tissue stripe which can be confused with the hemidiaphragm. Differentiation from the hemidiaphragm is made by viewing serial scans. The abnormal fluid will always maintain contact with the chest wall. The diaphragm will change in position on successive caudal scans.

Inversion of the Hemidiaphragm

Large pleural effusions are capable of inverting the hemidiaphragm [32]. The area of the hemidiaphragm most inverted will relate to the location of the largest portion of the fluid collection. In most situations, fluid accumulates maximally in the posterior and dependent portions of the pleural spaces. On the left side, the abdominal viscera

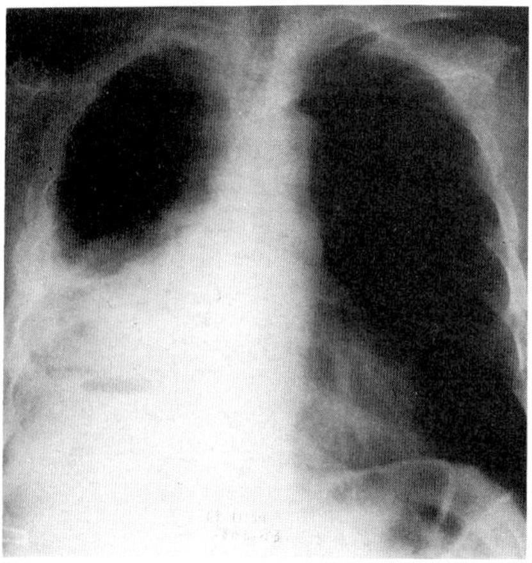

(a)

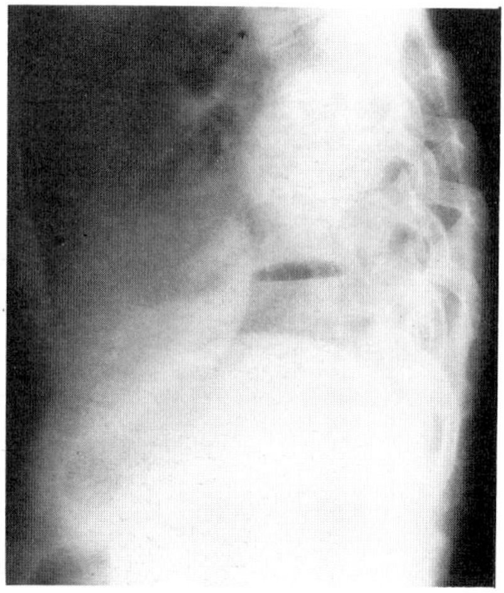

(b)

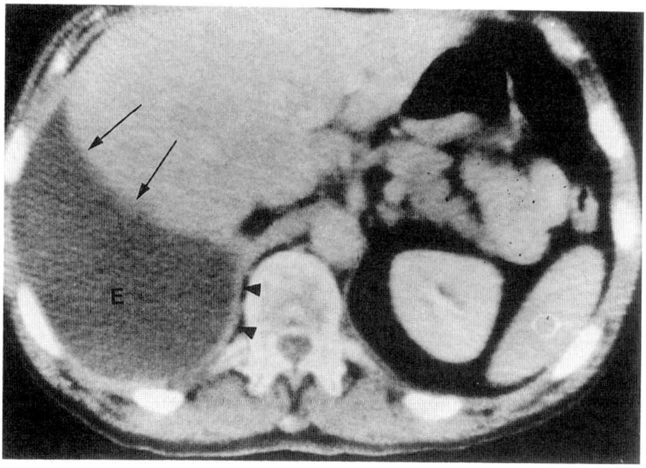

(c)

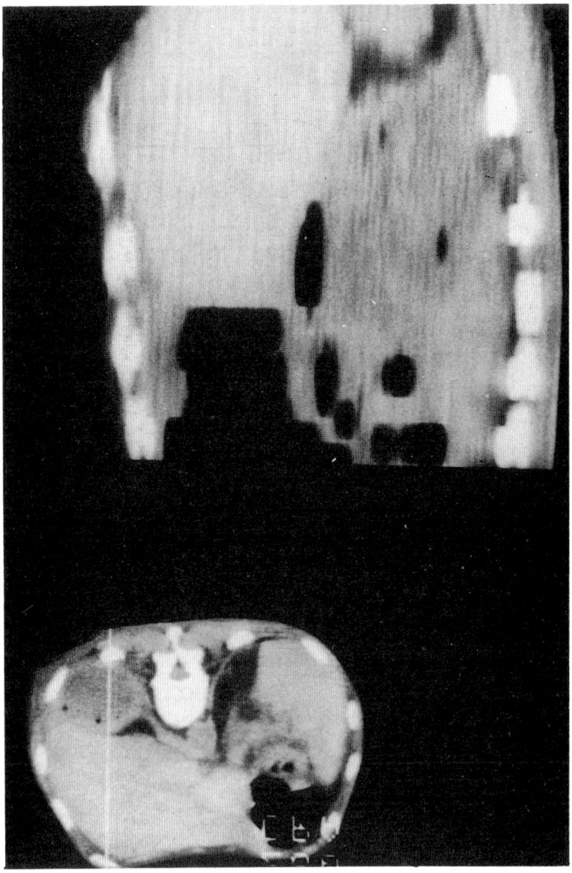

Figure 15. *LARGE EMPYEMA WITH INVERSION OF THE RIGHT HEMIDIAPHRAGM. (a and b) Frontal and lateral projections demonstrate a large area of increased density in the lower portion of the right hemithorax. Note that the air fluid level on the orthogonal projections is approximately equal which should favour an intrapulmonary process. (c) Transaxial section at the level of the tip of the spleen (cursor). Note that the pleural fluid (E) resides inside the right hemidiaphragm (arrowheads) as opposed to the usual situation in the absence of inversion of the hemidiaphragm. Note also the lack of sharpness of the border of the liver, again favouring a pleural collection. (d) Axial and parasagittal reconstruction clearly demonstrate the split pleura sign in keeping with an empyema and on the sagittal reconstruction the collections of air and fluid entirely within the pleural space. There was no extension into the peritoneal cavity.*

is displaced primarily anteriorly and medially. On the right side, the liver will be displaced primarily to the left and somewhat anteriorly.

Cross-sectional imaging will show that the pleural fluid collection is bounded by the hemidiaphragm. The displaced viscera lie outside and anterior to this collection. The fluid collection within the outlines of the hemidiaphragm will appear to be subphrenic whereas in reality it lies within the pleural space (Fig. 15). Correct identification of an inverted hemidiaphragm is facilitated by examination of serial sections. In the caudad direction, the diameter of the pleural fluid collection will become progressively smaller as one reaches the 'apex' of the inverted hemidiaphragm. Conversely, examination of serial sections in a cephalad direction will show continuity of the fluid collection with obvious fluid within the remainder of the pleural space [7,24].

In summary, knowledge of the anatomy of the diaphragm and application of the four signs discussed above will generally result in the accurate differentiation of pleural effusion/empyema from ascites/subphrenic abscess. One must, however, be cognizant of the potential pitfalls as described.

References

1. VanSonnenberg E, Nakamotol SK, Mueller PR, Kasola G, Neff CC, Friedman PJ, Ferrucci JT, Simeone JF. CT and ultrasound guided catheter drainage of empyemas after chest tube failure. *Radiology* 1984;**151**:349-353.
2. Westcott JL. Percutaneous catheter drainage of pleural effusion and empyema. *AJR* 1985;**144**:189-193.
3. Schmitt GS, Ohar JM, Ranter KR, Naunheim KS. Indwelling transbronchial catheter drainage of pulmonary abscess. *Ann Thor Surg* 1988;**45**:43-47.
4. Parker LA, Melton JW, Delany DJ, Yankaskas BC. Percutaneous small bore catheter drainage in the management of lung abscesses. *Chest* 1987;**92**:213-218.
5. Ball WS, Bisset GS, Towbint RB. Percutaneous drainage of chest abscesses in children. *Radiology* 1989;**171**:431-434.
6. Warwick R, Williams PL. *Gray's Anatomy.* 35th ed. pp 1190-1194. Edinburgh: Longman Group Ltd, 1973.
7. Proto AV, Rost RC. CT of the thorax. *Radiographics* 1985;**5**:784-800.
8. Robbins SL. *Pathologic Basis of Disease.* pp 86,816-818,842. Philadelphia: W.B. Saunders, 1974.
9. Maier HC, Haight C. Large infected solitary pulmonary cysts simulating empyema. *J Thor Surg* 1940;**91**:471-494.
10. Friedman PJ, Hellekant CAG. Radiologic recognition of bronchopleural fistula. *Radiology* 1977;**124**:289-295.

11. Bressler EL, Frances IR, Glazer GM, Gross EH. Bolus contrast medium enhancement for distinguishing pleural from parenchymal lung disease: CT features. *JCAT* 1987;**11**:436-440.
12. Pugatch RD, Saling LJ, Rohbins AH, Snider GL. Differentiation of pleural and pulmonary lesions using computed tomography. *JCAT* 1978;**2**:601-606.
13. Baber C, Hedlund LW, Oddson TA, Putman CE. Differentiating empyemas and peripheral pulmonary abscesses. The value of computed tomography. *Radiology* 1980;**135**:755-758.
14. Shin MS, Ho KJ. Computed tomographic characteristics of pleural empyema. *CT:JCT* 1983;**7**:179-182.
15. Williford ME, Hidalgo H, Putman CE, Korobkin M, Ram PC. Computed tomography of pleural disease. *AJR* 1983;**140**:909-914.
16. Stark DD, Federle MP, Goodman PC, Podrasky AE, Webb WR. Differentiating lung abscess and empyema: radiography and computed tomography. *AJR* 1983;**141**:163-167.
17. Stark P, Gadziala N, Greene R. Fluid accumulation in pre-existing pulmonary airspaces. *AJR* 1980;**134**:701-706.
18. Zinn WL, Naidich DP, Whelan CA, Litt AW, McCauley DI, Ettenger NA. Fluid within preexisting pulmonary airspaces: a potential pitfall in the CT differentiation of pleural from parenchymal disease. *JCAT* 1987;**11**:441-418.
19. von Sinner WN, Linjawi T, Al Watban J. Mediastinal hydatid disease: report of three cases. *JCAR* 1990;**41**:79-82.
20. Warwick R, Williams PL. *Gray's Anatomy.* 35th ed. pp 516-518. Edinburgh: Longman Group Ltd, 1973.
21. Kollins SA. Computed tomography of the pulmonary parenchyma and chest wall. *Radiol Clin N Am* 1977;**15**:297-308.
22. Dwyer A. The displaced crus; a sign for distinguishing between pleural fluid and ascites on computed tomography. *JCAT* 1978;**2**:598-599.
23. Teplick JG, Teplick SK, Goodman L, Haskin ME. The interface sign: a computed tomographic sign for distinguishing pleural and intra-abdominal fluid. *Radiology* 1982;**144**:359-362.
24. Alexander ES, Proto AV, Clark RA. CT differentiation of subphrenic abscess and pleural effusion. *AJR* 1983;**140**:47-51.
25. Griffin DJ, Gross BH, McCracken S, Glazer GM. *JCAT* 1984;**8**;24-28.
26. Callen PW, Korobkin M, Isherwood I. Computed tomographic evaluation of the retrocrural prevertebral space. *AJR* 1977;**129**:907-910.
27. Callen PW, Filly RA, Korobkin M. Computed tomographic evaluation of the diaphragmatic crura. *Radiology* 1978;**126**:413-416.
28. Halvorsen RA, Fosterr WL, Pedyshin PJ, Thompson WM, Korobkin M. Ascites or pleural effusion? CT differentiation: four useful criteria. *Radiographics* 1986;**6**:135-149.
29. Halvorsen RA, Fedyshin PJ, Korobkin M, Thompson WM. CT differentiation of pleural effusion from ascites. An evaluation of four signs using blinded analysis of 52 cases. *Invest Radiol* 1986;**21**:391-395.
30. Silverman PM, Baker ME, Mahony BS. Atelectasis in subpulmonic fluid: a CT pitfall in distinguishing pleural from peritoneal fluid. *JCAT* 1985;**9**:763-766.
31. Federle MP, Mark AS, Guillaumin ES. CT of subpulmonic pleural effusions and atelectasis; criteria for differentiation from subphrenic fluid. *AJR* 1986;**146**:685-689.
32. Rigby M, Zylak CJ, Wood LDH. The effect of lobar atelectasis on pleural fluid distribution in dogs. *Radiology* 1980;**130**:603-607.

Computer tomography and magnetic resonance imaging for staging of lung cancer

Charles V. Zwirewich and Nestor L. Müller
Department of Radiology, University of British Columbia and Vancouver General Hospital, Vancouver, Canada

Introduction

Lung cancer is the most common fatal malignancy worldwide [1] and approximately 90% of patients who develop lung cancer will die of their disease [2]. While the incidence of almost all other malignancies is declining or remaining steady, the incidence of bronchogenic carcinoma continues to rise, particularly among women [3]. Of all lung cancers 80 - 90% are directly attributable to cigarette smoking [4,5], the incidence in smokers being 10- to 25-fold greater than among non-smokers [6]. Adenocarcinoma is now the most common cell type accounting for 35% of cases; squamous cell carcinoma accounts for 25% of cases, small cell carcinoma for 20%, and large cell undifferentiated carcinoma for 15% [5].

The 5-year survival is only 10 - 15% because most bronchogenic carcinomas are unresectable when first diagnosed. Complete surgical excision of the tumour remains the most effective form of therapy and offers the patient the only reasonable hope of cure. Recent advances in surgical technique including methodical resection of the primary tumour combined with meticulous intra-operative mediastinal lymph node dissection offer the potential for improved survival in a selected group of patients. These advances have important implications for the continually evolving role of computed tomography (CT) and magnetic resonance imaging (MRI) in the staging of lung cancer.

This chapter will review: (1) The new International Staging System for Lung Cancer and its implications for surgical therapy in non-small cell tumours, (2) the complementary role of CT, MRI and invasive techniques in the staging of lung cancer, and (3) the current limitations of invasive and non-invasive staging techniques in the evaluation of the extent of primary tumour, nodal and metastatic disease.

The International Staging System for Lung Cancer

Clinical staging has been defined as the best estimate of the extent of disease in a patient with malignancy made prior to institution of therapy [7] and generally stops when enough information is available to determine an appropriate course of treatment [8,9]. The Tumour - Nodal involvement - Metastasis (TNM) staging system is the most widely employed. Originally described by Denoix [10] this system describes the extent of the primary tumour by the letter T; the letter N denotes the absence or presence of regional lymph node metastases with appropriate subscripts; and the letter M indicates the absence or presence of distant metastases. The advantage of the TNM system lies in the fact that survival data for bronchogenic carcinoma is related to the extent of primary tumour (T), lymph node metastases (N) and the presence of distant metastases (M). The original Task Force for Lung Cancer combined the TNM subsets into three distinct stages which formed the basis of the two most widely used staging systems prior to 1986, those of the American Joint Committee on Cancer (AJCC) [11] and the Union Internationale Contre Cancer (UICC) [12].

In 1986, Mountain [13] proposed a new staging system for lung cancer. The goal of this system was to emphasize the anatomic extent of disease in the selection of therapy [1] make the staging of lung cancer reflect recent advances in surgical therapy, and resolve differences between the AJCC and UICC staging systems. This staging system has subsequently been accepted by the AJCC and UICC as the new International Staging System for Lung Cancer [13].

Primary Tumour (T) Subsets

T defines the primary tumour and its local extent (Tables 1 and 2).

Table 1. *Primary tumour (T)*

TX	Tumour proven by the presence of malignant cells in bronchopulmonary secretions but not visualized roentgenographically or bronchoscopically, or any tumour that cannot be assessed as in a retreatment staging.
T0	No evidence of primary tumour.
TIS	Carcinoma in situ.
T1	A tumour that is 3.0 cm or less in greatest dimension, surrounded by lung or visceral pleura, and without evidence of invasion proximal to a lobar bronchus at bronchoscopy.*
T2	A tumour more than 3.0 cm in greatest dimension, or a tumour of any size that either invades the visceral pleura or has associated atelectasis or obstructive pneumonitis extending to the hilar region. At bronchoscopy, the proximal extent of demonstrable tumour must be within a lobar bronchus or at least 2.0 cm distal to the carina. Any associated atelectasis or obstructive pneumonitis must involve less than an entire lung.
T3	A tumour of any size with direct extension into the chest wall (including superior sulcus tumours), diaphragm or the mediastinal pleura or pericardium without involving the heart, great vessels, trachea, oesophagus or vertebral body, or a tumour in the main bronchus within 2 cm of the carina without involving the carina.
T4	A tumour of any size with invasion of the mediastinum or involving heart, great vessels, trachea, oesophagus, vertebral body or carina or presence of malignant pleural effusion.*

* See Table 2. Reproduced with permission from ref. 13

T1 lesions include those measuring 3 cm or less in diameter and which are surrounded by lung or visceral pleura. This category includes the majority of small peripheral cancers. T2 lesions are tumours greater than 3 cm in diameter or tumours associated with atelectasis or postobstructive pneumonitis involving less than the

Table 2. *Footnote to TNM definitions*

T1*	The uncommon superficial tumour of any size with its invasive component limited to the bronchial wall which may extend proximal to the main bronchus is classified as T1
T4*	Most pleural effusions associated with lung cancer are due to tumour. There are, however, some patients in whom cytopathological examination of pleural fluid (on more than one specimen) is negative for tumour, the fluid is non-bloody and is not an exudate. In such cases where these elements and clinical judgement dictate that the effusion is not related to the tumour, the patients should be staged T1, T2, or T3, excluding effusion as a staging element.

* See Table 1.
Reproduced with permission from ref. 13

whole lung. T3 lesions include those involving the chest wall, tumours extending into diaphragm, mediastinal pleura or pericardium without invasion of the heart, great vessels, trachea, oesophagus or vertebral body. Tumours within 2 cm of but not involving the tracheal carina are included in the T3 descriptor, as are superior sulcus tumours with invasion of the chest wall. T4 designates those primary tumours which are so locally extensive that curative surgery is generally not feasible. These include primary tumours with invasion of the heart, great vessels, trachea, oesophagus, vertebral body and those with a malignant pleural effusion.

Lymph Node Metastasis (N) and Distant Metastasis (M) Subsets

The incidence of lymph node metastases increases with increasing primary tumour size, ranging from 31 to 71% in patients undergoing curative resection [14] and 75 - 94% in autopsy series [15,16]. The presence of mediastinal lymph node metastases is one of the most important factors determining prognosis [14,17].

N0 describes those patients with no lymph node metastases. Only 10 - 15% of patients are N0 at diagnosis. N1 indicates intrapulmonary or hilar lymph node metastases (Table 3). The N2 descriptor defines subcarinal and ipsilateral mediastinal lymph node metastases; these are potentially resectable for cure. N3 defines the presence of contralateral mediastinal lymph node metastases, as well as ipsilateral or contralateral scalene or supraclavicular nodal involvement. N3 status contraindicates curative resection [1] and portends a poor outcome.

Table 3. *Nodal involvement (N)*

N0	No demonstrable metastasis to lymph nodes
N1	Metastasis to lymph node in the peribronchial or the ipsilateral hilar region, or both, including direct extension
N2	Metastasis to ipsilateral mediastinal lymph nodes and subcarinal lymph nodes
N3	Metastasis to contralateral mediastinal lymph nodes, contralateral hilar lymph nodes, ipsilateral or contralateral scalene or supraclavicular lymph nodes

Reproduced with permission from ref. 13.

Consistency in reporting the location of lymph node metastases has been greatly improved through the use of lymph node mapping schemes such as those proposed by the American Thoracic society (ATS) [7] and by Naruke et al [14]. The ATS node map is designed to facilitate and standardize the description of nodal station involvement and is based on the relationship of lymph nodes to major anatomical structures within the pulmonary hilum and mediastinum (Fig. 1). This scheme provides clear separation between critical node stations using fixed anatomic landmarks which are easily identified by the radiologist on chest radiographs and CT scans and by the surgeon at mediastinoscopy and thoracotomy (Table 4). The ATS node map is routinely used in the prethoracotomy assessment of mediastinal lymph nodes on CT and at mediastinoscopy at our institution.

The M descriptor remains unchanged from the original TNM classification. M0 defines the subset of patients with no demonstrable distant metastases and M1 those patients with proven distant metastases (Table 5).

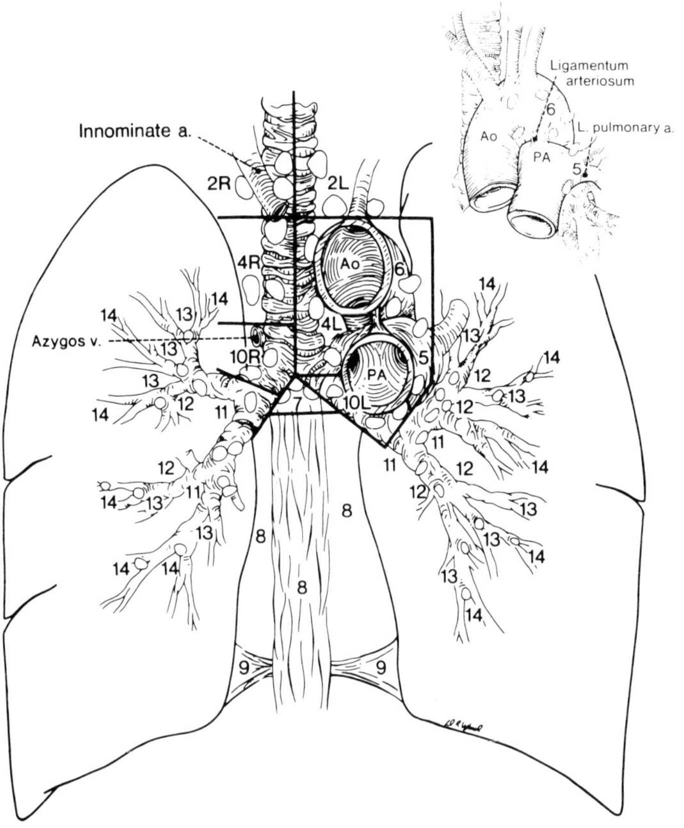

Figure 1. *THE AMERICAN THORACIC SOCIETY (ATS) NODE MAP. Critical landmarks which separate nodal stations include the ligamentum arteriosum, azygos vein, origin of the innominate artery and upper lobe bronchi (Table 4). AO = Aortic arch, PA = main pulmonary artery. Modified and reproduced with permission from ref. 7.*

Guidelines for Patient Management and Prognosis by Stage Grouping

Surgical resection remains the only reliable method of curing lung cancer, but there is considerable controversy as to what constitutes the optimal surgical approach to lung cancer. Selection criteria for surgical candidates have changed as advances in treatment and new

Table 4. *Definitions of regional nodal stations*

X	Supraclavicular nodes.
2R	Right upper paratracheal (supra-innominate) nodes: nodes to the right of the midline of the trachea between the intersection of the caudal margin of the innominate artery with the trachea, and the apex of the lung. (Includes highest R mediastinal node.) (Radiologists may use the same caudal margin as in 2L.)
2L	Left upper paratracheal (supra-aortic) nodes: nodes to the left of the midline of the trachea between the top of the aortic arch and the apex of the lung. (Includes the highest L mediastinal node.)
4R	Right lower paratracheal nodes: nodes to the right of the midline of the trachea between the cephalic border of the azygos vein and the intersection of the caudal margin of the brachiocephalic artery with the right side of the trachea. (Includes some pretracheal and paracaval nodes.) (Radiologists may use the same cephalic margin as in 4L.)
4L	Left lower paratracheal nodes: nodes to the left of the midline of the trachea between the top of the aortic arch and the level of the carina, medial to the ligamentum arteriosum. (Includes some pretracheal nodes.)
5	Aortopulmonary nodes: subaortic and para-aortic nodes, lateral to the ligamentum arteriosum or the aorta or left pulmonary artery, proximal to the first branch of the LPA.
6	Anterior mediastinal nodes: nodes anterior to the ascending aorta or the innominate artery. (Includes some pretracheal and pre-aortic nodes.)
7	Subcarinal nodes: nodes arising caudal to the carina of the trachea but not associated with the lower lobe bronchi or arteries within the lung.
8	Para-oesophageal nodes: nodes dorsal to the posterior wall of the trachea and to the right or left of the midline of the oesophagus. (Includes retrotracheal but not subcarinal nodes.)

Table 4 *continued*

9	Right or left pulmonary ligament nodes: nodes within the right or left pulmonary ligament.
10R	Right tracheobronchial nodes: nodes to the right of the midline of the trachea from the level of the cephalic border of the azygos vein to the origin of the right upper lobe bronchus.
10L	Left peribronchial nodes: nodes to the left of the midline of the trachea between the carina and the left upper lobe bronchus, medial to the ligamentum arteriosum.
11 - 14	Intrapulmonary nodes removed in the right or left lung specimen plus those distal to the mainstem bronchi or secondary carina. These include stations 11 (interlobar), 12 (lobar), 13 (segmental), and 14 (subsegmental).

Reproduced with permission from ref. 7

Table 5. *Distant metastasis (M)*

M0	No (known) distant metastasis
M1	Distant metastasis present - specify site

Reproduced with permission from ref. 13.

surgical techniques extend the limits of technical resectability [9]. Technical resectability refers to the surgeon's ability to remove all known tumour disease during thoracotomy and lymph node dissection.

Confirmation of a complete or 'curative' resection is based largely upon pathological analysis of the resected lung specimen and is defined as one in which: (1) the surgeon is certain that the procedure has removed all known disease; (2) the most proximal resection margins are free of tumour; (3) the most distal nodes within the lymphatic drainage of the region are free of tumour; and (4) the capsule of resected tumour-containing lymph nodes is intact with no evidence of perinodal tumour extension [9]. Several pre-operative criteria have been proposed to identify patients who are optimal candidates for curative surgical resection [1]. These include: (1) a primary tumour which is resectable (ideally T1 or T2); (2) the absence of distant metastases (MO); (3) ipsilateral mediastinal lymph node metastases (N2), if present, should involve only one node group, preferably the ipsilateral low paratracheal nodes; (4) the absence of extranodal tumor extension at mediastinoscopy; (5) squamous carcinoma histology; and (6) a patient who is a good surgical candidate from the functional standpoint.

Stage I

Stage I disease includes those patients with T1 or T2 tumours without any evidence of intrapulmonary or mediastinal lymph node metastasis or distant metastasis (N0M0, Table 6). These patients are candidates for curative surgical resection with a 5-year survival ranging from 60 to 85% [4,13,18] (Fig. 2). Unfortunately recurrence rates as high as

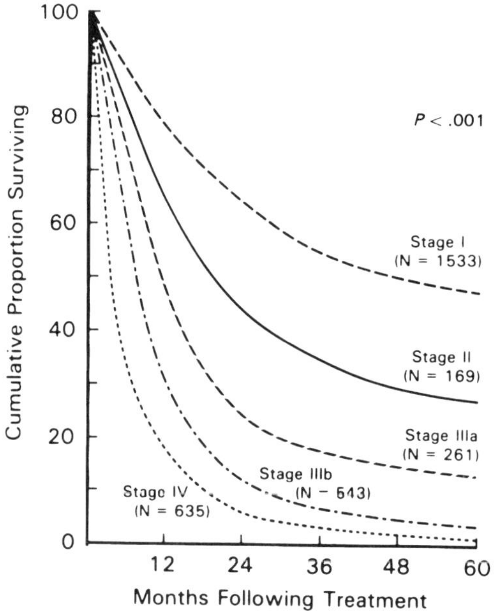

Figure 2. *CUMULATIVE PROPORTION OF PATIENTS SURVIVING 5 YEARS BY CLINICAL STAGE OF DISEASE. Reproduced with permission from ref. 13.*

45% have been reported in Stage I lung cancer, with the most common sites involving brain and lung [19]. Recurrence rates are also higher with non-squamous carcinoma histologies, and there is a 25% risk of developing a subsequent, second lung cancer in this group [17]. Although surgical lobectomy and full mediastinal lymph node dissection are the cornerstones of therapy in Stage I disease, preliminary evidence suggests that complete excision of these tumours by generous wedge resection or segmentectomy may be as effective as lobectomy [20,21] with survival rates equivalent to standard lobectomy without an increase in mortality.

Table 6. *Stage grouping of TNM subsets*

	Stage groupings		
Occult carcinoma	TX	N0	M0
Stage 0	TIS	Carcinoma in situ	
Stage I	T1	N0	M0
	T2	N0	M0
Stage II	T1	N1	M0
	T2	N1	M0
Stage IIIa	T3	N0	M0
	T3	N1	M0
	T1 - 3	N2	M0
Stage IIIb	Any T	N3	M0
	T4	Any N	M0
Stage IV	Any T	Any N	M1

Reproduced with permission from ref. 13.

Stage II

Stage II defines those patients with T1 or T2 lesions with lymph node metastases limited to the peribronchial or ipsilateral intrapulmonary hilar nodes (N1). Curative surgery is preferred for Stage II disease and pneumonectomy may be required if intrapulmonary N1 disease (11R or 11L positions) is central. Therefore, some patients with borderline pulmonary function may not be candidates for curative resection. In the presence of N1 disease, 5-year survival is generally under 50% [22].

Stage IIIa

Patients with Stage III lung cancer have extrapulmonary spread of disease by direct extension alone or in combination with lymph node metastases, but lack evidence of distant metastases. Stage III disease is divided into a and b categories (Table 6). The principal determinants of resectability in patients with Stage III disease relate to the status of the primary tumour (T) and lymph node metastases (N).

Stage IIIa defines a subset of patients with limited circumscribed extrapulmonary extension of the primary tumour alone or in combination with regional lymph node metastases (T3N0 - N2). This category includes T3 cancers that may be cured with newer surgical techniques [13]. Five-year survival rates for Stage IIIa disease are in the range 20 - 40% if the tumour and regional lymph nodes are completely resected [1,4,9,13]. Included in this category are peripheral tumours with localized chest wall extension amenable to lobectomy or pneumonectomy in combination with *en bloc* resection of the chest wall and chest wall reconstruction. Although these patients constitute only 8% of those undergoing curative resection for lung cancer [2] their 5-year survival is primarily determined by nodal status and may be as high as 56% for T3N0M0 lesions [23,24].

Superior sulcus tumours are also considered operable Stage IIIa lesions if they have no clinical evidence of invasion into the vertebral body, other major mediastinal structures and no evidence of Pancoast or Horner's syndrome [9]. Superior sulcus tumours involving only mediastinal pleura and central tumours with limited pericardial invasion have been shown to have a 5-year survival ranging from 32 to 41% following resection [9].

Tumours involving the upper lobe or mainstem bronchi within 2 cm of the carina may be amenable to lobectomy with sleeve resection, a lung-sparing procedure [2,4]. With this technique, a portion of the mainstem bronchus is removed in continuity with the involved lobe, usually an upper lobe. This procedure is preferred to pneumonectomy in those patients who carry a poor surgical risk due to compromised pulmonary function [2,25]. There is no difference in either the morbidity or mortality between lobectomy with sleeve resection and pneumonectomy [26].

The other major determinant of resectability in Stage IIIa disease is nodal status. The majority of patients seen in clinical practice (35 - 45%) have N2 disease at presentation [2]. Using previous staging systems the presence of mediastinal lymphadenopathy generally indicated a poor prognosis with survival ranging from 5 to 30% at 5 years [15,27-30]. However in selected patients, N2 disease may be amenable to curative resection with or without adjuvant radiotherapy. Mountain reviewed the survival data in 69 patients with T3N0, T3N1 and T3N2 lesions. Five-year survival was 36% for the T3N0 and T3N1 groups, and was 26% for T3N2 lesions, with a more favorable outcome for squamous carcinomas [31]. Martini et al [22] and Kirsh et al [32] have reported similar survival data.

Although these data indicate that patients with limited mediastinal lymph node metastases have a more favorable outcome, Pearson has shown that not all patients with N2 disease benefit from surgery [33]. Among patients in whom nodal metastases were identified at mediastinoscopy, the 5-year survival was 9%, whereas patients with N2 disease discovered at thoracotomy following a negative mediastinoscopy had a 5-year survival rate of 24%. This study clearly indicates that survival is worse if N2 status is identified at mediastinoscopy rather than at thoracotomy.

Therefore if resection is feasible by T and M criteria, patients with N2 disease should undergo cervical mediastinoscopy alone or in combination with anterior mediastinotomy to assess by biopsy the condition of all accessible lymph nodes in order to determine resectability [9]. In the absence of evidence of N2 metastases on analysis of biopsy material obtained from all accessible nodes at mediastinoscopy, patients are considered resectable and may proceed to thoracotomy.

Stage IIIb and Stage IV

Stage IIIb describes tumours associated with extensive extrapulmonary spread (T4) and those with scalene, supraclavicular or contralateral mediastinal lymph node metastases (N3). It is important to document by biopsy the presence of nodal involvement because N3 disease is surgically unresectable and is associated with a 5-year survival of less than 20% [4]. While N3 lesions are unresectable, a small number of patients with highly localized tumours involving the proximal mainstem bronchi, carina or trachea (T4N0M0) may be amenable to resection with tracheobronchial reconstruction (Fig. 3). The absence of lymph node metastases and a favourable cell type

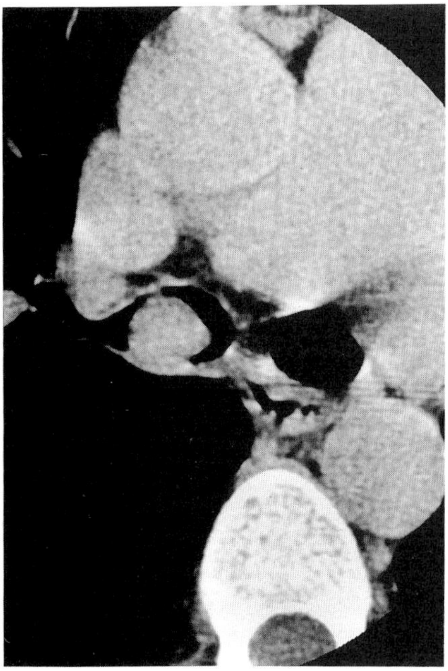

Figure 3. *CT SCAN DEMONSTRATES A 12 mm POLYPOID CARCINOID TUMOUR ORIGINATING FROM THE POSTERIOR WALL OF THE RIGHT MAINSTEM BRONCHUS (RMB). This lesion was successfully resected by right upper lobectomy with sleeve resection of the RMB and anastomosis of the bronchus intermedius to the RMB stump. Despite the central location of this tumour suggesting a T3 designation, only minimal submucosal invasion was evident at pathological examination, rendering this a T1 lesion by the International Staging System. No lymph node metastases were identified at thoracotomy. This is an uncommon example of stage I tumour (T1N0M0) involving the mainstem bronchus.*

(well-differentiated squamous) are necessary prerequisites for this surgery [9,34,35]. Patients with pathologically proven distant metastases are classified Stage IV regardless of T and N status, are considered unresectable and have a very poor prognosis.

CT, MRI Technique and Invasive Staging Procedures

The goal of pre-operative lung cancer staging is to identify distant metastases, N3 or unresectable N2 disease and T4 lesions, thereby sparing patients from the morbidity and potential mortality of unnecessary thoracotomy [36,37]. While considerable controversy exists regarding the roles of non-invasive imaging and invasive staging procedures (cervical mediastinoscopy and anterior mediastinotomy), it is clear that CT and MRI are useful in the pre-operative evaluation of bronchogenic carcinoma. Although CT remains the principal imaging technique used in the staging of lung cancer, MRI offers several potential advantages and has been shown to be superior to CT in the assessment of local vascular invasion, invasion of the chest wall, pericardium and heart, and in the assessment of metastatic disease.

In practice, the staging process generally begins with an evaluation for the presence of distant metastases; this includes obtaining a careful history and physical examination and judicious use of screening laboratory investigations which may guide further imaging techniques and biopsy. In the absence of detectable distant metastases, staging proceeds to the evaluation of mediastinal lymph node metastases and assessment of the extent of invasion of the primary tumour into the mediastinum, chest wall, or contiguous structures.

CT Technique

The CT techniques used in the evaluation of lung cancer varies from institution to institution. Many centres do not use intravenous contrast because it adds very little useful information in the assessment of the mediastinal nodes and adrenal glands. We routinely use a contrast enhanced scan protocol with 10 mm collimation scans through the chest and an incremental dynamic study of the liver to assess for mediastinal invasion, hilar adenopathy and hepatic metastases. A high-spatial frequency algorithm (such as the 'bone' algorithm available on the GE CT 9800 scanner) is routinely used for image reconstruction in the chest as this has been shown to improve spatial resolution [38]. Bolus contrast infusion administered via a selectable flow rate infusion pump is preferred because hilar lymphadenopathy can be more easily distinguished from vessels than on scans performed without contrast or with a slow continuous infusion of contrast.

In evaluating selected lesions which involve the distal trachea or proximal main bronchi, we often employ a dynamic contrast enhanced scan sequence consisting of two overlapping sets of six contiguous 5 mm scans obtained during a single breath-hold. The image data are reconstructed to a small display field-of-view (25 cm) affording improved spatial resolution. This technique is used to evaluate the relative extent of intra- and extraluminal tumour among patients who are candidates for lung-sparing surgery, or among candidates for palliative endoscopic laser therapy to alleviate atelectasis or pneumonia distal to an obstructing tumour (Fig. 4).

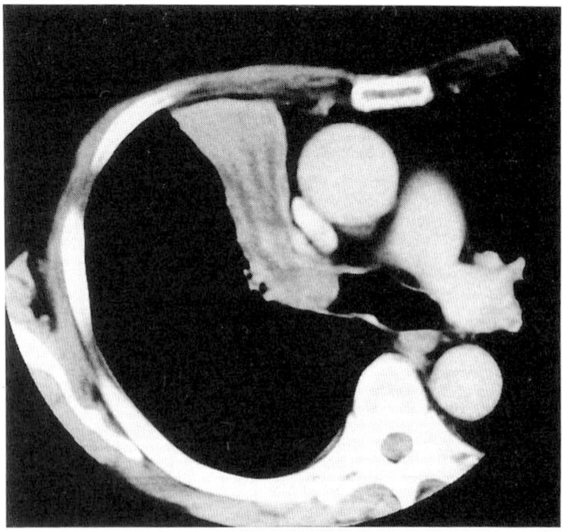

Figure 4. *CT OF A PREDOMINANTLY INTRALUMINAL TUMOUR CAUSING RIGHT UPPER LOBE ATELECTASIS. An endobronchial mass completely obstructs the origin of the bronchus to the right upper lobe, which is collapsed. The mass extends to within 1 cm of the carina. If unresectable by other N or M criteria, this patient would be an ideal candidate for palliative laser photoresection alone or in combination with radiotherapy. Reproduced with permission from ref. 145.*

MRI Technique

MRI scanning technique typically includes a T1-weighted coronal localizing sequence (short TR, short TE) which is performed initially to survey the chest and guide the positioning of subsequent transverse, coronal or sagittal image planes. T1-weighted images optimize contrast between high-signal fat, low signal flowing blood in vessels, and intermediate-signal masses and lymph nodes [39]. Dual echo spin-echo techniques yield balanced T1 and T2 or proton density images (long TR, short TE) and T2-weighted images (long TR, long TE). Balanced or proton-density images are preferred for detection of lung nodules and parenchymal changes. The T2-weighted sequences facilitate further differentiation between tumour and adjacent structures, and enhance the visualization of pleural fluid [39].

Electrocardiogram (ECG) gating and respiratory-ordered phase encoding may be used to help suppress cardiac and respiratory motion artefacts which may degrade image quality. Spatial presaturation and gradient-moment-nulling algorithms are of additional benefit in reducing undesirable flow related signal [39]. Gradient-echo pulse sequences are particularly helpful in the evaluation of vessel patency and thrombosis, as rapidly flowing blood in patent vessels displays high signal intensity and can be separated from tumour or a bland thrombus on images acquired using this technique.

The selection of appropriate scanning planes is essential in MRI and should be tailored to the specific clinical indication following acquisition of a coronal localizing sequence. In general most patients are adequately evaluated using T1, balanced proton density and T2 weighted sequences in the transverse plane. Apical lesions are best studied using a surface coil and a small field-of-view [39] in the sagittal and coronal planes. Lesions with chest wall or suspected mediastinal, diaphragmatic or cardiac invasion may also benefit from sagittal and coronal scans in addition to conventional scans in the transverse plane.

Cervical Mediastinoscopy and Anterior Mediastinotomy

Many investigators have reported cervical mediastinoscopy to be the most reliable method for staging mediastinal lymph node metastases prior to thoracotomy [33,40-42]. In this procedure, a small incision is made just above the sternal notch through which a mediastinoscope is inserted. Separation of the mediastinal soft tissue planes is then performed by blunt dissection. Although mediastinoscopy is an invasive test and requires general anesthesia, Luke et al [43] observed an overall complication rate of only 2.3% in their series of 1 000 consecutive mediastinoscopies, with no mortality related to the procedure. Mediastinoscopy allows visualization of lymph nodes in the 2, 4 and 10 positions bilaterally, as well as in the anterior subcarinal space (position 7). Mediastinoscopy alone cannot identify anterior mediastinal nodes in front of the aortic arch (position 6), nodes in the aorticopulmonary window (position 5), along the course of the phrenic nerves, subaortic region and in the posterior subcarinal space (position 7) [44]. In patients with left upper lobe or left hilar tumours where metastases to the aortopulmonary window and anterior mediastinal nodes are common, a left anterior mediastinotomy is generally performed through the second intercostal space if cervical mediastinoscopy biopsy material is negative for malignancy [7].

Assessment of Mediastinal Lymph Nodes

The reported prevalence of lymph node metastases depends upon how thoroughly the mediastinum is sampled at mediastinoscopy and thoracotomy. Prevalence rates of lymph node metastases ranging from 4 to approximately 40% have been reported [33,45]. Studies in which complete resection of all accessible nodes was performed at thoracotomy tend to report a higher prevalence of metastatic disease [46-48] than those in which dissection was incomplete or in which only enlarged or palpably abnormal nodes were resected. Dales et al [49] reviewed 42 studies in the CT literature performed between 1980 and 1988 and found an average prevalence rate of lymph node metastases of 38%. While this is a representative figure, the actual prevalence rate in a given population of patients is also influenced by the histology and location of the primary tumour; lymph node metastases are more common among non-squamous histologies and central rather than peripheral tumours [49].

Computed Tomography

CT has been strongly advocated in the staging of mediastinal nodes because it is non-invasive and has been reported by some to have a high sensitivity in the detection of tumour-containing lymph nodes [52-56]. However, there is controversy regarding the role of CT in the evaluation of mediastinal lymph nodes. This is largely due to the wide range for sensitivity and specificity reported in the CT literature which in turn reflects the diversity of opinion regarding the size of normal mediastinal lymph nodes on CT, whether short axis or long axis should be used in measurement, and which threshold size is optimal.

The range of normal for mediastinal lymph node size has been reported to vary from less than 7 mm to greater than 11 mm [54,57]. However only a few studies have correlated node size with node location at mediastinal dissection in healthy patients without cancer [56-59]. Genereux [57] found that 95% of histologically normal nodes measured less than 11 mm using the CT long axis. Schnyder [56] reported that among normal volunteers, 93% of lymph nodes in the pretracheal retrocaval space were less than 10 mm and none measured more than 14 mm. Other studies [58-59] have demonstrated a significant range in size for normal lymph nodes depending on their position within the mediastinum. The largest nodes tend to be located in the subcarinal and right tracheobronchial regions (positions 7, 4R, and 10R) while upper paratracheal nodes tend to be smaller [58]. Kiyono et al [59] proposed an upper limit of normal of 12 mm for subcarinal nodes, 10 mm for lymph nodes in positions 4R and 10R, and 8 mm for nodes elsewhere. Kiyono's data deal with a small study group from rural Japan where there is a low prevalence of granulomatous disease and pneumoconioses; the results must therefore be applied with caution in North America and Europe where these afflictions are commonplace.

The use of long or short axis for CT measurement of lymphadenopathy is also controversial. Gross and Glazer [60] favour the use of the short axis measurement which is less influenced by node orientation within the mediastinum. They believe that transverse images yield an accurate long axis measurement only if a node is oriented with its long axis in the horizontal plane [46]. CT may therefore underestimate true node size if nodes are oriented vertically or obliquely. While short axis measurements are also affected by node orientation, the coefficient of variation of short axis measurements is lower [58] and short axis has therefore been proposed as a more discriminating measurement.

Glazer et al [46] performed a receiver-operator characteristic analysis and determined an optimal short axis measurement of between 1 and 1.5 cm, concluding that short axis longer than 1 cm is the preferred threshold in lymph node detection. Conversely, Staples' data [48] support the use of long axis as an appropriate measurement technique.

The optimal lymph node size threshold for CT analysis has also been debated; criteria used range from any visible node to only those measuring more than 2 cm [47,51]. In general, the smaller the diameter used as a threshold to separate malignant from benign lymph nodes, the greater the sensitivity and lower the specificity of CT in detecting metastases [61]. Approximately 25 - 30% of nodes measuring 1 - 2 cm contain malignancy, whereas 75% measuring more than 2 cm harbour cancer [61].

While a number of reports indicate that CT has a high sensitivity [51-55] and specificity in the detection of lymph node metastases based on size criteria alone, their results are difficult to interpret for a number of reasons. Most studies include a small number of patients,

Table 7. *CT of mediastinal lymph nodes*

				CT			
	Study size	Prevalance of metastases (%)	Node mapping used	Node axis used	Node size (mm)	Sens. (%)	Spec. (%)
Full nodal sampling not performed							
Baron [57]	94	41	NS	NS	≥ 10	95	80
Eckholm [143]	35	20	NS	NS	> 10	29	46
Faling [52]	49	18	NS	NS	≥ 15	88	94
Lewis [53]	75	NS	NS	NS	> 10	91	94
Matthews [144]	174	37	NS	Any	> 10	86	78
Osbourne [54]	42	43	NS	NS	$> 5 - 6$	94	62
Patterson [70]	84	37	NS	NS	> 10	71	88
Rendina [55]	171	NS	NS	NS	> 10	95	83

Table 7 *continued*

Full nodal sampling performed							
Glazer [46]	49	43	NS	Area	> 100 mm^2	95	64
				Short	≥ 5	≈ 94*	≈ 20*
				Short	≥ 10	≈ 94	≈ 64
				Short	≥ 15	≈ 80	≈ 95
Libshitz [47]	86	24	NS	Any	≥ 10	67	66
Libshitz [50]	50	26	NS	NS	≥ 10	54	76
McKenna [62]	102	25	Yes	Any	≥ 10	60	60
Staples [48]	151	37	Yes	Long	> 5	95	23
				Long**	> 10	79	65
				Long	≥ 15	61	93
				Short	> 10	61	93

NS = not specified by the authors.
* Estimated from ROC curve.
** Mediastinoscopy plus CT long-axis > 10 mm: sensitivity = 95%, specificity = 97%.

many having fewer than 50. A number of studies involved incomplete nodal dissection at thoracotomy or biopsy of only those nodes that were enlarged at mediastinoscopy (Table 7). Furthermore, few studies include full details of the CT scanning technique, use of intravenous contrast and specification of whether radiological and surgical analyses were performed in a blinded fashion [49]. For these reasons true disease extent has not always been well defined [49] and rigorous comparison between studies is often not feasible.

McKenna et al [62] and Libshitz [47,50] reported low sensitivities ranging from 54 to 67% in the CT assessment of mediastinal nodal metastases. Contrary to other studies, their data were based on full nodal sampling at thoracotomy and correlation of CT with histology by node groups. These data were confirmed by Staples et al [48] who performed a careful CT-pathological correlation in which multiple size and axis criteria were analyzed. All patients underwent cervical mediastinoscopy and a left anterior mediastinotomy was also performed in those with left upper lobe or left hilar tumours. Among those patients in whom findings at mediastinoscopy were negative, all accessible lymph nodes were either removed or sampled at thoracotomy. Pathologically proven nodal metastases were observed in 37% of cases. Lymph nodes on CT scans were analyzed using a variety of size criteria including long axis > 5 mm, > 10 mm, and ≥ 15 mm, as well as short axis > 10 mm. All lymph nodes were mapped to stations defined by the ATS node mapping scheme.

Staples's data indicate that a CT long axis threshold > 5 mm was associated with a high sensitivity (95%) but a low specificity (23%). Long axis measurement ≥ 15 mm and short axis > 10 mm were also associated with high specificity (93% for both) but demonstrated low sensitivity (61% for both). CT long axis > 10 mm was found to be the best size criterion on CT, yielding sensitivity equal to mediastinoscopy (79%) with an acceptable specificity of 65%. In seven of 44 patients (16%) with positive lymph nodes at thoracotomy, lymph nodes measuring > 10 mm long axis were identified on CT but tumour was present in normal-sized nodes in different locations [48]. This study supports the use of CT long axis > 10 mm as the best threshold for lymph node size measurement, while emphasizing the need for meticulous dissection at thoracotomy.

A number of studies have reviewed the relationship between small peripheral tumours and the frequency of lymph node metastases within the mediastinum. Several of these suggest a low prevalence of mediastinal lymph node metastases in patients with T1 or T2 lesions ranging from 4 to 11.5% and therefore question the necessity for CT in the pre-operative staging of the mediastinum [63,64]. In contrast, other studies show a higher prevalence rate of lymph node metastases among T1 lesions ranging from 19% to 31% [45,46,57,65,66].

Since the major determinant of metastatic involvement on CT is nodal size, there will always be a finite false positive rate which may range from 15 to 30% [53,67]. Therefore it is clear that the decision to label a patient as inoperable should never be based solely on the findings of enlarged nodes on CT [46,47]. The presence of tumour within the enlarged nodes should be confirmed by biopsy.

Magnetic Resonance Imaging

MRI has not been shown to differ significantly overall in the accuracy of detection of lymph node metastases when compared to CT [68-70]. However, the ability of MRI to image in multiple planes may be helpful in evaluation of specific anatomic areas. The coronal plane is useful in the evaluation of the aortopulmonary window and subcarinal areas [71-73]. Calcification is not easily detected within nodes at MRI [8] and therefore identification of calcified lymphadenopathy secondary to granulomatous disease may be difficult or impossible.

Preliminary attempts to differentiate normal from tumour-containing lymph nodes based on T1 and T2 characteristics have been limited by considerable overlap in the T1 and T2 relaxation times between normal and abnormal nodes [74,75]. The longer scan times, higher unit examination cost and the more limited availability of MRI are additional drawbacks [39]. For these reasons, we do not routinely use MRI in evaluation of mediastinal lymph nodes but reserve it for selected cases such as those with indeterminate findings on CT, and in patients with previous severe allergic reaction to contrast media.

Mediastinoscopy

Cervical mediastinoscopy has been advocated as a routine procedure in patients with potentially resectable disease prior to thoracotomy [40-43] as it allows identification and biopsy of potentially tumour-containing nodes in the majority of patients with N2 disease [53]. Tumours involving the left upper lobe or left hilum metastasize to the left anterior mediastinal lymph nodes in 10 - 15% of cases [33] and in these patients left anterior mediastinotomy is usually performed.

Mediastinoscopy and anterior mediastinotomy became widely accepted by surgeons once it became clear that they reduce the incidence of unnecessary thoracotomy from 40% to approximately 10% in patients with advanced N2 or N3 disease [53].

The major advantage of mediastinoscopy over imaging techniques is the fact that it does not rely simply on node size to assess mediastinal involvement. The sensitivity of mediastinoscopy has been reported to be as high as 94 - 97% [36] with a specificity approaching 100% [70]. Therefore many surgeons strongly defend the role of routine mediastinoscopy in most patients [70,75,76] as there is a 95% chance that the carcinoma will prove resectable at thoracotomy if mediastinoscopy is negative for nodal metastases [7].

The high sensitivity in some of these studies may have been misleading because nodal sampling of the mediastinum was incomplete at thoracotomy. When complete dissection of all accessible nodal stations is used as a reference, the sensitivity for mediastinoscopy is approximately 80% [48]. The major disadvantages of mediastinoscopy are the requirement for general anaesthesia and the inability to identify inferior mediastinal and posterior subcarinal nodes which, if involved with tumour, herald a higher risk of N3 disease [14,15,77] and hence a poor prognosis. Despite these limitations, however, mediastinoscopy remains indispensable in the staging of patients with suspected mediastinal lymph node metastases.

It is clear, however, that even surgical staging with mediastinoscopy often misses disease and therefore we believe that CT and mediastinoscopy are complementary and that both should be performed in most patients with bronchogenic carcinoma who are considered candidates for surgical resection. CT identifies the precise anatomical location of enlarged nodes and guides the selection of the most useful staging technique, providing useful information including possible sites of nodal involvement that are not accessible to mediastinoscopy and that require biopsy by other means. Although it has significant limitations, CT is the best non-invasive staging technique available. CT remains the method of choice where mediastinoscopy is not readily available and is cost effective when the prevalence of nodal metastases exceeds 6% [78].

Evaluation of Mediastinal and Chest Wall Invasion

Limited chest wall and mediastinal invasion is now classified as Stage IIIa lung cancer; although this is considered technically resectable, it often necessitates en bloc resection which is associated with greater morbidity and mortality.

CT has been shown to be effective in predicting chest wall invasion only if there is definite rib destruction [79] (Fig. 5) or an obvious chest wall mass [61] (Fig. 6). In the absence of these

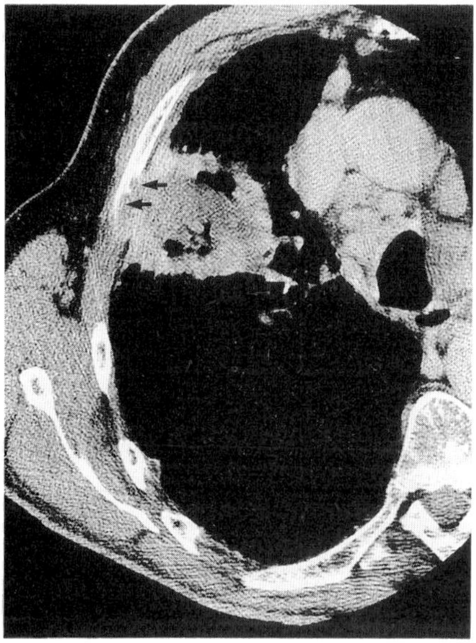

Figure 5. *STAGE IIIA (T3N2M0) POORLY DIFFERENTIATED ADENOCARCINOMA INVADING THE CHEST WALL. CT demonstrates a cavitating mass in the right upper lobe contacting the pleural surface and invading the adjacent rib (arrows). Multiple enlarged right paratracheal (4R) nodes are present. Nodal biopsy at mediastinoscopy was negative for malignancy. At thoracotomy adenocarcinoma was identified on frozen section biopsy material from the 4R and subcarinal (7) nodes, establishing the presence of N2 disease. The patient was deemed unresectable due to the extent of mediastinal lymph node involvement.*

findings CT is of limited value [79-81] (Fig. 7). Scott et al [82] reviewed 23 patients with resectable Stage IIIa lung cancer and found definite chest wall invasion on CT in only 20% of cases in which it

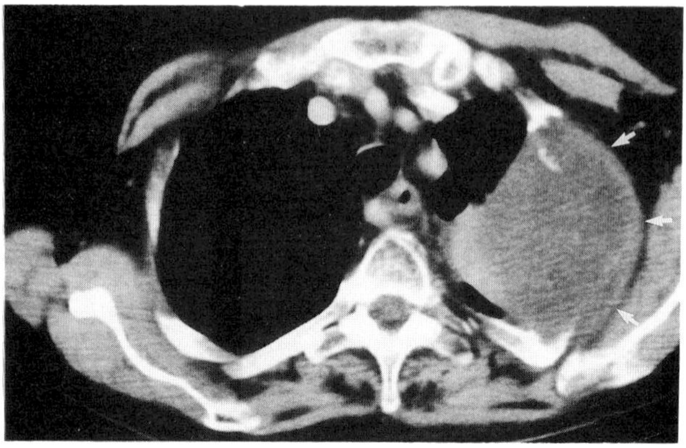

Figure 6. *CHEST WALL INVASION IN AN UNRESECTABLE STAGE IIIB (T4N0M0) SQUAMOUS CARCINOMA. The large left upper lobe tumour directly invades the chest wall (arrows). Rib destruction is evident. Direct mediastinal invasion was identified on scans obtained at a lower level.*

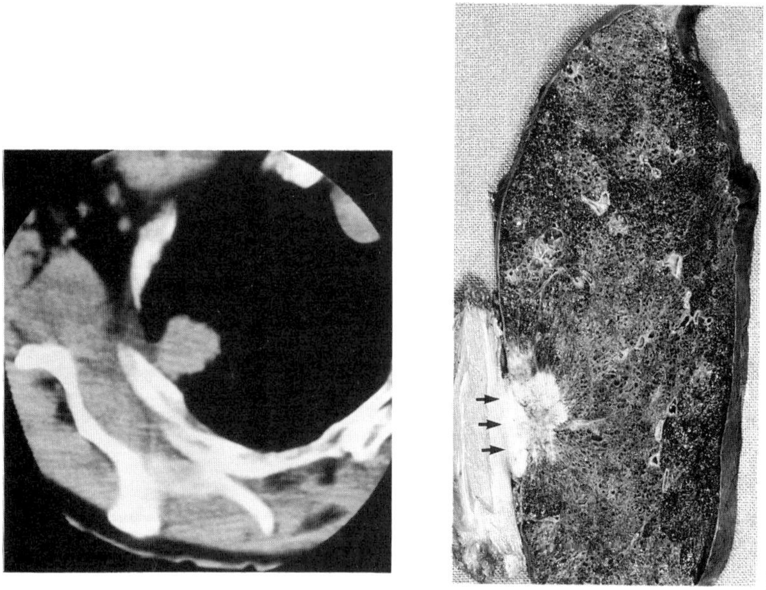

(a) (b)

Figure 7. *RESECTABLE STAGE IIIA (T3N1M0) ADENOCARCINOMA WITH LIMITED CHEST WALL INVASION. (a) Typical CT appearance of a peripheral tumour abutting the chest wall. The tumour is contiguous with pleura but no rib destruction or chest wall mass is identified. (b) Pathologic specimen demonstrates the peripheral tumour with localized chest wall extension over a distance of approximately 4 mm (arrows). Ribs were not invaded. Only N1 nodes were involved and resection was complete. Reproduced with permission from ref. 82.*

proven surgically. Glazer et al [80] studied CT scans in 47 patients with peripheral tumours contacting the chest wall or pleural surface. The presence of an obtuse angle between the mass and pleura, pleural contact over a distance greater than 3 cm and associated pleural thickening yielded a sensitivity of 87% for chest wall invasion with a specificity of only 59%. The presence of focal chest wall pain, while not as sensitive as CT, was highly specific for invasion [80]. Evidence of vertebral body destruction generally indicates unresectable disease and can be readily identified with CT [83]. Extension into the neural foramen of the vertebral body also precludes resection (Fig. 8).

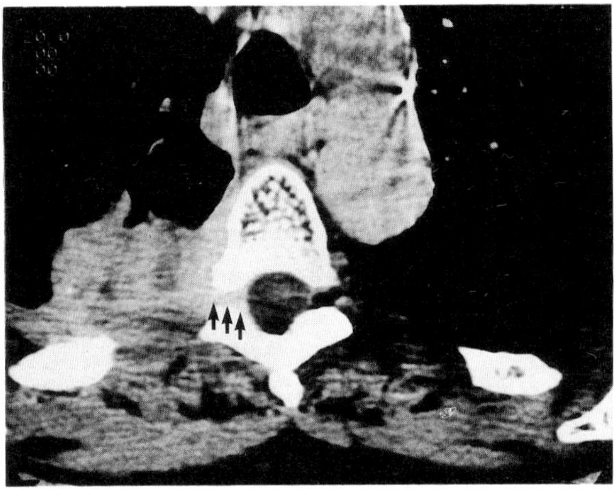

Figure 8. *UNRESECTABLE STAGE III SQUAMOUS CARCINOMA. The right upper lobe tumour extends into the paraspinal soft tissue and neural foramen at this level, where it produces extensive, dense enhancement of the epidural fat (arrows). There is no distortion of the thecal sac or evidence of vertebral body invasion. At mediastinoscopy all accessible lymph nodes were free of tumour. This lesion was considered unresectable due to the extensive infiltration of tumour into the neural foramen.*

Superior sulcus tumours (Pancoast tumour) are a subset of lung cancers which arise in the extreme apices of the lung and have a propensity for early invasion of the neck, brachial plexus, subclavian vessels and spine [84,85]. If diagnosed early, many of these tumours are amenable to treatment with en bloc resection and adjuvant preoperative radiotherapy. Both CT and MRI have been shown to be of value in the detection of resectability of superior sulcus tumours.

MRI is superior to CT in the assessment of apical invasion due to its ability to image in the sagittal and coronal planes [82,86], making it the imaging procedure of choice for superior sulcus tumours [87-89]. MRI is superior to CT in identifying unresectable invasion of the brachial plexus [39], vertebral body marrow, neural foramina, spinal canal, and to confirm inoperable vascular involvement [9,39,86] (Figs. 9 and 10). Furthermore, the superior contrast resolution of MRI may better demonstrate subtle chest wall invasion by distinguishing between tumour and muscle on T2-weighted images [69,90].

Mediastinal invasion which may be technically resectable includes limited invasion of the pericardium, mediastinal pleura or fat, pulmonary veins, and vagus and phrenic nerves [91]. More extensive invasion of the mediastinum with involvement of the heart, great vessels, oesophagus and trachea as well as vertebral body invasion are classified Stage IIIb and are generally considered unresectable.

The CT and MRI criteria which indicate unresectable mediastinal invasion include interdigitation of tumour into mediastinal fat, encasement of mediastinal great vessels, the mainstem bronchi, and trachea [91]. Vascular invasion can be confidently diagnosed if there is circumferential encasement of the vessel or circumferential tapering or abrupt truncation (Fig. 11). Partial volume averaging on CT may simulate vessel narrowing caused by tumour encasement but scalloping of the vessel wall and lumen is a specific feature of tumour encasement [92].

The identification of limited and potentially resectable mediastinal invasion is more difficult. Findings on CT which have been shown to be unreliable in predicting resectability include mass effect upon mediastinal structures, focal obliteration of mediastinal fat planes, and pericardial or mediastinal pleural thickening [91]. Three signs are helpful in suggesting that a tumour abutting the mediastinum or descending aorta is potentially resectable. These include the presence of a fat plane between the tumour and mediastinum, contact of 3 cm or less between the tumour and mediastinum and less than 90° of arc contact between the tumour and descending thoracic aorta [91]. Of resectable masses 97% exhibited one or more of these features and CT helped predict technical resectability in 45% of patients. Although these features are helpful, they still leave a large number of patients in whom the CT findings are indeterminate.

CT is also a poor predictor of the need for pneumonectomy versus lobectomy in central lung masses [93]. Quint has shown that central

(a)

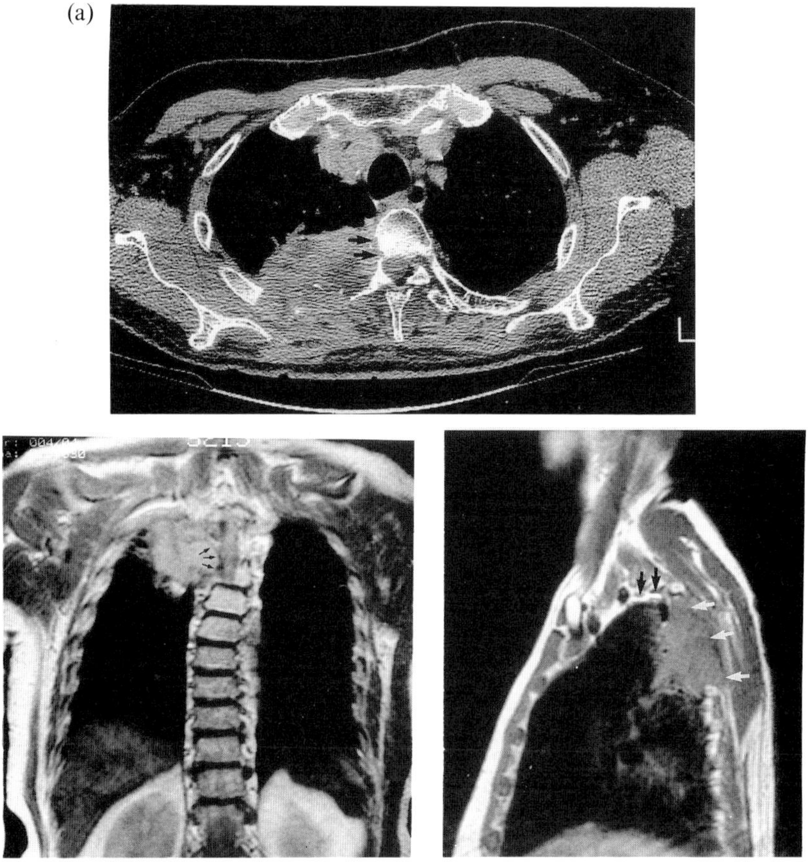

(b) (c)

Figure 9. *STAGE IIIB (T4N0M0) SQUAMOUS CARCINOMA WITH CHEST WALL AND VERTEBRAL BODY INVASION. (a) CT scan 1.5 mm collimation demonstrates an inhomogeneous mass arising in the posterior segment of the right upper lobe invading the right fourth rib and the posterolateral aspect of the T4 vertebral body (arrows). The peripheral extent of the chest wall mass is difficult to ascertain by CT. No enlarged mediastinal lymph nodes were identified. (b) Coronal and (c) sagittal T1-weighted MR images (TR = 800 msec, TE = 20 msec) confirm direct extension into the T4 vertebral body (arrows, b) without involvement of the spinal canal. The sagittal MR image demonstrates the extensive nature of chest wall invasion. Normal extrapleural fat over the lung apex (black arrows, c) is obliterated where the intercostal musculature is infiltrated by tumour (white arrows, c). Destruction of the right third and fourth ribs is evident. This lesion was not resected.*

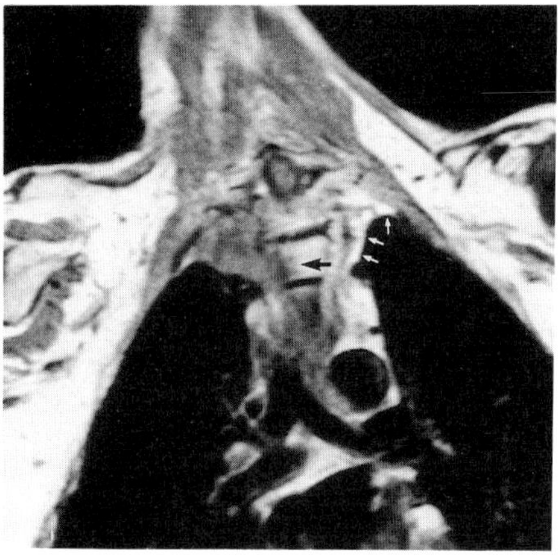

Figure 10. *CORONAL T1-WEIGHTED MR IMAGE (TR = 840 msec, TE = 20 msec) OF STAGE IIIB (T4N0M0) SUPERIOR SULCUS TUMOUR. The right apical mass directly invades the vertebral body marrow (black arrow). Extrapleural fat adjacent to the cupola of the lung is clearly visible on the left (white arrows) but is obliterated on the right indicating invasion of the thoracic outlet. Biopsy showed undifferentiated large cell carcinoma. Clinically the patient had Pancoast syndrome.*

bronchial, pulmonary arterial involvement and transfissural spread which may necessitate extended lobectomy or pneumonectomy is identified by CT in only approximately 50% of patients (Fig. 12) [93].

As with CT, MRI is poor at distinguishing contiguity of tumour from true invasion of mediastinal pleura or fat [68,69,90] but is superior to CT in identifying vascular invasion especially when aortic invasion or superior vena cava obstruction are present [86,94-97]. Identification of pericardial tumour invasion has traditionally been diagnosed by positive cytology obtained at pericardiocentesis. Although it has been suggested that pericardial effusions are a common feature of neoplastic invasion [98], Dawson et al recently reviewed 23 patients with pericardial tumour invasion and found effusion in only 26% [99]. On CT, 91% had focal or nodular pericardial thickening > 2 mm and only 9% demonstrated diffuse thickening. CT was judged superior to echocardiography in the assessment of pericardial tumour invasion due to the low incidence of effusions in this series. MRI is generally superior to CT in the assessment of pericardial and cardiac invasion [86,94-97] and may be helpful in the assessment of pulmonary venous invasion as well.

(a)

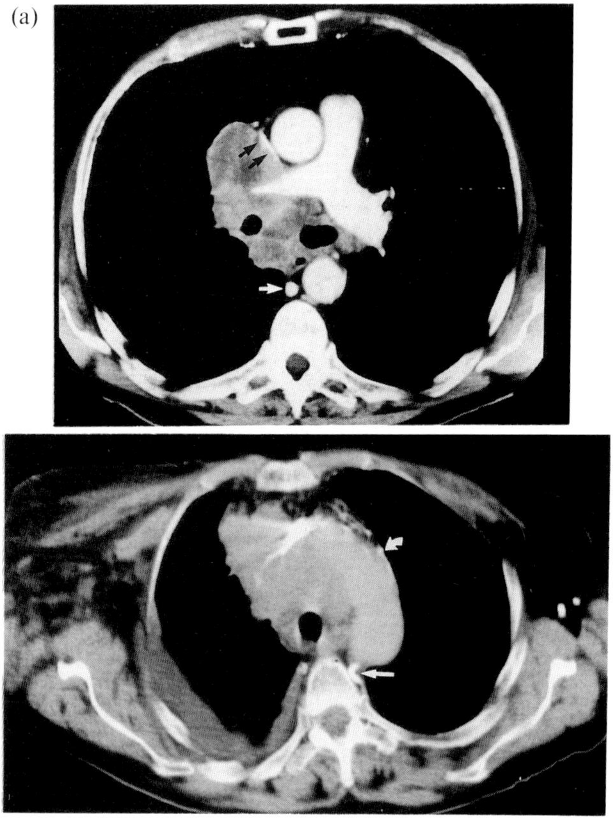

(b)

Figure 11. *CT OF SUPERIOR VENA CAVA (SVC) OBSTRUCTION IN TWO PATIENTS WITH EXTENSIVE UNDIFFERENTIATED SMALL CELL CARCINOMA. (a) A mediastinal mass consisting of enlarged right hilar, azygous and subcarinal lymph nodes encases the bronchus intermedius, left main bronchus and right pulmonary artery which is compressed but not occluded. The SVC is grossly distorted and almost completely occluded by tumour (black arrows), and densely opacified venous blood in the azygous vein (white arrow) indicates collateral venous return. (b) Enlarged tumour containing lymph nodes encase and deform the left innominate vein and SVC which was occluded below this level. Left axillary, superior hemi-azygous (arrow) and superior intercostal (curved arrow) venous collaterals are opacified.*

(a)

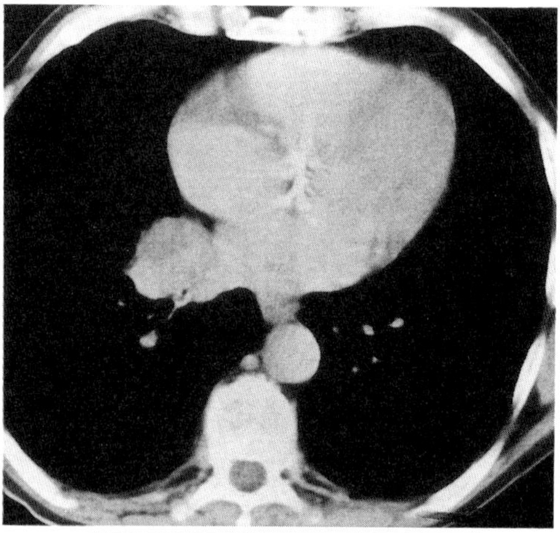

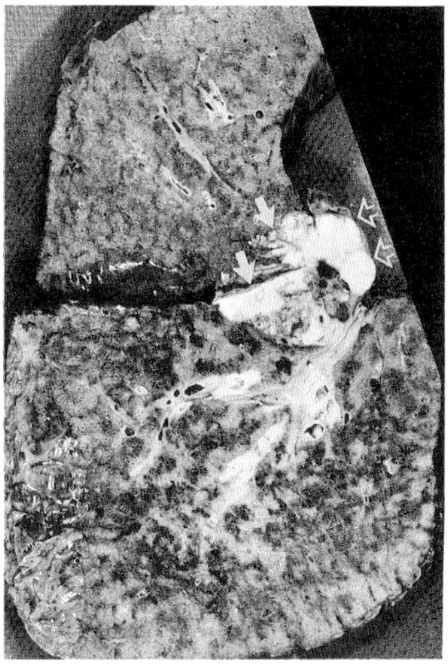

(b)

Figure 12. *RESECTABLE STAGE IIIA (T3N1M0) ATYPICAL CARCINOID TUMOUR WITH PERICARDIAL INVASION AND TRANSFISSURAL EXTENSION. (a) CT scan shows a mass at the junction of the right lower and middle lobes abutting the mediastinum at the level of the inferior pulmonary vein. CT did not reliably assess the degree of extension. (b) Pathological specimen demonstrates a 6 cm hilar lesion (T3) involving both the middle and right lower lobes by transfissural extension (arrows). Pleural perforation with involvement of the pericardium (open arrows) was present. This lesion was completely resected en bloc and only N1 nodes were positive. Reproduced with permission from ref. 146.*

Assessment of Multicentric Lung Cancer

Multicentric bronchogenic carcinoma has previously been considered uncommon, with a reported incidence ranging from 0.2 - 1.8% [100]. Multicentricity has been reported most commonly with squamous and bronchiolo-alveolar cell types [100-102]. Recently, McElvaney et all [101] reported multicentricity in 19% of 62 consecutive lung resections for bronchogenic adenocarcinoma. Many of these tumours were missed pre-operatively by CT.

Using widely accepted criteria to exclude metastatic disease [103] Zwirewich et al [104] recently performed a CT - pathological correlation in 88 patients with adenocarcinoma and found a 22% prevalence rate of multicentricity among the surgical specimens. Two or more tumours were identified on CT for a sensitivity of 63% and a specificity of 86% in detecting multicentricity. The appearance of multicentricity on CT varied from the presence of multiple well-defined nodules to hazy areas of ill-defined air-space opacification simulating pneumonitis (Fig. 13). Five patients had 10 or more tumours in the resected lung and all of these were bronchiolo-alveolar carcinomas. In the majority of these patients, the tumours were very small, frequently measuring < 5 mm, and most were undetectable on CT. In a subset of these patients, bronchiolo-alveolar cell adenomas were present within the resected lung specimen, and it appears that these adenomas may represent an early, premalignant phase of glandular neoplasia with a potential for evolution to carcinoma [105]. The presence of multicentric lung cancer raises important issues regarding tumour staging and management. The method by which these patients are staged has not been specifically addressed in standard staging guidelines. Our policy is to treat and stage two or more dominant histologically dissimilar primary tumours independently and to view the prognosis as probably most dependent on the tumour which has the highest stage. Since the likelihood of additional lesions in the non-resected lung appears high [101,106] multicentric lung cancer is staged as TX (tumour that cannot be assessed).

Bewtra [107] indicates that the detection of two or more tumours in a patient should not be grounds for ruling out surgery as complete resection affords a survival rate that is similar to resection of a solitary tumour. Pneumonectomy for synchronous primary tumours in separate lobes of the same lung has been recommended by Ferguson et al [108]. In patients with bilateral tumours Ferguson recommends

(a)

(b)

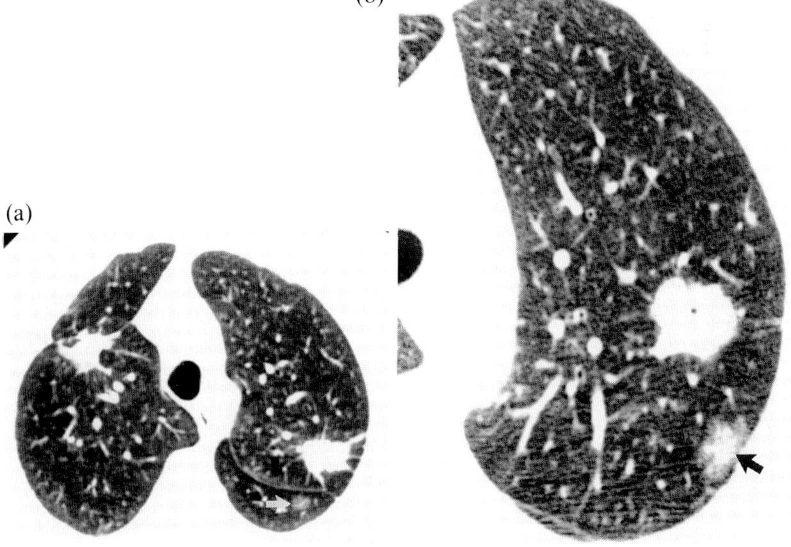

Figure 13. *CT DEMONSTRATION OF MULTICENTRIC BRONCHIOLO-ALVEOLAR CARCINOMAS. (a) Bilateral tumours appear as well-defined mass lesions in this patient. Florid multicentricity was present in the right upper lobe at pathological sectioning but no additional tumours were evident on CT images even in retrospect. The small opacity in the superior segment of the left lower lobe (arrow) was not resected. (b) 1.5 mm collimation CT scan through left upper lobe in a different patient with florid multicentric disease. The dominant tumour measured 2.3 cm. Despite the presence of well over 10 additional tumours within the resected specimen, only a single additional nodule was evident on the scan (arrow). This lesion demonstrates a hazy ill-defined contour simulating pneumonitis, and had a sponge-like, lacy appearance at pathological sectioning. Reproduced with permission from ref. 104.*

sequential resections starting with the most advanced lesion [108]. It is our practice to resect the dominant lesion and at the time of thoracotomy remove by wedge excision any additional smaller nodules which are palpable. Survival in this group of patients has yet to be adequately defined.

Assessment of Extrathoracic Metastatic Disease

The presence of metastatic disease places the patient in the Stage IV category and precludes curative resection. Metastases are most frequently seen among patients with small cell carcinoma, 70 - 90% having evidence of mediastinal or distant metastatic disease at the time of diagnosis [5]. Overall, the prevalence rate of extrathoracic metastases among non-small cell tumours is approximately 30% for single organ involvement and 12% for multi-organ involvement at the time of diagnosis [116]. Brain, liver, adrenal, bone and soft tissue metastases account for the majority of cases [109,110] and among patients with normal-sized mediastinal lymph nodes at CT, distant metastases were observed in 25% in one series [110]. Clinically silent metastases are uncommon [110].

Among patients with non-small cell carcinoma, adenocarcinoma has the highest tendency to metastasize early with a predilection for the central nervous system and adrenal glands[5]. Adenocarcinoma is more aggressive than squamous cell carcinoma and at autopsy frequently involves regional lymph nodes (80%), pleura (60%) and the contralateral lung (40%) [111,112]. It is important to recognize that the rate of metastases for adenocarcinoma and large cell carcinoma (which together account for approximately 50% of lung cancers) is greater than for squamous carcinoma and does not correlate with the TN staging in contrast to metastases from squamous cancer [109].

Several studies have demonstrated that the routine use of bone, brain and liver - spleen scans is unnecessary and potentially misleading [113-115]. The best screen for extrathoracic spread of tumour continues to be a thorough history and physical examination along with laboratory data including serum calcium, bilirubin, trans-aminases, lactate dehydrogenase and alkaline phosphatase tests [116]. CT scanning is superior to ultrasound in the assessment of the liver and adrenal glands for metastatic disease [117,118] and can be accomplished at the time of the chest CT scan. A dynamic incremental CT protocol is advocated for detection of hepatic metastases using CT [119-121], but this technique is less sensitive than CT arterial portography [122,123]. MRI sensitivity has been shown to exceed that of conventional or dynamic hepatic CT [124,125].

By weight the adrenal glands show a higher incidence of metastases than any other organ [126]. The frequency of adrenal metastases ranges from 3 - 8% in clinical series [109] and is as high as 38% in autopsy series [126]. Perhaps more alarming are the data reported by Pagani [127] who found a 12% prevalence rate of metastases in morphologically normal glands biopsied percutaneously under CT guidance.

Adrenal masses seen at CT have been reported in 21% of patients evaluated for non-small cell carcinoma [128] and more than two-thirds of these lesions are benign [129]. Most represent non-functioning adrenal adenomas [130]. The majority of adrenal metastases are asymptomatic and adrenal insufficiency, even with complete replacement of both glands with metastatic disease, is very unusual [131]. Therefore the presence of an adrenal mass demonstrated by CT during the staging of lung cancer can pose a significant diagnostic dilemma. An adrenal mass with a thick enhancing rim, irregular or poorly defined margins, inhomogeneous enhancement and a mass greater than 3 cm favours malignancy, whereas homogeneous adrenal masses measuring less than 2 cm in size demonstrating CT attenuation values equivalent to muscle and showing absent or only minimal homogeneous enhancement are more consistent with adrenal adenomas [132].

While adrenal metastases have a higher signal intensity on T2-weighted images on MRI than adenomas, there is considerable overlap and differentiation is not always possible [133,134]. Contrast enhanced MRI scanning with gadolinium-DPTA may prove to be of value in this regard [135]. In a patient with an underlying malignancy and an adrenal mass without evidence of metastatic disease elsewhere, CT-guided adrenal biopsy is indicated to exclude metastatic disease [136].

Contrast enhanced brain CT or MRI is recommended for all patients with known or suspected lung cancer who have neurological symptoms, and in those patients with small cell carcinoma and adenocarcinoma who are asymptomatic. Although brain metastases are often symptomatic, approximately 21% have been reported to be asymptomatic at the time of diagnosis [109] and silent brain metastases have been observed in 5 - 10% of CT examinations in patients with lung cancer [137-139]. Contrast enhanced MRI using gadolinium-DTPA affords a higher sensitivity in the detection of intraparenchymal brain metastases than contrast enhanced CT [140].

Whole body radionuclide scintigraphy is considered the best technique in detecting skeletal metastases [141-142]. False positive rates as high as 40% [109] are common and frequently relate to non-malignant causes such as arthritis or old fractures. Routine use of bone scanning in screening asymptomatic patients for metastatic skeletal disease therefore is not generally warranted as it may unnecessarily delay appropriate surgical therapy.

Summary

Lung cancer is now the commonest fatal malignancy among men and women. Although the overall mortality rate is high and most patients present with unresectable disease, advances in surgical therapy have prompted modifications in the staging which reflect improved survival among certain subsets of patients. The new International Staging System therefore has important implications for both the non-invasive imaging and invasive surgical techniques (mediastinoscopy and mediastinotomy) used in lung cancer staging. Although CT is a less than optimal technique for the evaluation of mediastinal lymph node metastases, having a false positive rate of approximately 10 - 15%, it remains the best non-invasive method of assessing the mediastinum.

CT is helpful in identifying potential sites of tumour involvement and in guiding invasivc biopsy procedures to suspicious-appearing node stations which may harbour tumour. Although mediastinoscopy has a very high specificity in the assessment of mediastinal lymph node metastases, it is an invasive procedure and is unable to identify lymph node in the posterior subcarinal, anterior mediastinal and aortocopulmonary window. Used alone, CT long axis > 10 mm yields a sensitivity equal to mediastinoscopy. The combination of CT long axis measurement > 10 mm and mediastinoscopy yields a sensitivity of 95% with a specificity exceeding 95%. CT is of additional benefit in identifying direct chest wall and mediastinal invasion which may not be evident at mediastinoscopy, and may therefore reduce morbidity and mortality from unnecessary thoracotomy in patients with unresectable disease.

Because of its multi-planar imaging capabilities and superior soft-tissue contrast, MRI is presently the non-invasive procedure of choice in evaluation of superior sulcus tumours and those lesions with suspected vascular, pericardial or cardiac invasion. MRI is complementary to CT in the evaluation of chest wall invasion and distant metastases.

References

1. Stitik FP, DiSantis DJ. Lung cancer staging. *Semin Roentgenol* 1990;**25**:34-44.
2. Karwande SV. Surgical advances in the treatment of lung cancer. *Semin US CT MR* 1988;**9**:27-33.
3. Silverberg E, Boring CC, and Squires TS. *Cancer statistics 1990* CA 1990;**40**:9-15.
4. Loeb LA, Ernster VL, Warner KE, Abbotts J, Laszlo J. Smoking and lung cancer. An overview. *Cancer Res* 1984;**44**:5940.
5. Filderman AE, Shaw C, Matthay RA. Lung cancer. Part I: Etiology, pathology, natural history, manifestations, and diagnostic techniques. *Invest Radiol* 1986;**21**:80-90.
6. Gazdar AF, Carney DN, Minna JD. The biology of non-small cell lung cancer. *Semin Oncol* 1983;**10**:3.
7. Tisi GM, Friedman PJ, Peters RM, Pearson G, Carr D, Lee RE, Selawry O. Clinical staging of primary lung cancer. *Am Rev Respir Dis* 1983;**127**:659-664.
8. Little AG, Stitik FP. Clinical staging of patients with non-small cell lung cancer. *Chest* 1990;**97**:1431-1438.
9. Mountain CF. Expanded possibilities for surgical treatment of lung cancer: Survival in Stage IIIa disease. *Chest* 1990;**97**:1045-1051.
10. Denoix PF. Enquete permanent dans les centres anticancereux. *Bull Inst Nat Hyg* 1946;**1**:70-75.
11. American Joint Committee on Cancer, Task Force on Lung. *Staging of Lung Cancer 1979.* Chicago: American Joint Committee on Cancer, 1979.
12. Harmer EM. *TNM classification of malignant tumours*, pp 41-45. Geneva: Union Internationale Contre le Cancer, 1978.
13. Mountain CF. A new international staging system for lung cancer. *Chest* 1986;**89(Suppl)**:225-233.
14. Naruke T, Suemasu K, Ishikawa S. Lymph node mapping and curability at various levels of metastasis in resected lung cancer. *J Thorac Cardiovasc Surg* 1978;**76**:832-839.
15. Bignall JR, Moon AJ. Survival after lung resection for bronchogenic carcinoma. *Thorax* 1955;**10**:183-190.
16. Gordon W. Lymphatic spread in the surgical treatment of lung cancer. *Am J Surg* 1962;**104**:866-868.
17. Martini N, Flehinger BJ, Zaman MB, Beattie EJjr. Prospective study of 445 lung carcinomas with mediastinal lymph node metastases. *J Thorac Cardiovasc Surg* 1980;**80**:390-399.
18. Mann H, Karwande SV. The new proposed international staging system for lung cancer. *Semin US CT MR* 1988;**9**:34-39.
19. Martini N, Flehingerr BJ, Zaman MB, Beattie EJjr. Results of surgieal treatment in N2 lung cancer. *World J Surg* 1981;**5**:675-679.
20. Errett LE, Wilson J, Shiu RC. Wedge resection as an alternative procedure for peripheral bronchogenic carcinoma in poor-risk patients. *J Thorac Cardiovasc Surg* 1985;**90**:656.
21. Stair JM, Womble J, Schaefer RF, Read RC. Segmental pulmonary resection for cancer. *Am J Surg* 1985;**150**:659-664.
22. Martini N, Flehinger BJ, Zaman MB, Beattie EJjr. Results of resection in non-oat cell carcinoma of the lung with mediastinal lymph node metastases. *Ann Surg* 1983;**198**:386-397.
23. Trastek VF, Pairolero PC, Piehler JM. Enbloe (non-chest wall) resection for bronchogenic carcinoma with parietal fixation. Factors affecting survival. *J Thorac Cardiovasc Surg* 1984;**87**:352-358.

24. McCaughan BC, Martini N, Bains MS. Chest wall invasion in carcinoma of the lung. Therapeutic and prognostic implications. *J Thorac Cardiovasc Surg* 1985;**89**:836-841.
25. Lowe JE, Bridgeman AH, Sabiston DC. The role of bronchoplastic procedures in the surgical management of benign and malignant pulmonary lesions. *J Thorac Cardiovasc Surg* 1982;**83**:227-234.
26. Weisel RD, Cooper JD, Delarue NC, Theman TE, Todd TRJ, Pearson FG. Sleeve lobectomy for carcinoma of the lung. *J Thorac Cardiovasc Surg* 1970;**78**:839.
27. Little AG, DeMeester TR, MacMahon H. The staging of lung cancer. *Semin Oncol* 1983;**10**:56-70
28. Williams DE, Pairolero PC, Davis CS. Survival of patients surgically treated for stage I lung cancer. *J Thorac Cardiovasc Surg* 1981;**82**:70-76.
29. Feld R, Rubinstein LV, Weisenberg TH. Sites of recurrence in resected stage I non-small cell lung cancer: a guide for future studies. *J Clin Oncol* 1984;**2**:1352-1358.
30. Martini N, Beattie EJjr. Results of surgical treatment in stage I lung cancer. *J Thorac Cardiovasc Surg* 1977;**74**:499-505.
31. Mountain CF. The biological operability of stage III non-small cell lung cancer. *Ann Thorac Surg* 1985;**40**:60-64.
32. Kirsh MM, Rotman H, Argenta L, Bove E, Cimmino V, Tashian J, Ferguson P, Sloan H. Carcinoma of the lung: results of treatment over ten years. *Ann Thorac Surg* 1976;**21**:371-377.
33. Pearson FG, DeLarue NC, Ilves R, Todd TRJ, Cooper JD. Significance of positive superior mediastinal nodes identified at mediastinoscopy in patients with resectable cancer of the lung. *J Thorac Cardiovasc Surg* 1982;**83**:1-11.
34. Grillo HC. Carinal reconstruction. *Ann Thorac Surg* 1982;**34**:356-373.
35. Dartevelle PG, Khalife J, Chapelier A, Marzelle J, Navajas M, Levasseur P, Rojas A, Cerrina J. Tracheal sleeve pneumonectomy for bronchogenic carcinoma: report of 55 cases. *Ann Thorac Surg* 1988;**46**:68-72.
36. Backer CL, Shields TW, Lockhart CG, Vogelzang R, LoCicero JIII. Selective preoperative evaluation for possible N2 disease in carcinoma of the lung. *J Thorac Cardiovasc Surg* 1987;**93**:337-343.
37. Libshitz HI. CT of mediastinal lymph nodes in lung cancer: is there a 'state of the art'? *AJR* 1983;**141**:1081-1085.
38. Zwirewich CV, Terriff B, Müller NL. High-spatial-frequency (bone) algorithm improves quality of standard CT of the thorax. *AJR* 1989;**153**:1169-1173.
39. Gefter WB. Magnetic resonance imaging in the evaluation of lung cancer. *Semin Roentgenol* 1990;**25**:73-84.
40. Carlens E. Appraisal of choice and results of treatment for bronchogenic carcinoma. *Chest* 1974;**65**:442-445.
41. Trinkle JK, Bryant LR, Hiller AJ, Playforth RH. Mediastinoscopy: experience with 300 consecutive cases. *J Thorac Cardiovasc Surg* 1970;**60**:297-300.
42. Coughlin M, Deslauriers J, Beaulieu M. Role of mediastinoscopy in pretreatment staging of patients with primary lung cancer. *Ann Thorac Surg* 1985;**40**:556-560.
43. Luke WP, Todd TRJ, Cooper JD. Prospective evaluation of mediastinoscopy for assessment of carcinoma of the lung. *J Thorac Cardiovasc Surg* 1986;**91**:53-56.
44. Pearson FG. Lung cancer: the past twenty-five years. *Chest* 1986;**89(Suppl)**:200-205.
45. Heavey LR, Glazer GM, Gross BH, Franeis IR, Orringer MB. The role of CT in staging radiographic T1N0M0 lung caneer. *AJR* 1986;**146**:285-290.
46. Glazer GM, Orringer MB, Gross BH, Quint LE. The mediastinum in non-small cell lung cancer: CT-surgical correlation. *AJR* 1984;**142**:1101-1105.
47. Libshitz HI, McKenna RJjr. Mediastinal lymph node size in lung cancer. *AJR* 1984;**143**:715-718.

48. Staples CA, Müller NL, Miller RR, Evans KG, Nelems B. Mediastinal nodes in bronehogenic carcinoma: comparison between CT and mediastinoscopy. *Radiology* 1988;**167**:367-372.
49. Dales RE, Stark RM, Raman S. Computed tomography to stage lung cancer: approaching a controversy using meta-analysis. *Am Rev Respir Dis* 1990;**141**:1096-1101.
50. Libshitz HI, McKenna RJjr, Haynie TP, McMurtrey MJ, Mountain CT. Mediastinal evaluation in lung cancer. *Radiology* 1984;**151**:295-299.
51. Baron RL, Levitt RG, Sagel SS, White MJ, Roper CL, Marbarger JP. Computed tomography in the preoperative evaluation of bronchogenic carcinoma. *Radiology* 1982;**145**:727-732.
52. Faling LJ, Pugatch RD, Jung-Legg Y, Daly BDT, Hong WK, Robbins AH, Snider GL. Computed tomographic scanning of the mediastinum in the staging of bronchogenic carcinoma. *Am Rev Respir Dis* 1981;**124**:690-695.
53. Lewis JWjr, Madrazo BL, Gross SC, Eyler WR, Magilligan DJjr, Kvale PA, Rosen RA. The value of radiographic and computed tomography in the staging of lung cancer. *Ann Thorac Surg* 1982;**34**:553-558.
54. Osborne DR, Korobkin M, Ravin CE, Putman CE, Wolfe WG, Sealy WC, Young WG, Breiman R, Heaston D, Ram P, Halber M. Comparison of plain radiography, conventional tomography, and computed tomography in detecting intrathoracic lymph node metastases from lung carcinoma. *Radiology* 1982;**142**:157-161.
55. Rendina EA, Bognolo DA, Mineo TC, Gualdi GF, Caterino M, DiBiasi C, Facciolo F, Ricci C. Computed tomography for the evaluation of intrathoracic invasion by lung cancer. *J Thorac Cardiovasc Surg* 1987;**94**:57-63.
56. Schnyder PA, Gamsu G. CT of the pretracheal retrocaval space. *AJR* 1981;**136**:303-308.
57. Genereux GP, Howie JL. Normal mediastinal lymph node size and number: CT and anatomic study. *AJR* 1984;**142**:1095-1100.
58. Glazer GM, Gross BH, Quint LE, Francis IR, Bookstein FL, Orringer MB. Normal mediastinal lymph nodes: number and size according to American Thoracic Society mapping. *AJR* 1985;**144**:261-265.
59. Kiyono K, Sone S, Sakai F, Imai Y, Watanabe T, Izuno I, Oguchi M, Kawai T, Shigematsu H, Watanabe M. The number and size of normal mediastinal lymph nodes: a postmortem study. *AJR* 1988;**150**:771-776.
60. Gross BH, Glazer GM, Orringer MB, Spizarny DL, Flint A. Bronchogenic carcinoma metastatic to normal-sized lymph nodes: frequency and significance. *Radiology* 1988;**166**:71-74.
61. Libshitz HI. Computed tomography in bronchogenic carcinoma. *Semin Roentgenol* 1990;**25**:64-72.
62. McKenna RJJr, Libshitz HI, Mountain CE, McMurtrey MJ. Roentgenographic evaluation of mediastinal nodes for preoperative assessment in lung cancer. *Chest* 1985;**88**:206-210.
63. Pearlberg JL, Sandler MA, Beute GH, Madrazo BL. T1N0M0 bronchogenic carcinoma: assessment by CT. *Radiology* 1985;**157**:187-190.
64. Smith SR, Hooper RG, Beechler CR, Whitcomb MF. Indications for mediastinal lymph node evaluation. *Chest* 1982;**81**:599-604.
65. Conces DJJr, Klink JF, Tarver RD, Moak GD. T1N0M0 lung cancer: evaluation with CT. *Radiology* 1989;**170**:643-646.
66. Hutchinson CM, Mills NL. The selection of patients with bronchogenic carcinoma for mediastinoscopy. *J Thorac Cardiovasc Surg* 1976;**71**:768-773.
67. Whittlesey D. Prospective computed tomographic scanning in the staging of bronchogenic cancer. *J Thorac Cardiovasc Surg* 1988;**95**:876-882.

68. Webb WR, Jensen BG, Sollitto R, de Geer G, McCowin M, Gamsu G, Moore E. Bronchogenic carcinoma: staging with MR compared with staging with CT and surgery. *Radiology* 1985;**156**:117-124.
69. Musset O, Grenier P, Carette MF, Frija G, Hauuy MP, Desbleds MT, Girard P, Bigot JM, Lallemand D. Primary lung cancer staging: prospective comparative study of MR imaging with CT. *Radiology* 1986;**160**:607-611.
70. Patterson GA, Ginsberg RJ, Poon PY, Cooper JD, Goldberg M, Jones D, Pearson FG, Todd TR, Waters P, Bull S. A prospective evaluation of magnetic resonance imaging, computed tomography and mediastinoscopy in the preoperative assessment of mediastinal node status in bronchogenic carcinoma. *J Thorac Cardiovasc Surg* 1987;**94**:679-684.
71. Webb WR, Magnetic resonance imaging of the hilla and mediastinum. *Cardiovasc Intervent Radiol* 1986;**8**:306-313.
72. Webb WR, Jensen BG, Gamsu G, Sollitto R, Moore EH. Coronal magnetic resonance imaging of the chest: normal and abnormal. *Radiology* 1984;**153**:729-735.
73. Webb WR, Moore EH. Differentiation of volume averaging and mass on magnetic resonance images of the mediastinum. *Radiology* 1985;**155**:413-416.
74. Glazer GM, Orringer MB, Chenevert TL, Borrello JA, Penner MW, Quint LE, Li KC, Aisen AM. Mediastinal lymph nodes: relaxation time/pathologic correlation and implications in staging of lung cancer with MR imaging. *Radiology* 1988;**168**:429-431.
75. Dooms GC, Hricak H, Moseley MR, Bottles K, Fisher M, Higgins CB. Characterization of lymphadenopathy by magnetic resonance relaxation times: preliminary results. *Radiology* 1985;**155**:691-697.
76. Ginsburg RJ, Rice TW, Goldberg M, Waters PF, Schmocker BJ. Extended cervical mediastinoscopy. *J Thorac Cardiovasc Surg* 1987;**94**:673-678.
77. Paulson DL. Selection of patients for operation in the treatment of bronchogenic carcinoma. *Dallas Med J* 1974;**60**:173.
78. Black WC, Armstrong P, Daniel TM. Cost effectiveness of chest CT in T1N0M0 lung cancer. *Radiology* 1988;**167**:373-378.
79. Pearlberg JL, Sandler MA, Beute GH, Lewis JWJr, Madrazo BL. Limitations of CT in evaluation of neoplasms involving chest wall. *J Comput Assist Tomogr* 1987;**11**:290-293.
80. Glazer HS, Duncan-Meyer J, Aronberg DJ, Moran JF, Levitt RG, Sagel SS. Pleural and chest wall invasion in bronchogenic carcinoma: CT eyaluation. *Radiology* 1985;**157**:191-194.
81. Shin MS, Anderson SD, Myers J, Ho K. Pitfalls in CT evaluation of chest wall invasion by lung cancer. *J Comput Assist Tomogr* 1986;**10**:136-138.
82. Scott IR, Müller NL, Miller RR, Evans KG, Nelems B. Resectable stage III lung cancer: CT, surgical, and pathologic correlation. *Radiology* 1988;**166**:75-79.
83. O'Connell RS, McLoud TC, Wilkins EW. Superior sulcus tumour: radiographic diagnosis and workup. *AJR* 1983;**140**:25-30.
84. Johnson DH, Hainsworth JD, Greco FA. Pancoast's syndrome and small cell lung cancer. *Chest* 1982;**82**:602-606.
85. Rockoff SD. Apical lung cancer masquerading as a Pancoast tumour. *AJR* 1982;139:163-165.
86. Naidieh DP, Sussman R, Kutcher WL, Aranda CP, Garay SM, Ettenger NA. Solitary pulmonary nodules: CT-bronchoscopic correlation. *Chest* 1988;**93**:595-598.
87. Takasugi J, Rapoport S, Shaw C. Superior sulcus tumours: the role of imaging. *J Thorac Imag* 1989;**4**:41-48.
88. Castagno AA, Shuman WP. MR imaging in clinically suspected brachial plexus tumour. *AJR* 1987;**149**:1219-1222.

89. Rapoport S, Blair DN, McCarthy SM. Brachial plexus: correlation of MR imaging with CT and pathologic findings. *Radiology* 1988;**167**:161-165.
90. Webb WR. MR imaging in the evaluation and staging of lung cancer. *Semin US CT MR* 1988;**9**:53-66.
91. Glazer HS, Kaiser LR, Anderson DJ, Molina PL, Emami B, Roper CL, Sagel SS. Indeterminate mediastinal invasion in bronchogenic carcinoma: CT evaluation. *Radiology* 1989;**173**:37-42.
92. Gay SB, Black WC, Armstrong P, Daniel TM. Chest CT of unresectable lung cancer. *Radiographics* 1988;**8**:735-748.
93. Quint LE, Glazer GM, Orringer MB. Central lung masses: prediction with CT of need for pneumonectomy versus lobectomy. *Radiology* 1987;**165**:735-738.
94. McMurdo KK, de Geer G, Webb WR, Gamsu G. Normal and occluded mediastinal veins: MR imaging. *Radiology* 1986;**159**:33-38.
95. Weinreb JC, Mootz A, Cohen JM. MRI evaluation of mediastinal and thoracic inlet venous obstruction. *AJR* 1986;**146**:679-684.
96. Barakos JA, Brown JJ, Higgins CB. MR imaging of secondary cardiac and paracardiac lesions. *AJR* 1989;**153**:47-50.
97. Winkler M, Higgins CB. Suspected intracardiac masses: evaluation with MR imaging. *Radiology* 1987;**165**:117-122.
98. Moncada R, Baker M, Salinas M, Demos TC, Churchill R, Love L, Reynes C, Hale D, Cardoso M, Pifarre R, Gunnar RM. Diagnostic role of computed tomography in pericardial heart disease: congenital defects, thickening, neoplasms, and effusions. *Am Heart J* 1982;**103**:263-282.
99. Dawson WB, Mayo JR, Muller NL. Computed tomography of cardiac and pericardial tumours. *J Can Assoc Radiol* 1990;**41**:270-275.
100. Rohwedder JJ, Weatherbee L. Multiple primary bronchogenic carcinoma with a review of the literature. *Am Rev Respir Dis* 1974;**109**:435-445.
101. McElvaney G, Miller RR, Müller NL, Nelems B, Evans KG, Ostrow DN. Multicentricity of adenocarcinoma of the lung. *Chest* 1989;**95**:151-154.
102. Wu SC, Lin ZQ, Xu CW, Koo KS, Huang OL, Xie DQ. Multiple primary lung cancers. *Chest* 1987;**92**:892-896.
103. World Health Organization. The World Health Organization histologic typing of lung tumours. *Am J Clin Pathol* 1982;**77**:123-136.
104. Zwirewich CV, Miller RR, Müller NL. Multicentric adenocarcinoma of the lung: CT-pathologic correlation. *Radiology* 1990;**176**:185-190.
105. Miller RR. Bronchioloalveolar cell adenomas. *Am J Surg Pathol* 1990;**14**:904-912.
106. Miller RR, Nelems B, Evans KG, Müller NL, Ostrow DN. Glandular neoplasia of the lung: a proposed analogy to colonic tumours. *Cancer* 1988;**61**:1009-1014.
107. Bewtra C. Multiple primary bronchogenic carcinomas, with a review of the literature. *J Surg Oncol* 1984;**25**:207-213.
108. Ferguson MK, DeMeeste TR, DesLauriers J, Littel AG, Piraux M, Golomb H. Diagnosis and management of synchronous lung cancers. *J Thorac Cardiovasc Surg* 1985;**89**:378-385.
109. Salvatierra A, Baamonde C, Llamas JM, Cruz F, Lopez-Pujol J. Extrathoracic staging of bronchogenic carcinoma. *Chest* 1990;**97**:1052-1058.
110. Sider L, Horejs D. Frequency of extrathoracic metastases from bronchogenic carcinoma in patients with normal-sized hilar and mediastinal lymph nodes on CT. *AJR* 1988;**151**:893-895.
111. Woodring JH, Stelling CB. Adenocarcinoma of the lung: a tumour with a changing pleomorphic character. *AJR* 1983;**140**:657.
112. Matthews MJ. Morphology of lung cancer. *Semin Oncol* 1974;**1**:175.

113. Hooper RG, Beechler CR, Johnson MC. Radioisotope scanning in the initial staging of bronchogenic carcinoma. *Am Rev Respir Dis* 1978;**118**:279.

114. Ramsdell JW, Peters RM, Taylor AT, Alazraki NP, Tisi GM. Multiorgan scans for staging lung cancer. Correlation with clinical evaluation. *J Thorac Cardiovasc Surg* 1977;**73**:653-659.

115. Turner P, Haggith JW. Preoperative radionuclide scanning in bronchogenic carcinoma. *Br J Dis Chest* 1981;**75**:291.

116. Filderman AE, Shaw C, Matthay RA. Lung cancer. Part II. Staging and therapy. *Invest Radiol* 1986;**21**:173-185.

117. Alderson PO, Adams DF, McNeil BJ. Computed tomography, ultrasound, and scintigraphy of the liver in patients with colon or breast carcinoma: a prospective comparison. *Radiology* 1983;**149**:225-230.

118. Knopf DR, Torres WE, Fajman WJ, Sones PJ. Liver lesions: comparative accuracy of scintigraphy and computed tomography. *AJR* 1982;**138**:623-627.

119. Malt RA. Medical intelligence: current concepts - surgery for hepatic neoplasms. *N Engl J Med* 1985;**313**:1591-1596.

120. Borg SA, Rubin P, DeWys WD. Metastases and disseminated disease. In *Clinical Oncology: A Multidisciplinary Approach.* 6th ed.,pp 498-515. New York: American Cancer Society, 1983.

121. Finlay IG, Meek DR, Gray HW, Duncan JG, McArdle CS. Incidence and detection of occult hepatic metastases in colorectal carcinoma. *Br Med J* 1982;**284**:803-805.

122. Miller DL, Simmons JT, Chang R, Ward BA, Shawker TH, Doppman JL, Chang AE. Hepatic metastasis detection: comparison of three CT contrast enhancement methods. *Radiology* 1987;**165**:785-790.

123. Matsui O, Takashima T, Kadoya M, Suzuki M, Hirose J, Kameyama T, Choto S, Konishi H, Ida M, Yamaguchi A, Izumi R. Liver metastases from colorectal cancers: detection with CT during arterial portography. *Radiology* 1987;**165**:65-69.

124. Stark DD, Wittenberg J, Butch RJ, Ferrucci JTJr. Hepatic metastases: randomized, controlled comparison of detection with MR imaging and CT. *Radiology* 1987;**165**:399-406.

125. Curati WL, Halevy A, Gibson RN, Carr DH, Blumgart LH, Steiner RE. Ultrasound, CT, and MRI comparison in primary and sccondary tumours of the liver. *Gastrointest Radiol* 1988;**13**:123-128.

126. Glomset DA. The incidence of metastases of malignant tumours to the adrenals. *Am J Cancer* 1938;**32**:57-61.

127. Pagani JJ. Non-small cell lung carcinoma adrenal metastases: computed tomography and percutaneous needle biopsy in their diagnosis. *Cancer* 1984;**53**:1058-1060.

128. Nielson MEJr, Heaston DK, Dunnick NR, Korobkin M. Preoperative CT evaluation of adrenal glands in non-small cell bronchogenic carcinoma. *AJR* 1982;**139**:317-320.

129. Oliver TW, Bernardino ME, Miller JI, Mansour K, Greene D, Davis WA. Isolated adrenal masses in non small-cell bronchogenic carcinoma. *Radiology* 1984;**153**:217-218.

130. Commons RR, Callaway CP. Adenomas of the adrenal cortex. *Arch Intern Med* 1948;**81**:37-41.

131. Mittman C, Bruderman I. Lung cancer: to operate or not? *Am Rev Respir Dis* 1977;**116**:477-496.

132. Berland LL, Koslin DB, Kenney PJ, Stanley RJ, Lee JY. Differentiation between small benign and malignant adrenal masses with dynamic incremented CT. *AJR* 1988;**151**:95-101.

133. Glazer GM, Woolsey EJ, Borrello J, Francis IR, Aisen AM, Bookstein F, Amendola MA, Gross MD, Bree RL, Martel W. Adrenal tissue characterization using MR imaging. *Radiology* 1986;**158**:73-79.

134. Chezmar JL, Robbins SM, Nelson RC, Steinberg HV, Torres WE, Bernardino ME. Adrenal masses: characterization with T1-weighted MR imaging. *Radiology* 1988;**166**:357-359.
135. Krestin GP, Steinbrich W, Friedman G. Adrenal masses: evaluation with fast gradient-echo MR imaging and gadolinium-DTPA enhanced dynamic studies. *Radiology* 1989;**171**:675-680.
136. Dunnick NR. CT and MRI of adrenal lesions. *Urol Radiol* 1988;**10**:12-16.
137. Butler AR, Leo JS, Lin JP, Boyd AD, Kricheff II. The value of routine cranial computed tomography in neurologically intact patients with primary carcinoma of the lung. *Radiology* 1979;**131**:399-401.
138. Jacobs L, Kinkel WR, Vincent RG. 'Silent' brain metastases from lung carcinoma determined by computerized tomography. *Arch Neurol* 1977;**34**:690-693.
139. Mintz BJ, Tuhrim S, Alexander S, Yang WC, Shanzer S. Intracranial metastases in the initial staging of bronchogenic carcinoma. *Chest* 1984;**86**:850-853.
140. Sze G, Shin J, Krol G, Johnson C, Liu D, Deck MDF. Intraparenchymal brain metastases: MR imaging versus contrast-enhanced CT. *Radiology* 1988;**168**:187-194.
141. Donato AT, Ammerman EG, Sullesta O. Bone scanning in the evaluation of patients with lung cancer. *Ann Thorac Surg* 1979;**27**:300-304.
142. Citrin DL, Hougen C, Zweibel W, Schlise S, Pruitt B, Ershler W, Davis TE, Harberg J, Cohen AI. The use of serial bone scans in assessing response of bone metastases to systemic treatment. *Cancer* 1981;**47**:680-685.
143. Ekholm S, Albrechtsson U, Kugelberg J, Tylen U. Computed tomography in preoperative staging of bronchogenic carcinoma. *J Comput Assist Tomogr* 1980;**4**:763-765.
144. Matthews JI, Richey HM, Helsel RA, Grishkin BA. Thoracic computed tomography in the preoperative evaluation of primary bronchogenic carcinoma. *Arch Intern Med* 1987;**147**:449-453.
145. Zwirewich CV, Müller NL, Lam SC. Photodynamic laser therapy to alleviate complete bronchial obstruction: comparison of CT and bronchoscopy to predict outcome. *AJR* 1988;**151**:897-901.
146. Forster BB, Müller NL, Miller RR, Nelems B, Evans KG. Neuroendocrine carcinomas of the lung: clinical, radiologic, and pathologic correlation. *Radiology* 1989;**170**:441-445.

Computed tomography of mediastinal masses

Stuart S. Sagel
Mallinckrodt Institute of Radiology, Washington University Medical Center, St. Louis, Missouri, USA

Introduction

The relatively inexpensive and universally available standard chest radiograph remains the initial radiological examination in a patient with suspected intrathoracic disease. In the great majority of cases when the mediastinum is questionably or definitively abnormal on conventional radiographs, computed tomography (CT) is the next radiological technique employed when further evaluation is required. A few exceptions might include a suspected acute traumatic lesion of the aorta or great vessels in which aortography is primarily used, or probable oesophageal pathology which should be studied first with barium oesophography. Conventional tomography is only employed now when assessment of the trachea or major airway is required in selected instances (e.g. length of a stricture).

CT is the most appropriate initial tomographic study of the thorax in the majority of clinical situations because of the wide variety of information it can provide [1,2]. The mediastinum as well as the lungs, pleura, chest wall and hila all can be evaluated simultaneously. The size, homogeneity, site of origin, extent, and relation to normal mediastinal components of any abnormal mass usually can be defined [3]. Distinction between benign lipomatous, calcific, or serous fluid collections from lymphadenopathy, soft tissue masses, and vascular lesions and anomalies (Fig. 1) often is possible. It should be empha-

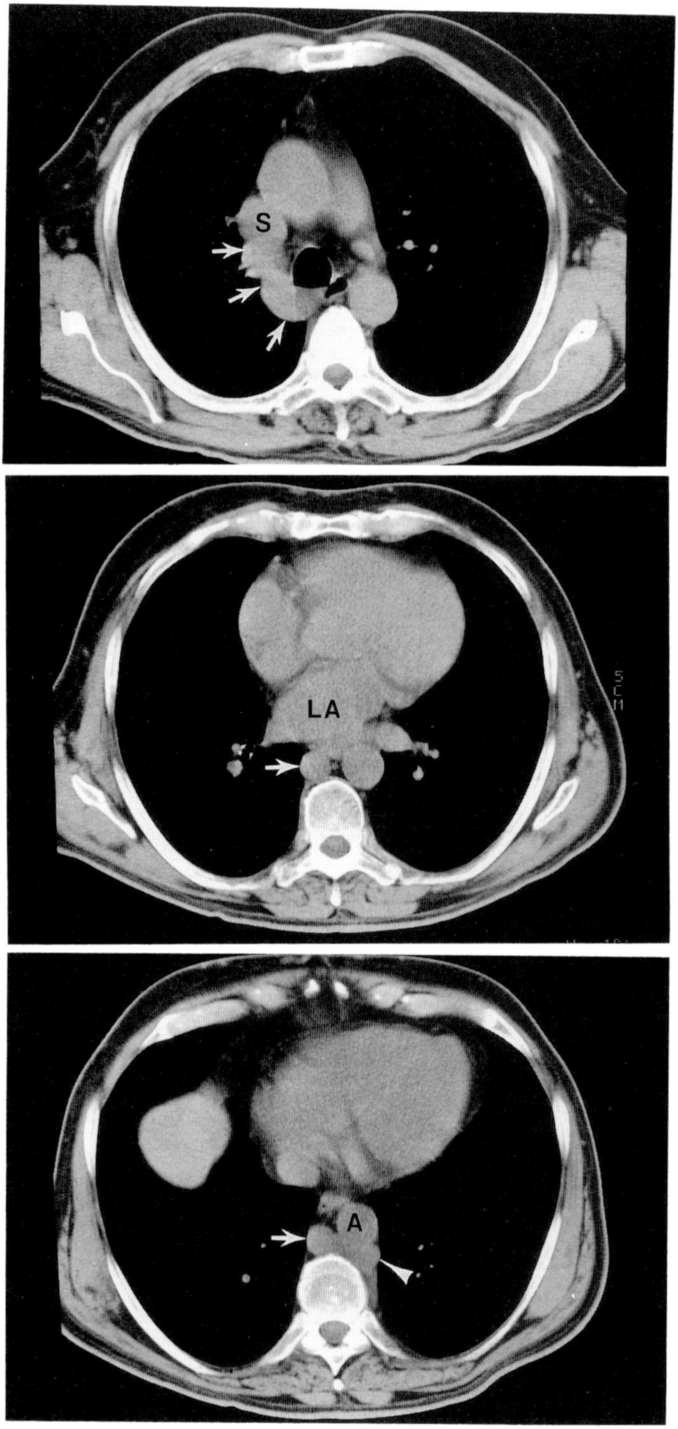

(a)

(b)

(c)

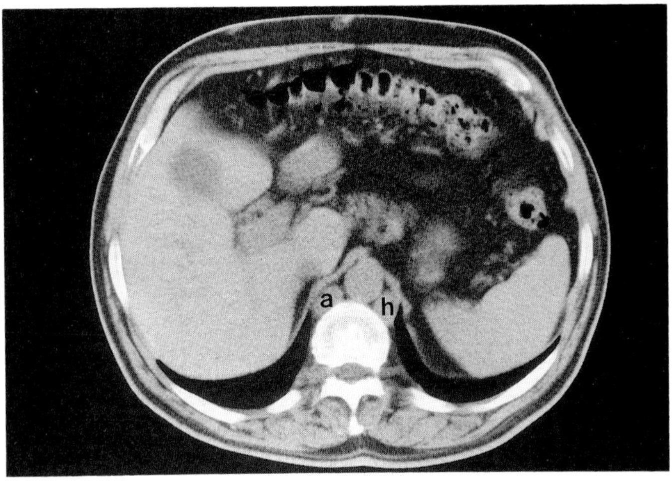

(d)

Figure 1. *AZYGOS CONTINUATION OF THE INFERIOR VENA CAVA. Even without intravenous contrast administration, definitive diagnosis of a vascular anomaly is often possible by analyzing the serial contiguous scans. (a) At the level of the aortopulmonary window, a markedly dilated azygos vein arch (arrows) drains into the superior vena cava (S). (b) Caudally, at the level of the left atrium (LA), a dilated azygos vein (arrow) is seen. (c) More caudad, the azygos vein (arrow) is noted to communicate with a dilated hemi-azygos vein (arrowhead) dorsal to the descending thoracic aorta* (**a**). *(d) More caudad, in the region of the retrocrural space, dilated azygos (a) and hemi-azygos* (**h**) *veins are responsible for the paraspinal line widening noted on a plain chest radiograph.*

sized that CT is basically a morphological and not a histological technique, and reliable distinction between benign and malignant soft tissues masses or enlarged lymph nodes generally is not feasible. Proper administration of intravenous contrast media helps distinguish vascular from non-vascular abnormalities (Fig. 2), or determine the effect of a pathological process on a major vessel. Demonstration of invasion into adjacent pleura, pericardium or lung, with or without constriction of nearby vessels and bronchi, does strongly suggest malignant neoplasm as the aetiology.

Although the various intrathoracic structures also can be imaged with magnetic resonance imaging (MRI), several pulse sequences usually are required to duplicate all of the comparable information available on a single CT study, and obtaining these multiple sequences can be time consuming. Compared to an MRI examination, a CT

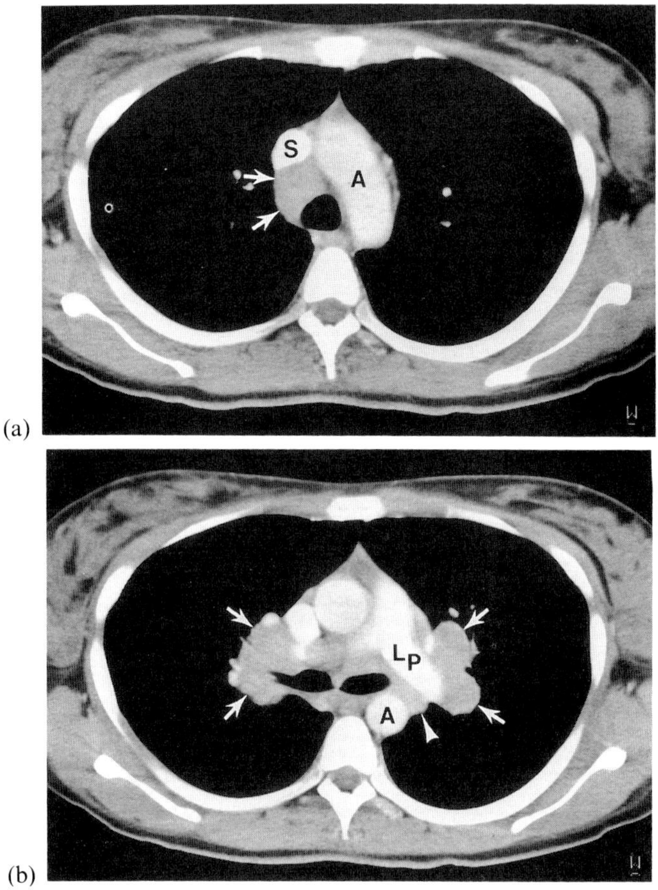

Figure 2. *MEDIASTINAL LYMPHADENOPATHY (SARCOIDOSIS); POST INTRAVENOUS CONTRAST ENHANCED CT IMAGES. (a) At the level of the aortic arch (A), right paratracheal lymphadenopathy (arrows) is easily recognized posterior to the superior vena cava (S), separate from the enhancing vessels of the mediastinum. (b) More caudad, bilateral hilar lymphadenopathy (arrows) as well as nodal enlargement (arrowhead) between the left pulmonary artery (LP) and descending thoracic aorta (A) can be distinguished.*

study is lower in cost, besides being more widely available and generally quicker and easier to perform [4]. In critically ill individuals requiring close monitoring or life-support equipment, or those with an implanted pacemaker, CT is the only option. The major advantage of MRI compared to CT is obviation of an intravenous contrast agent. It is rare that the coronal, sagittal, or another non-transaxial imaging plane provides vital clinically relevant data. Almost never is MRI more specific in affording histological distinction (e.g. separation of malignant neoplastic from benign inflammatory disease) of an enlarged lymph node or mediastinal mass. The inability of MRI to identify calcification (or high iodine content) within a mediastinal mass, sometimes the hallmark of a benign lesion, can be a considerable limitation. It is best to utilize MRI to evaluate one specific problem raised by the clinical, plain chest radiographic or a prior CT examination, rather than to use it to evaluate the entire thorax looking for a variety of possible abnormalities. While CT and MRI theoretically need not be considered competitive techniques, because each has its own particular strengths which may be advantageous in specific instances, it is not realistic to perform both in patients with intrathoracic disease in the hope that complementary information of clinical value will be provided. In most situations only one should be performed, and most times that is CT. MRI may be the imaging modality of choice in some selected circumstances, most relating to the diagnosis of a vascular lesion - especially if intravenous contrast media cannot be administered, or in a patient with a posterior mediastinal mass which is probably a neurogenic tumour because of the ability of MRI to show the relationship of the mass to the spinal canal without using intrathecal contrast media. Otherwise, MRI of the mediastinum generally should be used as a secondary technique when CT is problematic or not definitive.

CT also may be employed when the plain chest radiographs are normal but strong clinical suspicion of a mediastinal lesion exists. Pathology that may be detected with CT which is occult on conventional radiographs would include the demonstration of a small thymoma in a patient with myasthenia gravis, a mass responsible for recurrent laryngeal nerve paralysis, or an ectopic parathyroid adenoma in a patient with hyperparathyroidism (Fig. 3).

Determination of the attenuation value of a mediastinal mass by CT may permit a definitive non-invasive diagnosis [5,6]. Focal lesions which present with values characteristic of benign fatty tissue, (-80 to -120 Hounsfield units (HU), including a pericardial fat pad, and omental herniations through the foramens of Morgagni or Bochdalek, can usually be conclusively diagnosed on CT and no further diagnostic evaluation is indicated. Most benign cysts (pericardial, bronchogenic) have a near-water equivalent density, with an

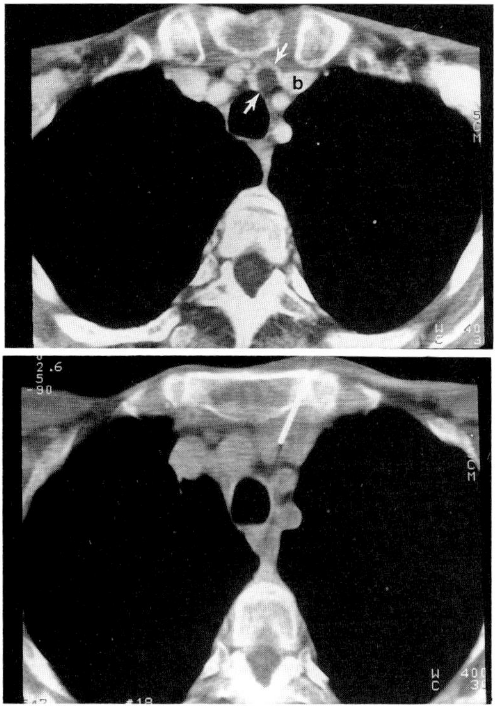

(a)

(b)

Figure 3. *ECTOPIC PARATHYROID ADENOMA IN SUPERIOR MEDIASTINUM. (a) A 1.5 cm ovoid mass with peripheral enhancement (arrows) is demonstrated just medial to the left brachiocephalic vein (b) in an elderly patient who had 'failed' neck surgery done previously for control of hyperparathyroidism. (b) Parathormone levels from the mass obtained via percutaneous needle aspiration, performed via an approach through the left sternoclavicular joint under CT guidance, were 2000 times higher than a simultaneous venous sample, corroborating that the mass represented an adenoma rather than incidental necrotic mediastinal lymph node.*

imperceptible wall. While malignant soft tissue density neoplasms, such as Hodgkin's disease, can undergo necrosis and contain areas of near water density, these lesions typically are either thick-walled or inhomogeneous, allowing distinction from benign cysts.

Abnormalities of the Mediastinal Fat

A lesion of pure fat density, with well defined margins, is almost invariably benign. In such cases, the CT diagnosis is usually conclusive and no further diagnostic evaluation is warranted.

Mediastinal Lipomatosis

This is a benign condition in which large amounts of histologically normal, unencapsulated fat accumulate in the mediastinum. It is most commonly associated with obesity or exogenous corticosteroid administration; it is less frequently seen with primary Cushing syndrome.

The excess fat deposition is mainly prominent in the upper mediastinum. Tracheal compression or displacement is uniformly absent. Less commonly, fat will accumulate preferentially in the paraspinal areas or near the cardiophrenic angles (pericardial fat pads). The fat in mediastinal lipomatosis should appear as uniform low density (-80 to -120 HU). If inhomogeneity is noted, an alternative diagnosis, such as liposarcoma, or superimposed processes, such as neoplastic infiltration, mediastinitis, or haemorrhage must be considered. Small foci of residual thymic tissue in the anterior mediastinum should not be mistaken for infiltrated fat.

Focal Fatty Masses

These are most frequently seen in the peridiaphragmatic areas, and usually represent herniations of abdominal fat. Omental fat can herniate through the foramen of Morgagni, almost always located on the right side, to create the appearance of a cardiophrenic angle mass. Fine linear densities can sometimes be seen within the herniated fat that represent small omental vessels, and their presence can help distinguish herniated fat through the foramen of Morgagni from a pericardial fat pad.

Fat herniation through the foramen of Bochdalek or a focal diaphragmatic defect (Fig. 4) is much more common on the left side, because the liver inhibits occurrence on the right. Herniation of perigastric fat through the oesophageal hiatus in the diaphragm may occur. Extension alongside the aorta can create widening of the paraspinal line(s) or simulate a retrocardiac mass on conventional radiography.

The malignant fatty tumours, even the well differentiated liposarco-

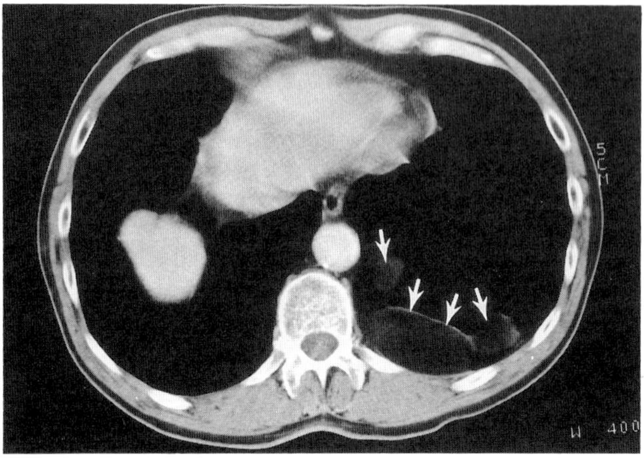

Figure 4. *EXTENSION OF RETROPERITONEAL FAT (arrows) INTO THE CAUDAL LEFT HEMITHORAX THROUGH A DEFECT IN (OR EVENTRATION OF) THE LEFT HEMIDIAPHRAGM.*

mas, tend to contain some soft tissue density elements besides the areas of fat density. Some liposarcomas have a predominantly soft tissue attenuation value rather than a fat density. An inhomogeneous fatty mass in the anterior mediastinum most likely represents a teratoma or a thymolipoma: the former may also contain some areas of calcification.

Lymphadenopathy

Normal lymph nodes are demonstrable on CT in most adult patients with even a modest amount of mediastinal fat [7]. The manifestations of lymphadenopathy (disease of lymph nodes) on both CT and MRI, consisting mainly of enlargement, are relatively straightforward, but generally non-specific as to aetiology. When a lymph node exceeds 1.0 cm in diameter, or in cross-section, recognized by direct measurement, it is considered pathological. Also, a localized cluster of lymph nodes of borderline enlarged size should be regarded as highly suspect of disease. Whether such enlargement is caused by metastatic neoplasm, lymphoma or inflammation usually cannot be ascertained by CT (or MRI) alone. Confirmation of abnormality and specific diagnosis may require histological examination of material from the lymph node(s) noted to be enlarged. Based upon the precise location of the involved lymph nodes, when clinically necessary, the most appropriate method of tissue sampling (e.g. transcervical mediastinoscopy, parasternal mediastinotomy, percutaneous or transbronchoscopic needle aspiration biopsy) can be selected.

Calcification within lymph node(s) generally connotes old granulomatous disease (Fig. 5). However, there are some rare exceptions

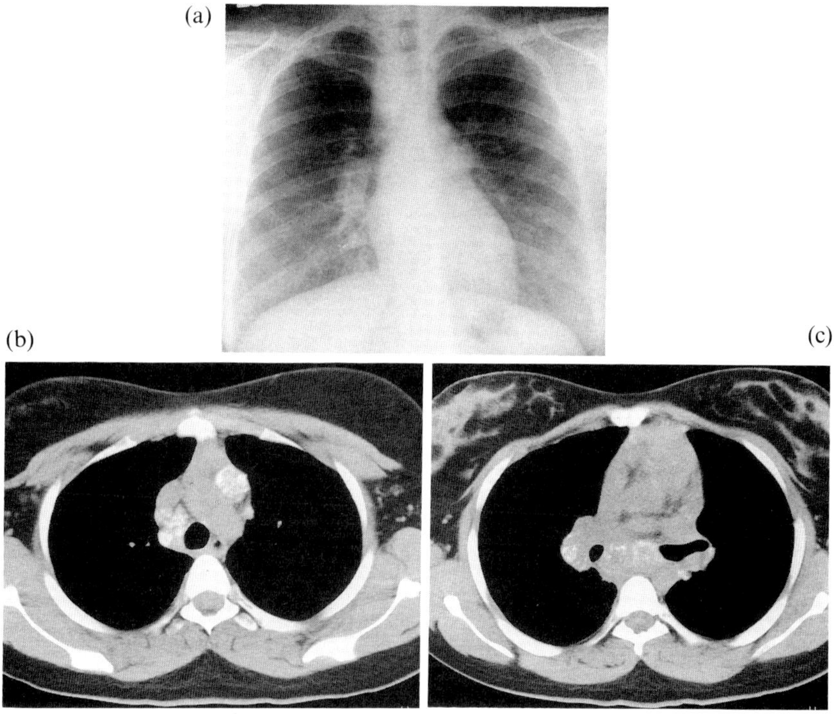

Figure 5. *CALCIFIED MEDIASTINAL LYMPH NODES DUE TO OLD HEALED HISTOPLASMOSIS. (a) Postero-anterior chest radiograph demonstrates paratracheal and hilar lymphadenopathy; no calcification within the lymph nodes could be discerned. (b and c) Non-contrast enhanced CT scans demonstrate faint diffuse calcification throughout the enlarged lymph nodes.*

due to metastatic neoplasm (e.g. mucinous ovarian carcinoma, bronchioloalveolar cell carcinomas); the clinical history and associated findings most often permit distinction (Fig. 6).

Necrosis within enlarged lymph nodes, resulting in low, near-water density central areas, usually with a preserved thick soft tissue density

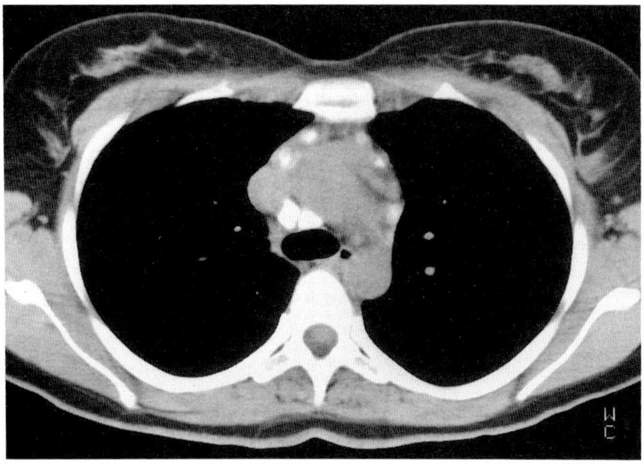

Figure 6. *CALCIFIED MEDIASTINAL LYMPH NODES DUE TO METASTATIC MUCINOUS ADENOCARCINOMA OF THE OVARY. These enlarged nodes regressed following chemotherapy.*

rim, can be seen with aggressive neoplastic involvement, but is occasionally encountered with granulomatous infection [8]. Also, low attenuation values within mediastinal lymph nodes, not due to necrosis, may occur secondary to involvement by metastatic testicular cancers.

Substantial enhancement of lymph node(s) after intravenous contrast administration may be noted, most typically with highly vascular metastatic neoplasm (e.g. renal cell or thyroid carcinoma). However, it also may be seen with benign conditions (e.g. angiofollicular lymph node hyperplasia). Also, non-lymph node masses in the mediastinum may exhibit marked contrast enhancement, such as intrathoracic goiter, paraganglioma, and haemangioma [9,10,11].

As disease advances in pathologically involved lymph nodes, the enlarged margins may lose their sharp definition and the surrounding mediastinal fat may increase in density. Such changes are due to extension of the disease process through the nodal capsule and an associated fibrotic or inflammatory reaction. When the disease process extends through the capsule of several adjacent nodes, a single larger coalescent mass may form. The resulting conglomerate mass may be difficult to ascribe confidently to lymphadenopathy, which, however, is the commonest cause of a soft tissue density mass in the middle mediastinum.

Lymphoma

Malignant lymphoma frequently involves the thorax; mediastinal lymphadenopathy is its most common intrathoracic manifestation. Lymphomatous masses are most commonly found in the anterior mediastinum in Hodgkin's disease; in the majority of cases this does not reflect lymphadenopathy but rather involvement of the lymphoid elements of the thymus (Fig. 7). Concomitant lymph node disease

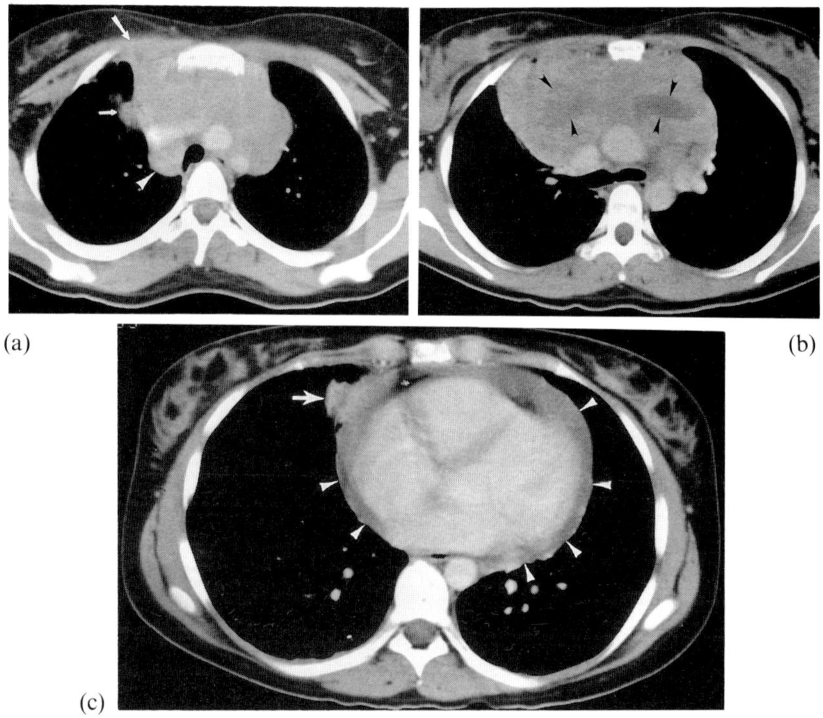

Figure 7. *THYMIC HODGKIN'S DISEASE (NODULAR SCLEROSING TYPE). (a) Postcontrast CT image demonstrates diffuse enlargement of the thymus, with extension of the neoplastic disease into the right anterior chest wall (large arrow) and right upper lobe (small arrow). Concomitant right paratracheal lymphadenopathy (arrowhead) also is present. (b) Caudad, at the level of the carina, which is displaced dorsally and compressed, necrotic ('cystic') areas (arrowheads) in the diffusely infiltrated thymus are demonstrated. (c) More caudad, neoplastic disease from the right lobe of the thymus (arrow) invades the pericardium, producing a pericardial effusion (arrowheads).*

elsewhere in the mediastinum (e.g. paratracheal, internal mammary, supra-diaphragmatic) is frequent [12,13]. Non-Hodgkin's lymphoma predominantly presents as enlargement of the middle mediastinal lymph nodes, but neither the localization pattern nor the appearance on CT of the abnormal nodes is distinct enough to play a vital role in differential diagnosis [14]. The size and appearance of involved lymph nodes in lymphoma span the entire spectrum, from well defined mildly enlarged lymph nodes in one region to large, conglomerate soft-tissue density masses in multiple areas. Typically, these nodal masses demonstrate little enhancement following intravenous contrast media administration: in fact, their central areas may become relatively quite hypodense.

CT also is helpful as a method of follow-up to assess treatment response. It may aid in the re-adjustment of therapy (e.g. reduction in radiation portal size as tumour bulk regresses). Relapse in the mediastinum may be detected when the plain chest radiograph is normal. Complete return to normal after successful treatment of mediastinal lymphadenopathy does not always occur. Follow-up CT examination may reveal some persistent, mildly-enlarged lymph nodes, even though they contain no viable neoplasm. These 'sterilized' nodes can pose a diagnostic and therapeutic dilemma. While percutaneous needle aspiration with cytological evaluation has been used, the cellular material obtained can be difficult to interpret after radiation or chemotherapy. Serial CT examinations, in patients otherwise doing well clinically after therapy, usually suffice to determine the adequacy of treatment. Recurrence or failure of the initial therapy should be diagnosed only if an increase in the size of the lymph nodes subsequently occurs. In selected cases, MRI may be able to differentiate post-therapeutic fibrosis (low signal intensity on both T1 and T2-weighted images) from lymphomatous involvement (high signal intensity on T2-weighted images).

Hilar Enlargement

Further assessment of an enlarged or questionably abnormal pulmonary hilum noted on plain chest radiography is a common radiological problem. Usually the major decision to be made is whether the prominence is due to a normal variation, enlargement of a pulmonary artery, enlargement of a lymph node(s), or a neoplastic mass commonly arising from a bronchus. CT is capable of allowing these distinctions.

The criteria for the diagnosis of hilar lymph node enlargement on non contrast CT scans are similar to those used for conventional radiography: the hilum is too big and its contour is too nodular. In addition, there may be obliteration of some normal anatomical interfaces, such as convex bulging into the azygo-oesophageal recess or the space between the left lower lobe pulmonary artery and the descending aorta. With advanced hilar nodal enlargement, the central bronchi may be distorted and compressed. If doubt remains as to whether hilar enlargement is due to a lymph node mass or a vessel, it can almost always be dispelled by scanning following a bolus injection of intravenous contrast media. MRI is considered a supplementary technique if the CT examination is equivocal: it may assume a more primary role if there is a known contra-indication to or the inability to use intravenous contrast media. When contrast media enhancement is used with CT, there is no difference in accuracy between the two techniques and CT is superior in assessing the adjacent bronchial tree, which may be very important in the evaluation of the hilum.

Mediastinal Cysts

Most cysts of the mediastinum are congenital in origin; they include aero-digestive tract duplications (bronchogenic, foregut), neurenteric, lymphogenous, and pleuropericardial. In adults, the majority are discovered as an incidental finding on a plain chest radiograph, and only rarely do they produce clinical findings. On CT they are typically sharply marginated and have a near-water equivalent density; they do not enhance after intravenous contrast administration. Generally, their appearance and attenuation values are so characteristic, that in an asymptomatic patient, surgery often may be avoided and the patient managed conservatively, with only plain radiograph follow-up being necessary to confirm their stability. Operation can be reserved for those unusually large cysts causing or potentially capable of compressing a major mediastinal structure, or when CT diagnosis is not definitive.

Bronchogenic Cysts

These result from abnormal budding of the tracheobronchial tree; approximately 90% are located within the middle mediastinum near the carina or along the right paratracheal wall. Bronchogenic cysts are lined by columnar respiratory epithelium, which may secrete a variety of fluids. Their contents can range from clear serous to a milky white to brown mucoid material, with variable viscosities. Consequently, different CT densities may be observed with bronchogenic cysts, depending upon their fluid composition. About half are of homogeneous, near-water density, reflecting their serous nature. This is the type of lesion, if relatively small, that can simply be followed radiologically. In the other half of cases, the density of a bronchogenic cyst can vary from the low soft tissue range to substantially higher than muscle, usually because of their viscid mucous proteinacious contents. Some cysts have very high attenuation values because the fluid contains calcium carbonate or calcium oxalate. Cysts in this density range generally are indistinguishable from solid soft tissue neoplasms, although their total lack of contrast enhancement may be a clue to the proper aetiology. MRI may be helpful and strongly suggest that these lesions are fluid-filled. While most bronchogenic cysts are low in signal intensity on T1-weighted MRI images, they are very high in signal intensity on T2-weighted images. Hemorrhagic or proteinaceous cysts may have a higher signal intensity than that of simple cysts on T1-weighted images.

Cystic Hygroma

These lymphogenous cysts typically occur in the superior mediastinum. On CT, they appear as round, occasionally multiloculated, smooth masses, with a homogenous attenuation value sometimes lower than water. They commonly compress surrounding tissues.

Pleuropericardial Cysts

They are most frequently located in the cardiophrenic angles. Typically, they have a near water attenuation value, with rare exceptions. Although sharply marginated, they are commonly not round, but rather somewhat triangular, conforming to the space afforded by the lower portion of the major fissure.

Mediastinal Abscess

CT can be valuable, especially in a febrile patient following median sternotomy, in detecting the presence and determining the extent of an abnormal mediastinal fluid collection. Reliable distinction between a diffuse mediastinitis and a drainable abscess is usually possible [15]. Sometimes pockets of air are seen within the mass, even though they cannot be recognized on plain radiographs, supporting the diagnosis of an abscess. Percutaneous needle aspiration, under CT guidance, may be required to distinguish an abscess (in which the attenuation values may vary from 10 - 40 HU) from an uninfected seroma or haematoma.

Thymic Mass

CT should be the imaging procedure of choice following standard chest radiography when thymic pathology is suspected [16,17,18]. Scanning at 5-mm intervals using 5-mm collimation, sometimes after intravenous contrast administration, may be valuable in selected cases when a small mass is suspected.

Thymoma

Thymomas are comprised of both epithelial cells and lymphocytes, the proportions varying, sometimes with a mosaic of compositions within the same neoplasm. This tumour is exceedingly rare before the age of 20 years; it occurs in association with myasthenia gravis or other less common conditions (red cell aplasia, hypogammaglobulinaemia) or sporadically.

Thymomas are present in 10 - 15% of patients with myasthenia gravis. Plain chest radiographs are relatively insensitive, since most of the neoplasms associated with this condition are relatively small and are hidden by the surrounding mediastinal vessels. CT is a sensitive procedure for the detection of these tumours; lesions as small as 1 cm in diameter can be reliably depicted [19,20]. A thymoma typically appears on CT as a soft tissue density mass, which is oval, round or lobulated and usually sharply demarcated. Most often the neoplasm grows asymmetrically to one side of the mediastinum. Focal areas of calcification may occur in about 25% of these tumours, which are usually also enhanced mildly and homogeneously after intravenous contrast administration. On MRI, fibrous septa may be recognized separating large groups of neoplastic cells, strongly supporting the diagnosis of a benign thymoma.

Approximately 10 - 15% of thymomas are classified as 'malignant'. Since the histological appearance of a thymoma does not permit reliable distinction between the benign and malignant forms, the term 'invasive' thymoma is generally preferred [21]. The presence of neoplastic growth through the capsule determines whether the tumour is 'invasive' ('malignant'). These neoplasms tend to be bulky and generally can be recognized on standard radiography. An invasive thymoma should be suspected on CT when, in addition to an anterior mediastinal mass in the vicinity of the thymus, infiltration into the surrounding mediastinal fat and fascia is seen (Fig. 8). This tumour further spreads by implanting along the nearby pleural and pericardial surfaces, most commonly on only one side of the thoracic cavity. Only rarely does it grow directly into the chest wall or

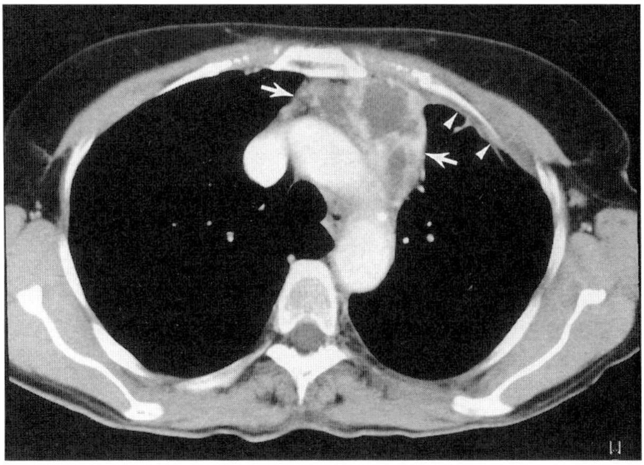

Figure 8. *INVASIVE ('MALIGNANT') THYMOMA. Postintravenous contrast CT scan demonstrates an irregularly marginated enhancing 7 cm anterior mediastinal mass (arrows) infiltrating the mediastinal fat and extending laterally (arrowheads) along the pleura.*

through the visceral pleura into the lung. Following growth along the pleura, an invasive thymoma may extend caudally and involve the diaphragm. The tumour can extend through a hiatus or gap and invade the abdomen (e.g., the posterior pararenal space, perigastric tissues, liver surface). CT excels at demonstrating these additional sites of disease, which are often hidden on conventional radiography.

About 65% of patients with myasthenia gravis and no thymoma have lymphoid hyperplasia of the organ. This is purely a histological diagnosis, characterized by numerous lymphoid follicles with active germinal centres in the medulla surrounded by a plasma cell and lymphocytic infiltration, because the total thymic weight is not altered and the thymus usually is not enlarged. In some cases, with CT, the hyperplastic thymus appears larger than for appropriate age-matched controls; this may result from delayed fatty involution, which increases the volume of fat-free thymic tissue and causes it to seem bigger. In most cases, lymphoid hyperplasia of the thymus is indistinguishable from a normal organ.

Lymphoma

The malignant lymphomas, particularly the nodular sclerosing form of Hodgkin's disease, commonly infiltrate and enlarge the thymus, creating an anterior mediastinal mass. Difficulty may arise in distinguishing de novo involvement from an invasive thymoma; even histological distinction may be a problem as a thymoma may contain abundant lymphocytes. On CT, the presence of lymph node enlargement elsewhere in the thorax (or abdomen) strongly favours a diagnosis of lymphoma, as does direct invasion of the anterior chest wall. Multiple pleural implants at separate locations would suggest a thymoma. Calcification within the thymic mass also is more compatible with a thymoma: it is rare in untreated lymphoma.

Rebound hyperplasia of the thymus is a well-recognized entity in children and young adults recovering from severe illness, including the administration of chemotherapy. The overgrowth is transient and usually disappears after several months. The diffuse enlargement of the thymus may simulate recurrent lymphoma [22] on conventional chest radiography or CT. If the patient is doing well clinically, and no recurrent or residual disease is evident in another location, repeat CT scanning in several months is an acceptable method of clarifying the cause of the enlargement without the need for percutaneous biopsy. A gradual reduction in size corroborates the benign cause of the enlargement.

Germ Cell Tumours

Derived from one to three of the primitive embryonic germ cell layers, most of these lesions in the thorax arise within the thymus. A variety of histological types are encountered.

Dermoid cysts (containing elements of the ectodermal layer of cells only) and benign teratomas (containing elements of more than one of the three germinal layers) account for the majority of these tumours. On CT, both types are well demarcated with a thick encapsulating wall; this rim may enhance after intravenous contrast administration. The internal contents of a benign teratoma are typically inhomogeneous, with a variable admixture of components exhibiting CT numbers in the range of fat, water and soft tissue density. They sometimes contain amorphous calcification, or malformed teeth or bone. A specific diagnosis may be made with CT when these pleomorphic tissue densities are recognized within an anterior mediastinal mass. Layering of fat and fluid within such a mass also is presumptive evidence for this tumour.

Local invasion is the only criterion that indicates a malignant neoplasm is present. For example, a malignant teratoma may be suggested on CT by irregular borders of the mass with infiltration of the mediastinal fat; compression or invasion of the mediastinal vessels and airways also may be present. The other rare malignant germ cell tumours (seminoma, embryonal cell carcinoma, choriocarcinoma, endodermal sinus) usually appear as irregular soft-tissue masses (Fig. 9), often with central areas of cyst formation or necrosis [23]. They may be indistinguishable in appearance from lymphoma or an invasive thymoma.

Thymolipoma

This entity is a rare, benign intrathymic neoplasm, which typically causes no symptoms. It can grow exceedingly large, and may extend caudally to the cardiophrenic angles. On CT, the thymic mass appears either entirely of near fat density, or it may contain some inhomogeneous areas of soft tissue. It does not compress or invade surrounding structures.

Carcinoid

A corticotropin producing (ectopic ACTH) carcinoid tumour may arise within the thymus, resulting in Cushing syndrome. The lesions

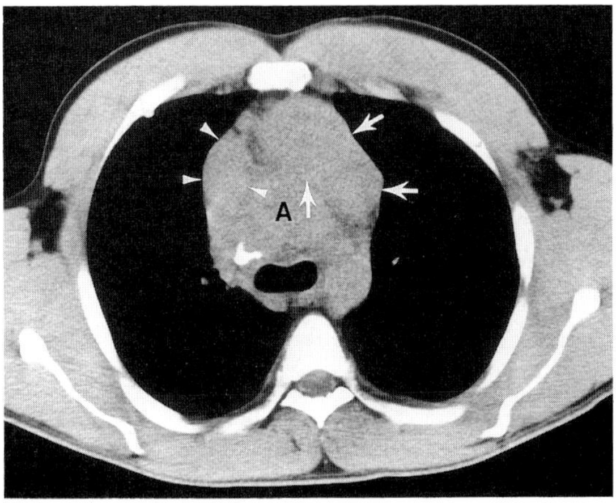

Figure 9. *PRIMARY GERM (EMBRYONAL) CELL CARCINOMA OF THE THYMUS. A large lobulated soft-tissue attenuation value mass is seen involving both the right (arrowheads) and left (arrows) lobes of the thymus. There is some concomitant right paratracheal lymphadenopathy; the nodal calcification in this area probably is the result of prior incidental healed granulomatous disease. A = ascending aorta.*

are often small and not detectable on plain chest radiographs. On CT, such a neoplasm appears identical with a small thymoma: distinction is based on the clinical findings.

Cyst

A rare lesion, which has features similar to a duplication or lymphogeneous cyst, except it is located within the thymus. Spontaneous haemorrhage into a thymic cyst may occur: pleuritic chest pain can result.

Thymic cysts also may occur in association with Hodgkin's disease; they are probably related to initial involvement of the organ with the disease rather than a consequence of radiotherapy or chemotherapy. Such cysts can persist or enlarge following successful treatment, while the lymphoma regresses, and they may simulate persistent or recurrent disease [24]. Their CT appearance, sometimes combined with percutaneous needle aspiration biopsy for corroboration, usually provides sufficient diagnostic information to obviate thoracotomy.

Posterior Mediastinal Masses

Oesophageal Hiatus Hernia

A common abnormality incidentally encountered on CT, oesophageal hiatus hernia appears as an air- and/or fluid-containing mass contiguous with the oesophagus and gastric fundus. If the diagnosis is not clear on a CT examination performed for evaluation of the thorax, the administration of oral contrast media permits the correct interpretation. Obviously, a barium oesophagogram, not CT, is the radiological procedure of choice for corroboration of the diagnosis if a question arises on a plain chest radiograph.

Neurogenic Tumours

These account for about 80% of posterior mediastinal neoplasms, the majority of which are discovered incidentally on plain chest radiographs. These tumours can originate from the nerve roots (schwannomas, neurilemmomas or neurofibromas) or from the sympathetic ganglia (neuroblastomas, ganglioneuromas or ganglioneuroblastomas).

Nerve root tumours usually are spherical and tend to occur near the junction of the vertebral body with the adjacent rib. Enlargement of an intervertebral foramen or pressure erosion of a rib is common. These neoplasms typically are sharply marginated, and of homogeneous soft tissue density on CT. Occasionally, they may be lower in attenuation value due to high amounts of lipids within the neural tissue (Fig. 10) [25]. Malignant neurogenic tumours tend to have poorly defined borders. Either MRI or CT (following opacification of the subarachnoid space with a non-ionic contrast agent) is crucial in determining whether an intraspinal component of the tumour is present.

Tumours arising from the sympathetic trunk tend to lie slightly anterior to the vertebral bodies and neural foramina. They are usually fusiform in shape in a cephalocaudal direction. On CT, they typically appear as a well circumscribed soft tissue density mass. Calcification occasionally occurs within them, especially the ganglioneuroblastoma.

Extramedullary Haematopoesis

This condition, usually secondary to a severe haemolytic anemia (e.g. thalassaemia major), may result in a paravertebral soft tissue density mass, that typically is bilateral along the lower thoracic spine. Associ-

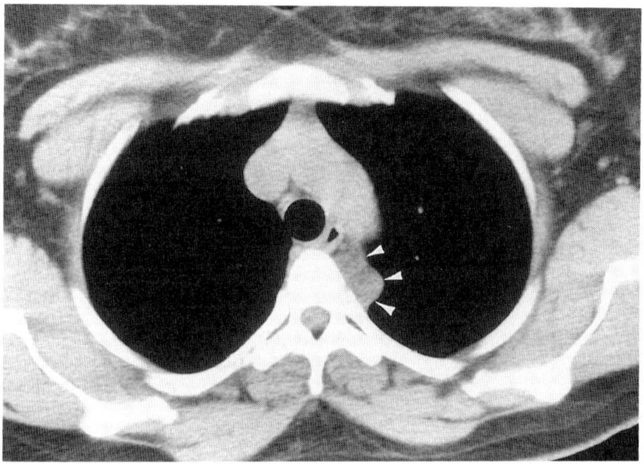

Figure 10. *NEURILEMMOMA OF THE POSTERIOR MEDIASTINUM. The mass (arrowheads) is slightly lower in attenuation value on this non-contrast enhanced CT scan than the blood in the mediastinal vessels and the chest wall musculature.*

ated expansion of the transverse processes of the vertebral bodies or of the ribs may be present.

Oesophageal Varices

These may occasionally enlarge sufficiently to produce a paraspinal mass near the distal oesophagus on conventional radiography. CT images after intravenous contrast administration generally permit definitive diagnosis; associated findings of cirrhosis and portal hypertension are usually present on other images through the upper abdomen.

Pancreatic Pseudocyst

An extrapancreatic fluid collection may spread into the posterior mediastinum from the retroperitoneum via either the aortic or oesophageal hiatus in the diaphragm. Typically, they are near-water density masses, but their attenuation values may be higher if haemorrhage or infection is superimposed. Usually, contiguity can be demonstrated on serial scans between the mediastinal fluid collection and peripancreatic inflammatory disease.

References

1. Baron RL, Levitt RG, Sagel SS, and Stanley RJ. Computed tomography in the evaluation of mediastinal widening. *Radiology* 1981;**138:**107-113.
2. Sones PJ, Torres WE, Colvin RS, Meier WL, Sprawls P, Rogers JV Jr. Effectiveness of CT in evaluating intrathoracic masses. *AJR* 1982;**139:**469-475.
3. Sagel SS, Glazer HS. Thorax: technique and normal anatomy and Mediastinum. Lee JKT, Sagel SS, Stanley RJ, eds. *Computed Body Tomography with MRI Correlation.* pp. 169-294. New York:Raven Press, 1989.
4. Aronberg DJ, Glazer HS, Sagel SS. MR and CT of the mediastinum: comparisons, controversies and pitfalls. *Radiol Clin N Amer* 1985;**23:**439-448.
5. Glazer HS, Siegel MJ, Sagel SS. Low-attenuation mediastinal masses on CT. *AJR* 1989;**152:**1173-1177.
6. Glazer HS, Molina PL, Siegel MJ, Sagel SS. High-attenuation mediastinal masses on unenhanced CT. *AJR* 1991;**156:**45-50.
7. Genereux GP, Howie JL. Normal mediastinal lymph node size and number: CT and anatomic study. *AJR* 1984;**142:**1095-1100.
8. Im J.-G, Song KS, Kang HS, Park JH, Yeon KM, Han MC, Kim C.-W. Mediastinal tuberculous lymphadenitis: CT manifestations. *Radiology* 1987;**164:**115-119.
9. Bashist B, Ellis K, Gold RP. Computed tomography of intrathoracic goiter. *AJR* 1983;**140:**455-460.
10. Glazer HS, Aronberg DJ, Sagel SS. Pitfalls in CT recognition of mediastinal lymphadenopathy. *AJR* 1985;**144:**267-274.
11. Spizarny DL, Rebner M, Gross BH. CT evaluation of enhancing mediastinal masses. *J Comput Assist Tomogr* 1987;**11:**990-993.
12. Heron CW, Husband JE, Williams MP. Hodgkin disease: CT of the thymus. *Radiology* 1988;**167:**647-651.
13. Hopper KD, Diehl LF, Lesar M, Barlles M, Granger E, Baumann J. Hodgkin disease: clinical utility of CT in initial staging and treatment. *Radiology* 1988;**169:**17-22.
14. Khoury MB, Godwin JD, Halvorsen R, Hanun Y, Putman CE. Role of chest CT in non Hodgkin lymphoma. *Radiology* 1986;**158:**659-662.
15. Carrol CL, Jeffrey RB Jr, Federle MP, Vernacchia FS. CT evaluation of mediastinal infection. *J Comput Assist Tomogr* 1987;**11:**449-454.
16. Baron RL, Lee JKT, Sagel SS, Levitt RG. Computed tomography of the abnormal thymus. *Radiology* 1982;**142:**127-134.
17. Molina PL, Siegel MJ, Glazer HS. Thymic masses on MR imaging. *AJR* 1990;**155:**495-500.
18. St. Amour TE, Siegel MJ, Glazer HS, Nadel SC. CT appearances of the normal and abnormal thymus in childhood. *J Comput Assist Tomogr* 1987;**11:**645-650.
19. Batra P, Herrmann C Jr, Mulder D. Mediastinal imaging in myasthenia gravis: correlation of chest radiography. CT, MR and surgical findings. *AJR* 1987;**148:**515-519.
20. Ellis K, Austin JHM, Jaretzki A III. Radiologic detection of thymoma in patients with myasthenia gravis. *AJR* 1988;**151:**873-881.
21. Zerhouni EA, Scott WW, Baker RR, Wharam MD, Siegelman SS. Invasive thymomas: diagnosis and evaluation by computed tomography. *J Comput Assist Tomogr* 1982;**6:**92-100.
22. Choyke PL, Zeman RK, Gootenberg JE, Greenberg JN, Hoffer F, Frank JA. Thymic atrophy and regrowth in response to chemotherapy: CT evaluation. *AJR* 1987;**149:**269-272.

23. Lee KS, Im J.-G, Han CH, Han MC, Kim C.-W, Kim WS. Malignant primary germ cell tumors of the mediastinum: CT features. *AJR* 1989;**153:**947-951.
24. Lindfors KK, Meyer JE, Dedlick CG, Hassell LW, Harris NL. Thymic cysts in mediastinal Hodgkin disease. *Radiology* 1985;**156:**37-41.
25. Cohen LM, Schwartz AM, Rockoff SD. Benign schwannomas: pathologic basis for CT inhomogeneities. *AJR* 1986;**147:**141-143.

Magnetic resonance imaging of mediastinal and hilar masses

David P. Naidich
Department of Radiology, New York Medical Center, New York, USA

Introduction

Despite tremendous initial enthusiasm the role of magnetic resonance imaging (MRI) in the evaluation of the mediastinum and hilum has been limited. The reasons for this are complex reflecting limitations in availability and cost, as well as the proven effectiveness of computed tomography (CT) to adequately assess most mediastinal and hilar abnormalities Nonetheless MRI has certain inherent properties that in many ways make it an ideal imaging modality to evaluate both the mediastinum and the hilum. In the first place, compared with CT, MRI offers significantly greater contrast resolution allowing differentiation between blood vessels and soft tissue masses without the need for administration of intravenous contrast medium (Fig. 1) [1-7]. Because it is sensitive to flow, MRI also has the potential to quantitate blood flow directly, and may be used to assess virtually all intra thoracic vascular pathology [8-13].

Secondly, MRI does not use ionizing radiation, a significant advantage in the paediatric population, as well as in cases requiring close repetitive monitoring, including patients following repair of aortic aneurysms, for example or patients with documented thoracic malignancies following therapy [1,14,15].

Thirdly, unlike CT, MRI scans can be obtained in virtually and plane allowing enhanced visualization of areas that often prove difficult to evaluate in cross-section, such as the aorticopulmonary

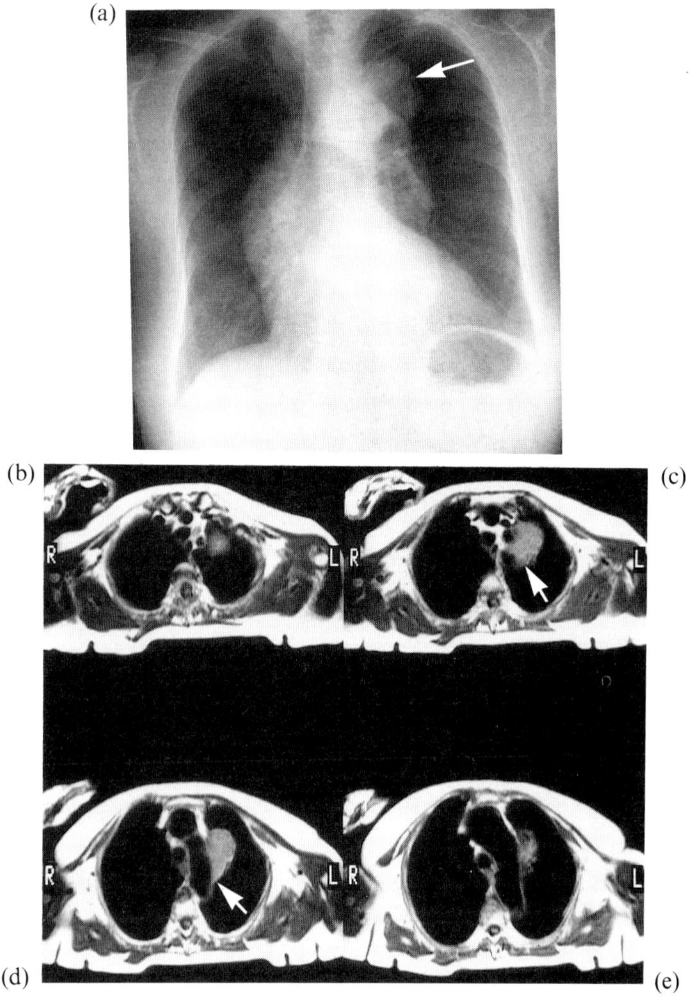

Figure 1. *(a) Postero-anterior radiograph shows marked tortuosity of the aorta. A soft tissue mass can be identified adjacent to the arch (arrow). Differentiation between an aneurysm and a lung mass is difficult. (b) - (e) Sequential T1-weighted axial MRI images clearly demonstrate the presence of a lung tumour in the left upper lobe abutting the mediastinum, arrows in (c) and (d). In the case, determination of mediastinal invasion is difficult.*

window (Fig. 2) [16-18]. Use of parasagittal images is especially valuable when assessing direct tumour invasion into the mediastinum.

Finally by differentiating between tissues with high versus low water content, MRI has the potential to specifically identify fluid-filled cysts and fat (Fig. 3) [5,6,19-21]. In select cases, MRI has the capability to differentiate fibrous tissue from tumour and/or inflammation [22]. This has proven especially valuable in assessing the response of patients with lymphoma to therapy [23-25].

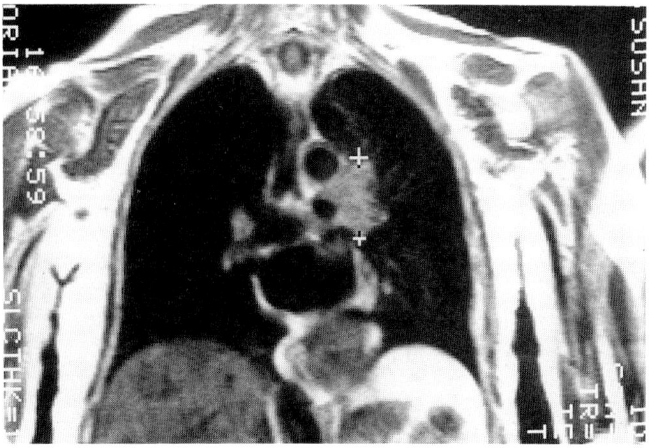

Figure 2. *MEDIASTINAL TUMOUR INVASION: MRI EVALUATION. T1-weighted, coronal MRI scan shows tumour in the left upper lobe with direct extension into the aorticopulmonary window (between crosshairs). Evaluation of mediastinal invasion is frequently made easier by use of parasagittal images.*

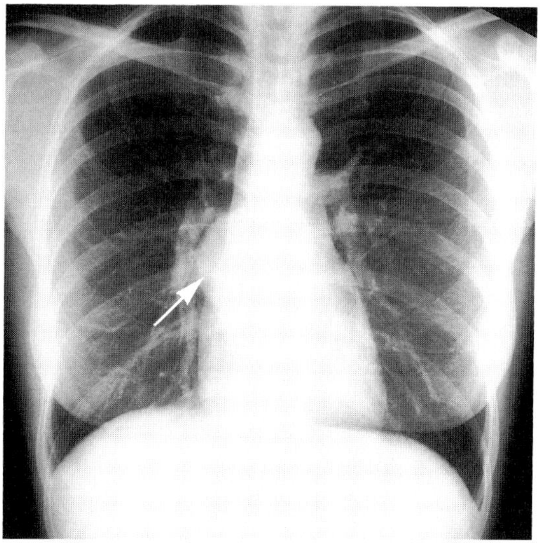

(a)

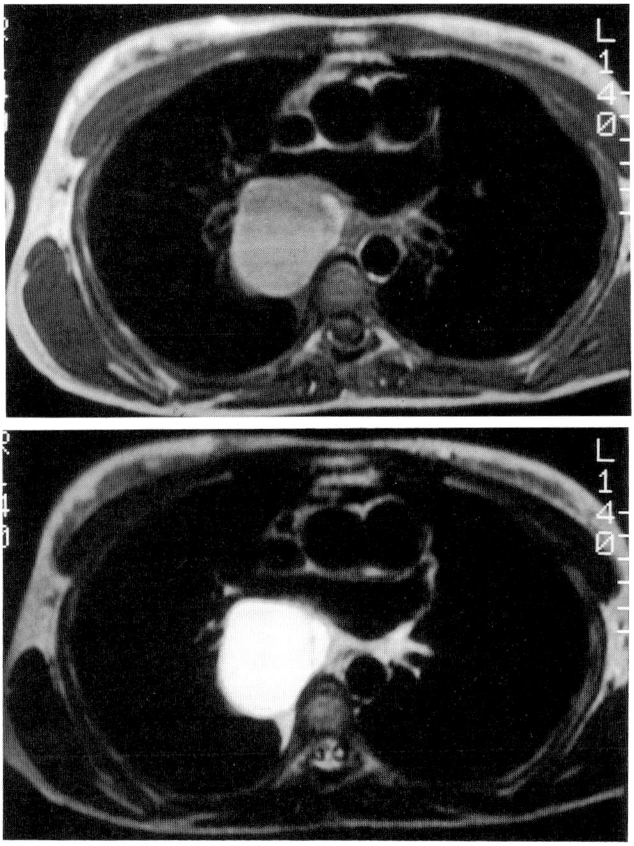

(a)

(b)

Figure 3. *BRONCHOGENIC CYST: MRI EVALUATION. (a) Postero-anterior radiography shows the presence of a smooth subcarinal mass (arrow). (b and c) T1 and T2-weighted axial images respectively confirm the presence of well-defined right hilar and subcarinal mass. Note that with T2-weighting the mass has a very high signal intensity, considerably greater than fat, indicative that this is a fluid-filled lesion. Intermediate signal intensity noted on the T1-weighted scan is due to the presence of an elevated protein content within this surgically-documented bronchogenic cyst.*

In our experience, MRI has functioned primarily as a problem solving device, especially for those cases in which CT cannot be performed, or is suboptimal [23,24]. The advantages and limitations of this technique, as well as current and potential indications for its use are the subject of this chapter.

Basic Principles and Technique

A complete review of the basic principles underlying MRI image formation is well beyond the scope of this chapter; this material has been covered in detail by others [1,4,5,7].

There is no standard MRI examination of the thorax: whenever possible, each case should be individualized. A significant exception is the use of cardiac gating, which should be utilized whenever possible to minimize image degradation due to motion artefacts. The choice of which pulse sequence(s) to utilize depends on the specific clinical problem(s) to be addressed. As a rule, an initial sequence of cardiac gated, SE T1-weighted axial sections are obtained in most patients through pre-selected regions of interest; only rarely is it necessary to obtain images throughout the entire thorax. This is because most pathological processes within the mediastinum result in regions of intermediate signal intensity which generally are easiest to identify when set against the bright signal background caused by mediastinal fat (Fig. 4). With gating, the effective TR is set by the heart rate. There is no indication for the routine use of coronal and/or parasagittal images; in our experience, these are generally best reserved for specific indications, such as analyzing the aorticopulmonary window, or the subcarinal space (Fig. 2) [16-18]. Coronal and/or parasagittal images may also be of value in assessing mediastinal invasion by lung tumours.

T2-weighted images are reserved specifically for those cases for which tissue characterization is required. These may be acquired either utilizing a prolonged TR (2000 ms) without cardiac gating, or preferentially utilizing cardiac gating (especially if the region of interest is adjacent to or involves the hila) with images obtained every second or third cardiac cycle (Fig. 3). In select cases, for example, evaluating mediastinal vessels to identify aneurysms or exclude thrombosis, gradient-refocused sequences with breath-holding can be employed to reduce scan time and optimize visualization of vascular pathology (Fig. 5) [29,39]. Recent interest has also focused on the use of short T1 inversion recovery (STIR) images to produce fat suppression and provide additive T1 and T2 effects to enhance the appearance of the lesion [30]. Although of interest, indications for routine use of these sequences has still to be established.

The role of Gadolinium-diethylenetriamine penta-acetic acid (Gd-DTPA) to evaluate thoracic lesions is also still under investigation.

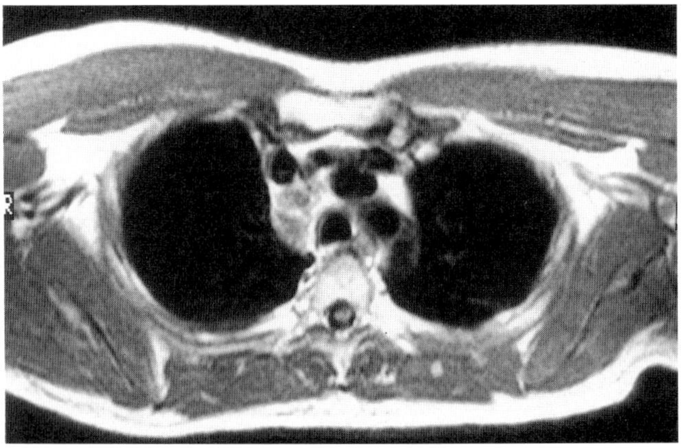

Figure 4. *MEDIASTINAL LYMPHADENOPATHY: MRI EVALUATION. T1-weighted axial section through the great vessels. Enlarged, discrete paratracheal lymph nodes can be identified as masses of intermediate signal intensity set off against high signal caused by mediastinal fat. In general, most mediastinal masses are easier to identify using T1-weighted images.*

Although Gd-DTPA has been used extensively to evaluate the central nervous system and spine, little attention has been paid to the potential use of this agent to evaluate mediastinal or hilar masses [31,32]. In doses of 0.1 mmol/kg administered intravenously, this paramagnetic contrast agent has the effect to shortening both T1 and T2 relaxation times of all perfused or vascularized tissues, including tumours. As a consequence, Gd-DTPA may be of value for assessing complex mediastinal or hilar masses, especially when these are associated with atelectasis in order to differentiate between central obstructing lesions and peripheral drowned lung.

Vascular Pathology

The ability of MRI to identify vascular pathology, both acquired and congenital, has been extensively documented [9-15]. Although this subject is considered in detail elsewhere in this volume, it cannot be over-emphasized that one of the most important indications for the use of MRI in the thorax is to differentiate vascular lesions, especially aneurysms, from mediastinal tumours or enlarged lymph nodes [33].

In older children and young adults in whom two-dimensional echocardiography is more difficult to perform, MRI has proven

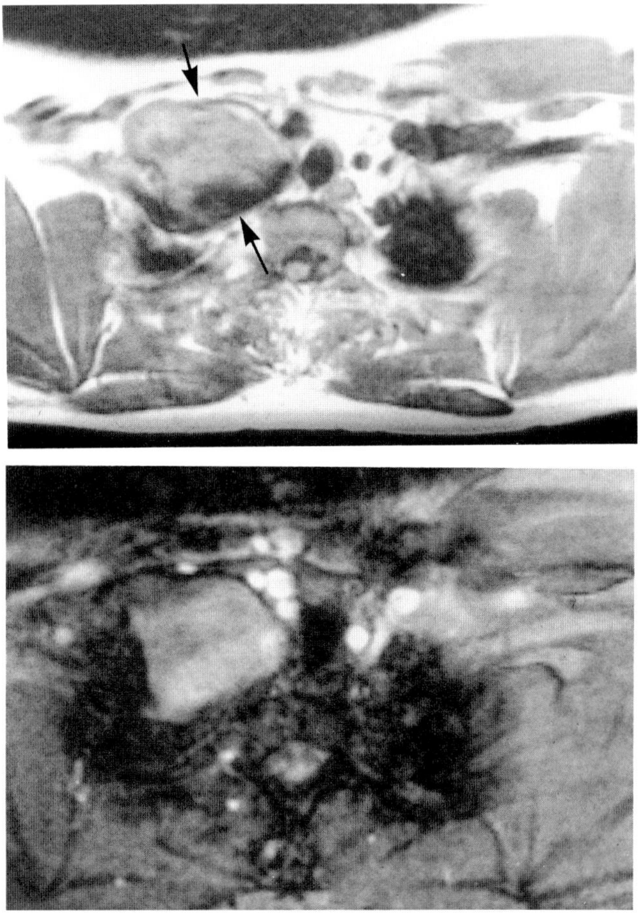

(a)

(b)

Figure 5. *SUBCLAVIAN ARTERY ANEURYSM: EVALUATION WITH GRADIENT-REFOCUSED ECHOES. (a) Axial T1-weighted MRI scan through the lung apex in a patient with a pulsatile right-sided neck mass shows a large, heterogeneous lesion (arrows) consistent with a subclavian artery aneurysm. Heterogeneous signal within suggested the possibility of thrombosis. (b) Section obtained at the same level using gradient-refocused echoes. Note that signal is present throughout the lesion, confirming free flow within the aneurysm. Gradient-refocused sequences are extremely flow sensitive and consequently are especially suited to evaluation of mediastinal vascular pathology. Case courtesy of Dr Elias Zerhouni, Baltimore, MD.*

particularly valuable in the diagnosis of anomalies of both the aortic arch and great vessels, including the pulmonary arteries [34-37]. Fletcher et al in a study of 19 patients suspected of having anomalies of the aorta or pulmonary arteries, found that in 11 patients, MRI demonstrated lesions that echocardiography either failed to visualize or were interpreted as non-diagnostic [34]. MRI has also proven useful in the evaluation of coarctation of the aorta, both pre- and post-repair [1,14,38]. Pre-operatively, MRI has been shown to be comparable to angiography and more accurate than two-dimensional echocardiography both for accurate display of aortic anatomy, as well as delineation of enlarged collateral vessels, the appearance of which may be mistaken for mediastinal masses on plain radiography.

Aortic aneurysms are particularly easy to identify with MRI. This is the result of the signal void characteristically produced by rapidly flowing blood [9-11,33]. Organized thrombi typically can be identified as areas of intermediate signal intensity, and usually are easily distinguishable from flowing blood within the residual aortic lumen [8]. Most important, MRI clearly demonstrates the relationship between aneurysms and surrounding mediastinal structures (Fig. 1).

MRI criteria for the diagnosis of aortic dissection are similar to those that have been defined for CT [9-11,40-42]. Most important is the detection of intimal flaps. These are identifiable as linear structures of intermediate signal intensity separating the true from the false lumen. In most series, CT an MRI have proven roughly comparable both in identifying as well as excluding aortic dissection. In fact, the sensitivity of MRI in detecting aortic dissection has been reported to be as high as 96%, provided considerable interpreter experience in accurately identifying flow-related signal changes and/or artefacts within the aorta [41].

MRI has proven extremely effective for evaluating mediastinal veins. Venous obstruction due to a variety of causes, both benign and neoplastic, are all easily detected with MRI [12,13,27,29]. In the setting of possible vena caval obstruction, multi planar image acquisition can be of particular value for differentiating between intrinsic and extrinsic causes of vena caval obstruction. Recently, attention has been paid to the use of MRI to establish the patency of mediastinal veins in the thoracic inlet especially using gradient-recalled pulse sequences [27,29]. Hansen et al, in an evaluation of 31 patients with suspected venous obstruction secondary to tumour invasion, extrinsic compression, coagulopathies and in-dwelling venous catheters found that MRI accurately identified abnormalities in 32 of 34 vessels (94%); there were no false negative studies [29]. MRI proved especially valuable in assessing the jugular veins and the superior vena cava. Similar results have been reported by Templeton et al [27].

Mediastinal Masses

Most mediastinal lesions are easily identified with MRI [1-5,19,20]. MRI has proven especially valuable in delineating the relationship between masses and adjacent vessels, including the pulmonary arteries. Tumour encasement, in particular, is easily assessed, as is the presence of tumour extension into the heart. As will be illustrated, on occasion, MRI may allow precise tissue characterization as well.

Mediastinal Adenopathy

Reports documenting the efficacy of MRI have found this modality to be comparable to CT in most cases, especially for identifying enlarged mediastinal lymph nodes in patients with bronchogenic carcinoma (Fig. 4) [1,4,43-48]. Although MRI is limited by poorer spatial resolution compared with CT, this is more than compensated for by far greater contrast resolution. Identification of mediastinal lymphadenopathy with MRI is enhanced when nodes are embedded in mediastinal fat or lie adjacent to mediastinal or hilar blood vessels. Not infrequently. MRI will disclose the presence of enlarged lymph nodes in locations otherwise difficult to assess with CT, including the region of the aorticopulmonary window, as well as areas such as the tracheo-oesophageal groove. As a consequence, MRI may be advantageous in assessing patients who present with symptoms suggestive of recurrent laryngeal nerve involvement (Fig. 6). Unfortunately, MRI is no more specific than CT in differentiating hyperplastic from malignant lymph nodes [49,50], a clear limitation, especially for routine staging of lung cancer. Furthermore, MRI is unable to detect calcification, making identification of granulomatous diseases more difficult, especially fibrosing mediastinitis (Fig. 7) [51,52].

Lymphoma

It is generally easy to identify intrathoracic pathology in patients with lymphoma using CT. With the development of effective therapies, however, a need has arisen for an accurate means of monitoring

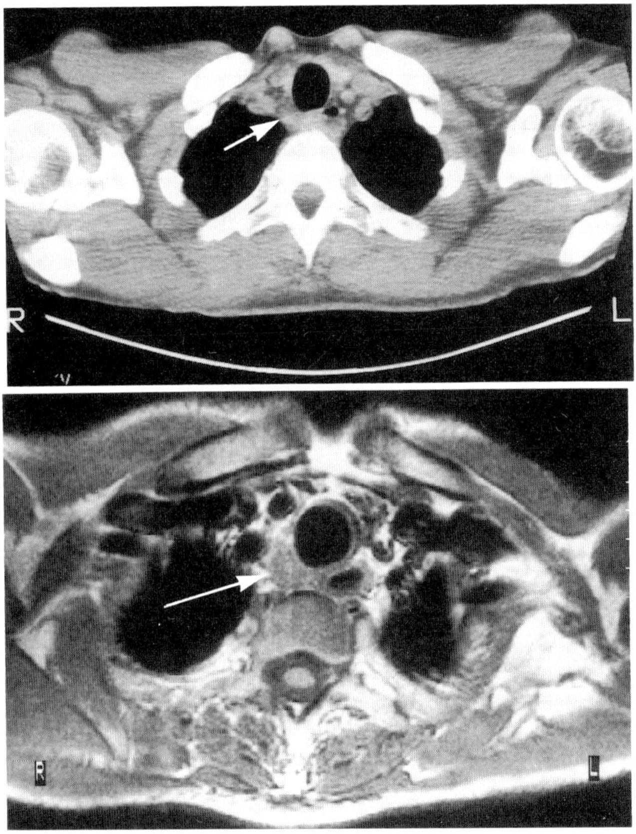

(a)

(b)

Figure 6. *MEDIASTINAL ADENOPATHY: CT/MRI CORRELATION. (a) Contrast-enhanced CT section through the lung apices in a patient with a history suggestive of recurrent laryngeal nerve pathology. There is a suggestion of a subtle soft-tissue density in the region of the tracheo-eosophageal groove (arrow). Prospectively, this abnormality was not identified. (b) T1-weighted axial MRI image at the same level as in (a). A mass of intermediate signal intensity is clearly identifiable (arrow) (compare with (a). In this case, identification of enlarged nodes was considerably easier with MRI.*

treatment response. Although reduction of tumour bulk can be satisfactorily monitored with CT, partial size regression is often observed, especially with Hodgkin's disease. These masses frequently contain residual fibrous tissue with no active lymphomatous component, representing so-called 'sterilized' lymphoma [53]. Unfortunate-

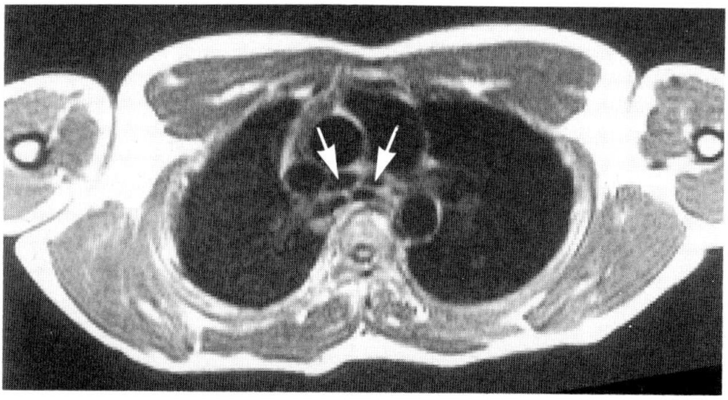

(a)

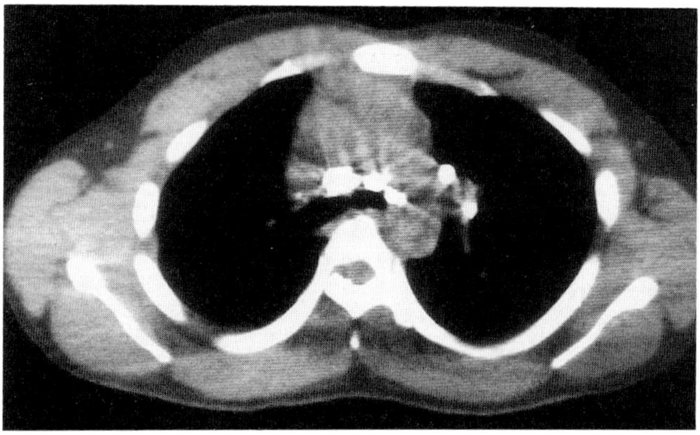

(b)

Figure 7. *MEDIASTINAL ADENOPATHY: CT/MRI CORRELATION. (a) Axial T1-weighted scan through the carina shows discrete low signal pre-carinal masses (arrow). Although suggestive of calcified nodes, this appearance is non-specific. (b) Non-enhanced CT scan at the same level as in (a) confirms the presence of densely-calcified lymph nodes in a patient subsequently proven surgically to have fibrosing mediastinitis. As shown by this case, calcifications are clearly easier to assess with CT. Case courtesy of Dr Jerry Patt, Baltimore, MD.*

ly, in a significant percentage of cases, active residual disease may still be present. Reports have documented this problem in differentiating residual active from inactive disease in nearly 90% of patients with Hodgkin's disease and 40% of patients with non-Hodgkin's lymphoma [54]. Using CT, masses containing active tumour are indistinguishable from residual fibrous tissue, since their densities are identical. Even tissue biopsies may prove non-diagnostic in these cases as marked cytological atypia in itself may result from chemotherapy or radiotherapy.

Preliminary data, while controversial, suggest that MRI can play a significant role in post-therapy tumour evaluation in patients with both Hodgkin's and non-Hodgkin's lymphomas [23,24,55-59]. Theoretically, this is based on the observation that lymphomatous cells contain a larger amount of water, with a relatively lower proportion of proteins, while mature fibrous tissue contains considerably less water by percentage and a high proportion of highly-polymerized proteins. These differences in composition between lymphoma and mature fibrous tissue lead to markedly different T2 relaxation times [59]. Although the number of cases reported to date has been small, it does appear that those lesions that are characterized by homogeneous low signal intensity both on T1 and T2-weighted images usually prove to be inactive (Fig. 8). In fact, whether or not this is actually due to the presence of mature fibrous tissue has yet to be determined. As recently reported by Negendank et al, in an evaluation of 32 patients with non-Hodgkin's lymphomas and 20 with Hodgkin's disease in whom histological correlation was available, lymphomas with dense fibrosis proved to have the brightest signal intensities on T2-weighted scans [58]. As the authors themselves note, the reason for this apparent paradox is unclear: in fact the high signal intensity observed in these cases may be caused by a process other than fibrosis, although no apparent cause could be identified pathologically. Regardless of the explanation, in our experience, the finding of uniform low-signal intensity within residual masses in patients with lymphomas can be interpreted as evidence of inactive disease. In fact, to date this has represented a small proportion of the studies we have performed in this population. It should be emphasized that high signal intensity, *per se*, within residual masses in patients with lymphomas should not be construed as indicative of tumour, as residual inflammation will cause the same appearance.

More recently, it has been suggested that the pattern of signal intensity on T1 and T2-weighted sequences may have predictive value in differentiating between low and high-grade non-Hodgkin's lymphomas. In as study of 50 patients with non-Hodgkin's lymphoma examined with MRI, Rhen et al showed that 63% of nodes in patients with high-grade non-Hodgkin's lymphoma had an inhomogeneous appearance while 90% of nodes in patients with low-grade non-Hodgkin's lymphoma proved to be homogeneous in appearance [56]. Unfortunately, these observations have not been consistently verified. Negendank et al in an evaluation of 32 patients with non-Hodgkin's

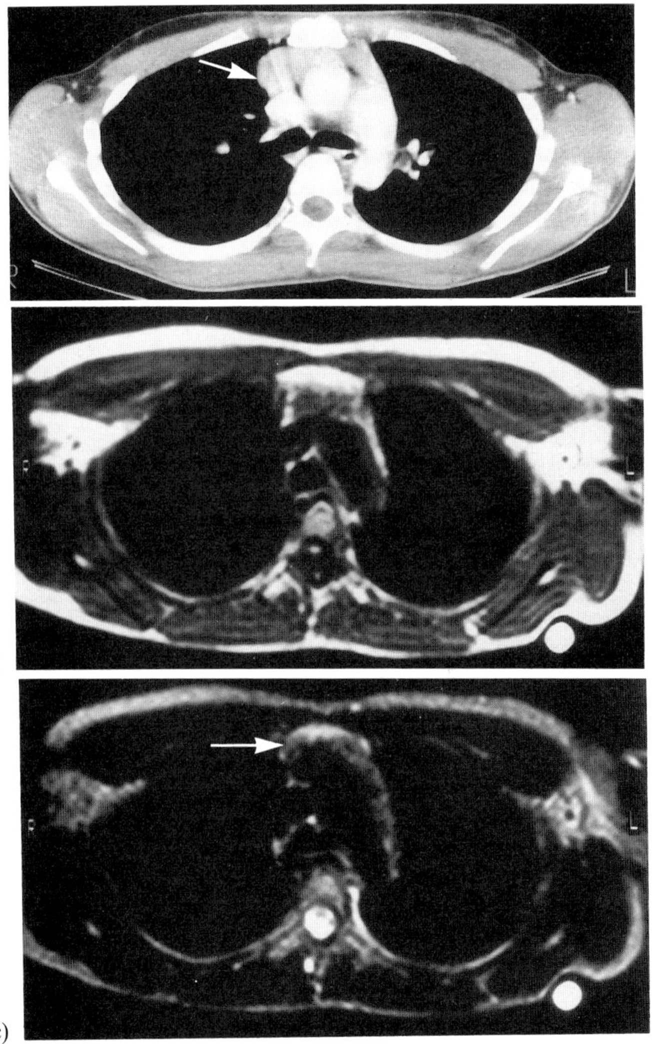
(a)
(b)
(c)

Figure 8. *HODGKIN'S DISEASE: ASSESSMENT OF RESPONSE TO THERAPY. (a) Contrast-enhanced CT shows a residual soft tissue mass within the anterior mediastinum (arrow) in a patient previously treated for Hodgkin's disease. This appearance is non-specific. (b) and (c) Axial T1 and T2-weighted scans, respectively, at the same level as shown in (a). Note that there is very little signal identifiable within the mass on the T2-weighted scan (arrow) consistent with the presence of a residual fibrotic mass. Subsequent follow-up examinations over a year have shown no change in appearance of this lesion.*

lymphoma found that in most cases, these tumours appeared relatively homogeneous both on T1 and T2-weighted scans; furthermore, in this population, low, intermediate and high-grade lymphomas have identical imaging characteristics [58]. It is apparent that the ability of MRI to accurately assess prognosis based on initial signal characteristics using routine spin-echo scans will require further evaluation.

Fatty lesions

Characteristically, well differentiated fat produces high signal intensity of T1-weighted scans. Although similar findings have been described in patients with haematomas or tumour with haemorrhage, in most cases, MRI accurately identifies most fatty lesions (Fig. 9) [6,19,21,60]. In an analysis of 17 patients with documented lipomatous tumours, Dooms et al reported that the fatty components in all except one of these tumours were well visualized with MRI [21]. Similarly, in an evaluation of 15 patients with documented liposarcomas, London et al showed that MRI correctly identified the presence of fat in all eight cases in which it was pathologically present [60]. Unfortunately, although MRI has proven no more accurate than CT in differentiating liposarcomas from benign lipomas, in most cases a presumptive diagnosis of benign lipoma can be made provided that the lesion is well-dcfined and is uniform and homogeneous without discernable internal architecture or septa. Although it might be anticipated that MRI would prove efficacious in diagnosing dermoid tumours and teratomas, especially those in which fat is demonstrable, experience with these tumours, in fact, is limited.

Mediastinal Cysts

MRI has been used successfully to diagnose a wide range of benign cystic lesions, including bronchogenic cysts, pericardial cysts, thymic cysts, colloid cysts within goitres, cystic hygromas and even mediastinal pseudocysts [1,5,6,19,20]. MRI is especially valuable in assessing complex cysts that do not appear fluid-filled on CT, especially when intravenous contrast cannot be administered (Fig. 3) [20]. Variable patterns of signal intensity can occur within cystic masses on T1-weighted sequences, presumably due to protein or haemorrhage within cysts; however, on T2-weighted sequences, considerable signal intensity almost invariably can be recognized [6]. MRI may also prove valuable by identifying solid components within the walls of

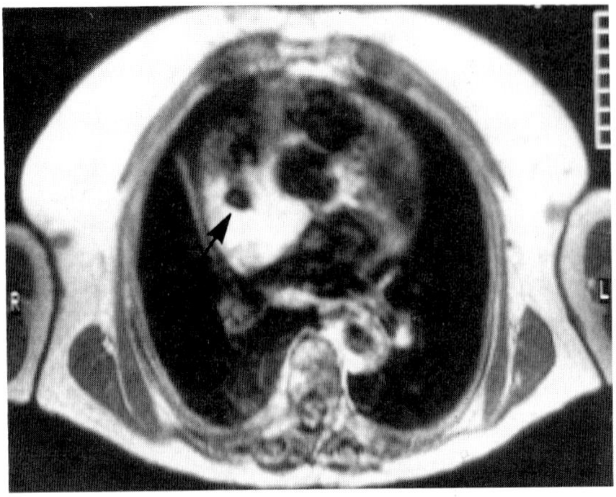

(a)

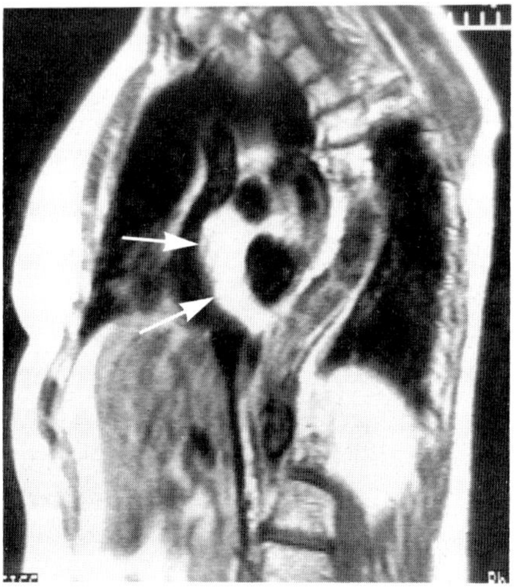

(b)

Figure 9. *INTRA-ATRIAL LIPOMATOSIS: MRI DIAGNOSIS. (a) and (b) T1-weighted axial and sagittal images, respectively, show the presence of a high signal intensity mass surrounding the superior vena cava (arrows in (a)), and extending inferiorly along the plane of the interatrial septum (arrows in (b)). Note that the signal intensity within the lesion is the same as subcutaneous fat. This appearance is characteristic of intra-atrial lipomatosis, and should not be confused with a primary cardiac or mediastinal tumour.*

lesions, suggesting possible malignancy. Identifications of intraparenchymal cystic or fluid-filled masses in association with anomalous vessels also has proven valuable in the diagnosis of pulmonary sequestration [20].

Thymus

To date, the role of MRI in the evaluation of the thymus has proven extremely limited. Characteristically, the thymus appears homogeneous, with intermediate signal intensity of both T1 and T2-weighted images (Fig. 10) [61-66]. Not surprisingly, the appearance of the thymus gland depends on the patient's age. Under 30 years of age, differentiation between the thymus and adjacent mediastinal fat is somewhat easier than in older patients; presumably identification of the thymus becomes more difficult with age secondary to progressive fatty replacement of the gland, rendering it the same density as adjacent mediastinal fat [62]. Occasionally, the signal intensity

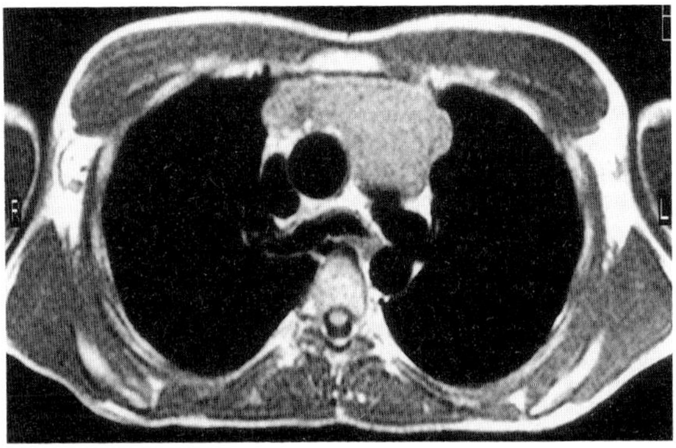
(a)

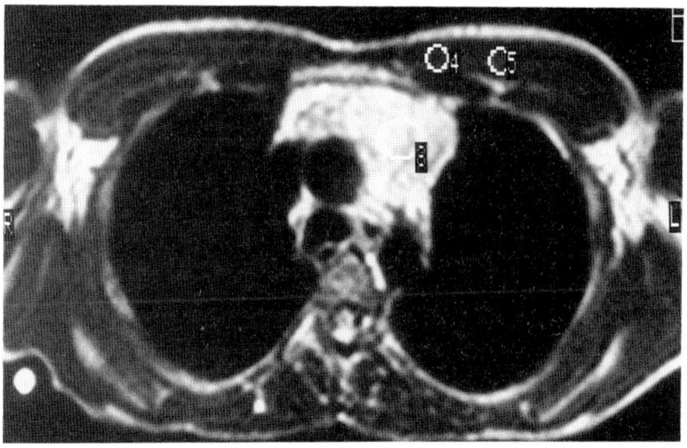
(b)

Figure 10. *THYMOMA. (a) and (b) T1- and T2-weighted axial images, respectively. A lobular anterior mediastinal mass is easily identifiable characterized by homogeneous signal intensity on both T1- and T2-weighted images. This appearance is entirely non-specific. Surgically confirmed non-invasive thymoma.*

characteristics of normal thymic tissue may be of value in identifying unusual configurations of the thymus, especially in children in whom posterior mediastinal extension between the superior vena cava and trachea is not uncommon [63]. MRI signal characteristics have also been reported of value in diagnosing a patient with a mediastinal thymolipoma which not surprisingly appeared as a fatty thymic tumour [64].

MRI evaluation of the thymus in patients with myasthenia gravis has been described; to date, the role of MRI in these patients has proven extremely limited. In a study of 16 patients with myasthenia gravis studied with both CT and MRI subsequently evaluated surgically, MRI provided little distinctive information [65]. In seven patients with histological evidence of thymic hyperplasia both CT and MRI displayed normal thymic morphology in five patients, and an enlarged and small thymus in one case each, respectively. Again, MRI signal intensities were of no value in differentiating thymic hyperplasia from normal glands. In our experience an important exception has been the use of MRI to evaluate patients with invasive thymomas, particularly those in whom vascular invasion is suspected when there is a contra-indication to the use of intravenous contrast media. In these cases, MRI can provide accurate delineation of the true extent of tumour, including identification of intracardiac extension of disease, findings that may significantly alter surgical approaches to therapy.

Thyroid

MRI has been shown to be a sensitive means for morphologically delineating the extent of the thyroid gland [1,5,19,67-75]. In addition, MRI allows precise delineation of associated abnormalities including the presence of cervical and/or mediastinal adenopathy, displacement of mediastinal organs such as the oesophagus, trachea, and great vessels, as well as loss of normal cervical and intrathoracic facial planes [67-75]. Unfortunately, MRI has proven to be of only limited value as a means for tissue characterization.

On T1-weighted images, the signal intensity within the normal thyroid gland is equal to or slightly greater than the adjacent sternocleidomastoid muscle. Signal intensity increases on T2-weighted scans [70,73,75], although not to the extent of most focal pathological processes, including adenomas, cysts and cancer which are easily identified on T2-weighted sequences because of their markedly prolonged T2 values. One exception appears to be functioning thyroid nodules, which have been reported to be iso-intense with normal thyroid tissue on both T1 and T2-weighted scans [72]. Multinodular goitres have been shown to be relatively hypo-intense as compared with normal thyroid tissue on T1-weighted images, except when there are foci of either haemorrhage or cysts, in which case focal areas of high signal intensity may be visualized. On T2-weighted images, multinodular goitres are typically heterogeneous, with high signal intensity noted throughout most of the gland (Fig. 11) [69-73]. Although it has been suggested that benign adenomas can be differentiated from follicular carcinomas based on the presence of an intact pseudocapsule surrounding adenomas, this finding has been insufficiently documented [73,74]; in most series, MRI has proven no more specific histologically than CT [66,70-72,75]. MRI has also proven of value in assessing postoperative patients [72,76-76]. Auffermann et al, in a series of 24 patients with primary thyroid carcinoma evaluated postoperatively found that MRI correctly diagnosed or excluded disease in 20 patients (83%); however, in this same series, MRI led to both false positive (n = 1) and false negative (n = 3) diagnoses, limiting its value [76].

Parathyroid Disease

Reports of the accuracy of MRI in evaluating parathyroid disease show that this modality is comparable to other non-invasive techniques for detecting parathyroid pathology [79-83]. The appearance of abnormal parathyroid glands on MRI has been well documented [5,19,68,69,75,79-83]. Similar to thyroid adenomas, most parathyroid adenomas show a marked increase in signal intensity on T2-weighted images; however, these findings also have been documented for parathyroid hyperplasia and carcinomas. In a small but significant percentage of cases, parathyroid adenomas fail to exhibit increased signal intensity. As documented by Auffermann et al, in a study of 30 patients with recurrent hyperparathyroidism, 13% of the abnormal glands failed to display high intensity on T2-weighted images [63]. Spritzer et al, using both T1- and T2-weighted scans to evaluate 23 patients with suspected disease reported an overall sensitivity of 76% and a specificity of 95% with a resulting overall accuracy of 90% [82]. Kneeland et al, evaluating 22 patients with hyperparathyroidism reported a sensitivity and specificity of MRI imaging of 74% and 66%, respectively [80]. As a consequence, following initial evaluation

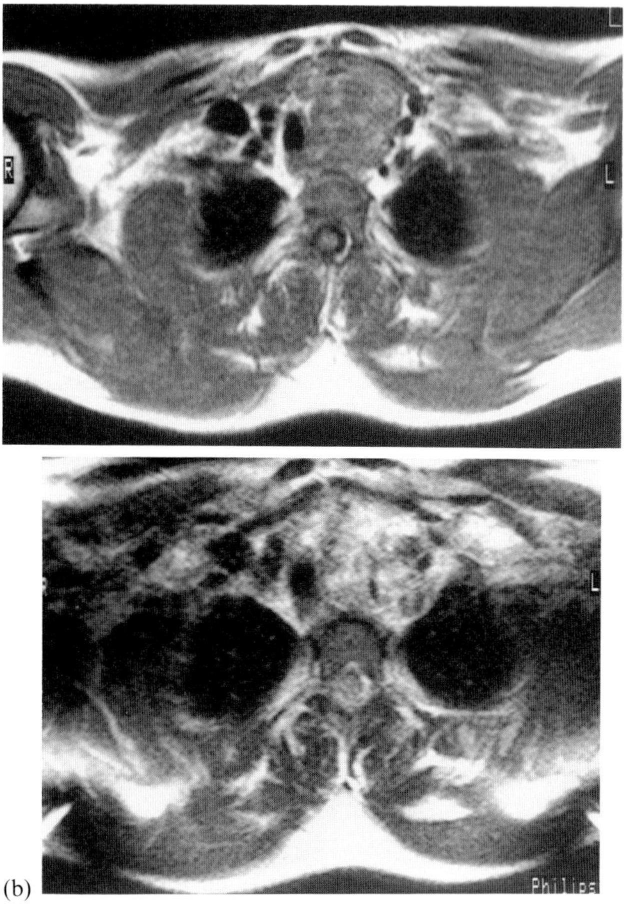

(a)

(b)

Figure 11. *MULTINODULAR GOITRE. MRI EVALUATION. (a) T1-weighted MRI image through the thoracic inlet shows typical appearance of a multinodular substernal goitre. Note that thyroid tissue is easily separable from adjacent mediastinal fat and vessels, displacing the trachea to the right. (b) T2 weighted MRI image obtained at a slightly higher level than in (a). There is considerable increase in signal within the goitre which appears markedly heterogeneous. On T2-weighted images, multinodular goitres are typically heterogeneous, with high-signal intensity identifiable throughout the gland. Reprinted with permission from ref. 25.*

with thallium scintigraphy, it can be recommended that MRI replace CT in the investigation of patients with recurrent hyperparathyroidism following surgery. CT is best reserved for those patients with suspected recurrent parathyroid carcinoma, especially to evaluate the lungs and the liver to rule out metastatic disease.

Paraspinal Pathology

MRI has several distinct advantages over other standard imaging modalities for imaging neurogenic tumours. MRI is most helpful in assessing intraspinal extension, as well as the presence and extent of associated spinal cord pathology. In this context, the ability of obtain multiplanar images is especially valuable as many of these tumours demonstrate longitudinal extension into structures along the axis of the spine (Fig. 12). As a consequence, MRI has essentially replaced CT as an initial imaging modality for the evaluation of patients with posterior mediastinal masses.

Typically, neurogenic tumours, both benign and malignant, have slightly greater signal intensity than muscle on T1-weighted images, and markedly increased signal intensity on T2-weighted images [84-87]. Unfortunately, MRI has proven no more specific than CT in differentiating benign from malignant lesions, necessitating histological evaluation in cases in which malignancy is suspected [87].

MRI of the Pulmonary Hila

Hilar Masses/Adenopathy

Numerous studies have compared the efficacy of CT with MRI in evaluating the pulmonary hila, especially in patients with bronchogenic carcinoma. These have consistently documented the two modalities to be essentially equivalent [43,44,46,49,88].

Musset et al in an analysis of 44 patients with bronchogenic carcinoma in whom tumour extent and nodal disease were prospectively evaluated, found no statistical difference between contrast-enhanced CT and MRI [44]. Glazer et al, in a prospective study comparing 55° oblique tomography, dynamic contrast-enhanced CT and MRI for evaluating the pulmonary hila in 19 patients with lung cancer in whom surgical confirmation was available, found no significant differences in the overall accuracy of these modalities [46]. It should be emphasized that while CT and MRI proved significantly more accurate than conventional 55° tomography, CT and MRI both proved to have relatively low specificity due to detection of

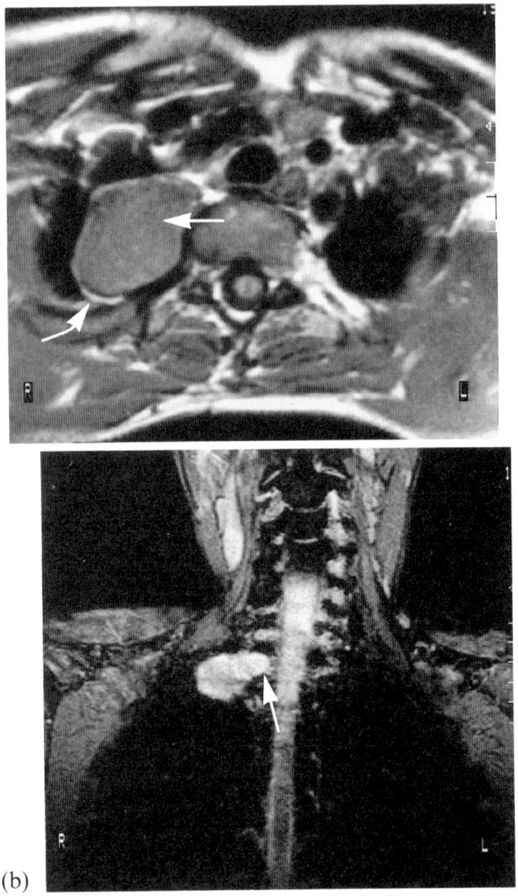

(a)

(b)

Figure 12. *NEUROGENIC TUMOUR: MRI ASSESSMENT. (a) T1-weighted axial section through the lung apices shows a well-defined mass of intermediate signal intensity adjacent to the spine (arrow). Note the presence of a thin rim of fat surrounding this lesion (curved arrow) confirming that it is extrapleural in location. (b) Coronal MRI image obtained using a gradient-recalled echo sequence shows the lesion is clearly extending into the neural foramina (arrow). Presumed neurofibroma, unchanged over several years observation. Reprinted with permission from ref. 25.*

minimally enlarged nodes that subsequently were proved surgically benign.

An important limitation of MRI compared with CT is that MRI cannot detect calcification, obviously limiting nodal evaluation

(Fig. 7). Furthermore, MRI is considerably less valuable than CT for identifying bronchial pathology (Fig. 13) [89]. In an evaluation of 29 patients suspected of having an endobronchial mass evaluated with both CT and MRI, Mayr et al, found that MRI could identify only 70% of pathologically confirmed abnormal airways, and only 45% of normal airways compared with near 100% accuracy with CT.

On routine cardiac gated, spin-echo scans most abnormalities within the hila are easily identifiable as foci of intermediate signal intensity, easily separable from normal hilar vessels and adjacent lung which are normally characterized by signal void may be seen at numerous levels in the normal hila: however, this rarely causes confusion diagnostically. Typically, signal that is present within normal hila rarely measures greater than approximately 1 cm in size, and presumably is due to normal-sized hilar lymph nodes. Partial volume artefacts resulting from small quantities of fat within the hilum also undoubtedly contribute, as well. Typically, abnormal nodes measure at least 1.5 cm in size, simplifying their identification. It should be emphasized that signal also may be present within normal hilar vessels, depending on the phase of the cardiac cycle at which images were acquired. This appearance rarely is a source of confusion.

Atelectasis

MRI may be of value in the assessment of patients with pulmonary atelectasis, especially to differentiate between central tumour an collapsed lung (Fig. 14) [4,45,90-93]. In a retrospective study of 18 patients with proximal bronchogenic carcinoma and postobstructive lobar collapse evaluated both with contrast-enhanced dynamic CT and MRI utilizing T2-weighted sequences, Tobler et al showed that differences between the signal intensity of tumour and the signal intensity of peripheral, collapsed lung could be identified in only five (50%) of 10 patients, while dynamic CT differentiated tumour from collapsed lung in eight (80%) of ten patients [92]. Of 18 patients evaluated with T1-weighted sequences, MRI accurately differentiated tumour from collapse in only one patient (5%). Despite these apparent differences, the authors concluded that there was no significant statistical difference between the two modalities. More recently, Herold et al have showed that MRI may be of value in differentiating between obstructive and non-obstructive atelectasis. Evaluated with T2-weighted sequences, the collapsed lung appeared hypo-intense,

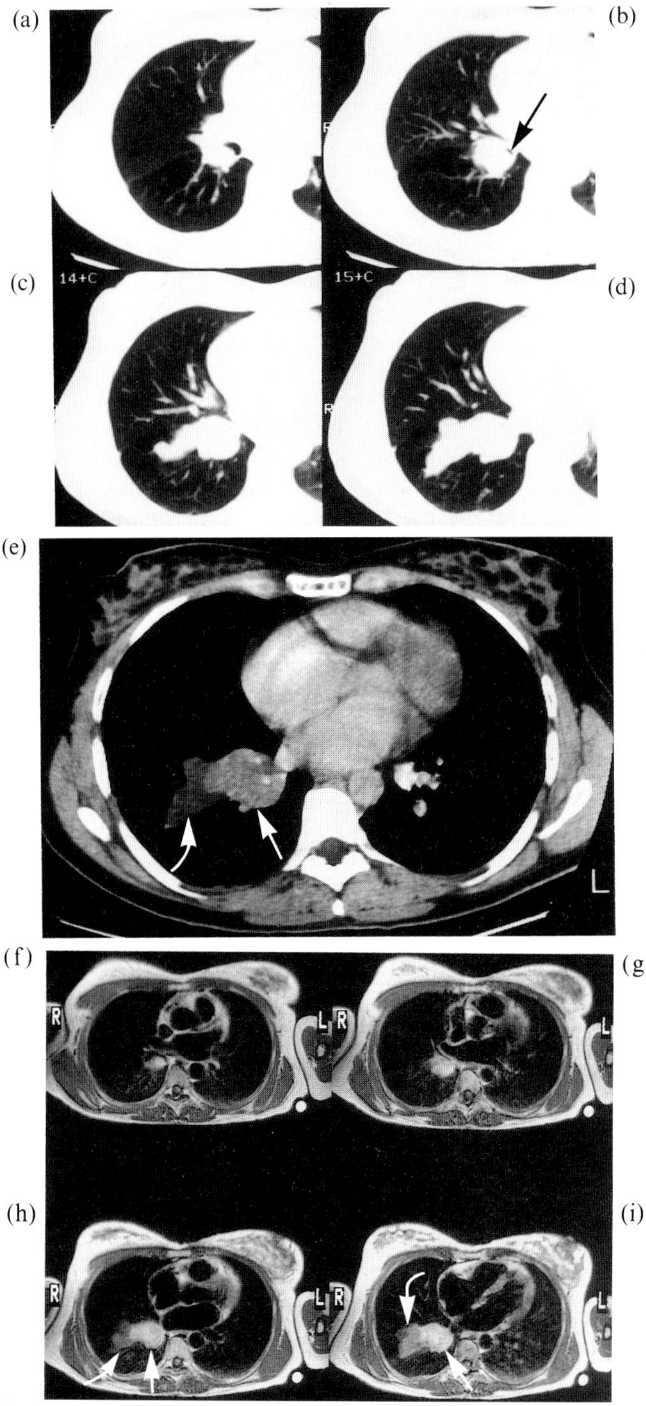
(a)
(b)
(c)
14+C
15+C
(d)
(e)
L
(f)
(g)
(h)
(i)
R
L

whereas atelectatic lung in all 17 patients with obstructive atelectasis appeared hyperintense. These authors postulated that low signal in non-obstructed lungs presumably reflected residual microscopic air causing magnetic susceptibility effects, unlike obstructed lungs in which there is a greater quantity of retained secretions.

These observations, while of interest, will require further investigation to be verified. Given the diversity of pathological changes found within tumour and collapsed lung, it may be anticipated that there will be considerable variation in the MRI appearance of atelectatic lungs. As documented by Burke and Fraser, in an evaluation of 50 consecutive patients undergoing pulmonary resection due to central, obstructing tumour, a wide spectrum of histological changes can be identified [94]. These range from initial accumulation of eosinophilic proteinaceous material within air-spaces, to the subsequent aggregation of lipid-laden macrophages and progressive lymphocytic infiltration and collagen deposition within the pulmonary interstitium (so-called lipid pneumonia), and finally, to the development of interstitial fibrosis. These factors clearly have implications for the potential role of both contrast-enhanced CT, and especially MRI for evaluating patients with pulmonary atelectasis. Interestingly, it has been shown that when tumour: fat and collapsed lung: fat MRI signal intensity ratios are calculated utilizing T2-weighted sequences, tumour could be differentiated from collapsed lung only in patients with collapsed lung: fat ratios greater than one. These preliminary findings suggest that MRI may be most useful in the subacute stage of collapse, in which lipid-laden macrophages are most conspicuous [92].

Figure 13. *CARCINOID TUMOUR: CT/MRI CORRELATION. (a) - (d) Enlargements of sequential CT sections through the right hilum imaged with wide (lung) windows show a mass obstructing the right lower lobe bronchus (arrow in b). (e) Contrast-enhanced CT scan shows that there is a mass in the right hilum inferiorly (arrow). Note the presence peripherally of obstructed branching, fluid-filled lower lobe bronchi (curved arrow). This constellation of findings is characteristic of a central carcinoid tumour, subsequently verified surgically. (f) - (i) Sequential axial MRI scans at the same levels as shown in (a) - (d), following injection of Gd-DTPA. A well-defined homogeneously enhancing hilar mass is easily identified (arrows in h and i). Dilated, fluid-filled bronchi are also easily identified peripherally (curved arrow in h and i) (compare with e). Note that although the mass is easily identified with MRI visualization of central bronchi is limited as compared with CT (compare with a - d).*

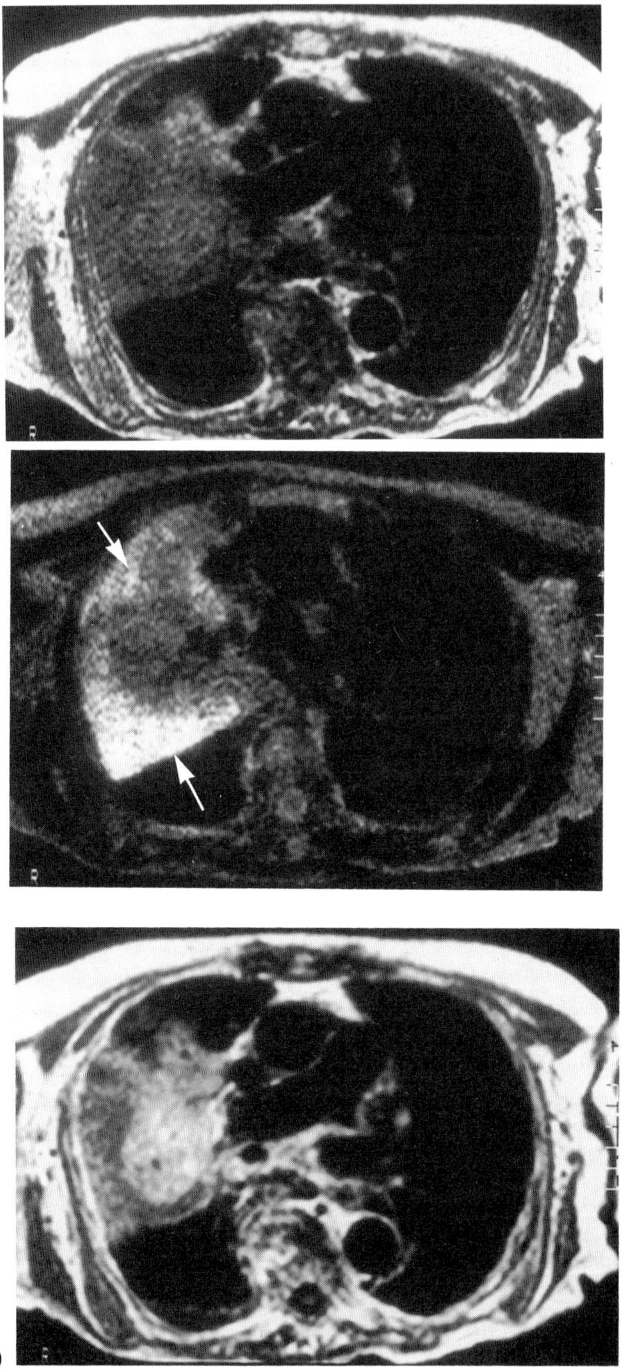

(a)

(b)

(c)

(d) (e)

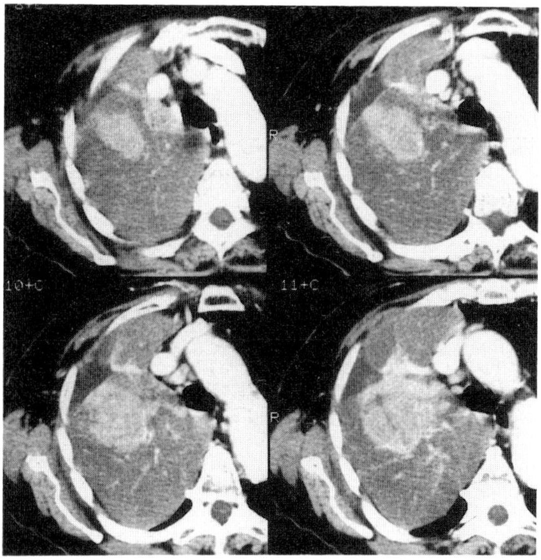

(f) (g)

Figure 14. *LOBAR ATELECTASIS: CT/MRI CORRELATIONS. (a) Axial T1-weighted MRI scan shows diffuse increased signal throughout the right lung. Differentiation between central tumour and peripheral lung is impossible. (b) T2-weighted scan at the same level as shown in (a). A low signal intensity central tumour mass can now be identified distinct from the high signal generated by fluid within collapsed, so-called, 'drowned' atelectatic lung (arrows). (c) T1-weighted scan obtained at the same level as shown in (a) and (b), following injection of Gd-DTPA. As compared with non-contrast enhanced images, central tumour is now identifiable as a mass of high signal intensity as compared with the lower signal generated by the peripheral collapsed lung (compare with a and b). This is because the mass is relatively well-vascularized as compared with the surrounding lung. (d) - (g) Enlargements of sequential contrast-enhanced CT scans at the same level as shown in (a), (b) and (c). In this case, tumour can be identified as a focal area of increased density, surrounded by low density within the fluid-filled, collapsed right upper lobe. These findings are identical to those seen with MRI. Reprinted with permission from ref. 26.*

It should be noted that the use of Gd-DTPA may obviate the need for T2-weighted sequences (Fig. 14). It has been shown that Gd-DTPA causes an immediate increase in the signal intensity of vascularized tumours, emphasizing their inhomogeneous structure [31,32]. Although collapsed lung also demonstrates signal enhancement, this is usually significantly less compared with tumour enhancement. Preliminary experience suggests that Gd-DTPA may ultimately prove to be the most efficacious manner to evaluate central obstructing tumours associated with pulmonary atelectasis.

Pulmonary Vascular Disease

The major indication for the use of MRI to evaluate the pulmonary hila is to differentiate between enlarged hilar nodes and/or hilar masses and enlarged or prominent pulmonary arteries. A wide variety of pathological changes within the pulmonary arteries can be identified with MRI, including identifying patients with pulmonary hypertension, with and without central pulmonary emboli [95-97]. In this setting, MRI has several inherent advantages compared with CT, including non-invasive evaluation of pulmonary blood flow, as well as simultaneous assessment of right ventricular function and morphology. In a retrospective study of 25 patients with documented pulmonary artery hypertension, with and without superimposed pulmonary emboli, Bouchard et al showed that the presence of intraluminal signal during systole correlated well with moderate to severe grades of pulmonary hypertension, identifiable in all patients with systolic pressures greater than 80 mmHg [95]. However, in patients with moderately severe degrees of pulmonary hypertension, including those with pressure between 65 and 80 mmHg, MRI proved positive in only three of five (60%) cases. MRI proved equality insensitive when mean pulmonary artery pressures were evaluated.

MRI can be used to measure right ventricular wall thickness, and paradoxical septal motion by assessing interventricular septal curvature; it is unlikely, however, that these measurements will prove of routine value in the detection of patients with early or mild pulmonary hypertension. MRI may be of considerable additional value in the identification of patients whose pulmonary hypertension secondary to intracardiac pathology.

In addition to identifying changes secondary to pulmonary hypertension, MRI may also be of value in establishing the presence of central pulmonary emboli (Fig. 15) [98-101]. Gamsu et al showed

Figure 15. *CENTRAL PULMONARY EMBOLI: CT/MRI CORRELATION. (a) and (b) Enlargements of sequential contrast-enhanced CT scans through the left hilum show a discrete filling defect within the left interlobar pulmonary artery (arrows). (c) and (d) T1-weighted axial scans at the same approximate levels as shown in (a) and (b), respectively, also show the presence of focal signal within the left interlobar pulmonary artery (arrows). Emboli subsequently confirmed angiographically (not shown).*

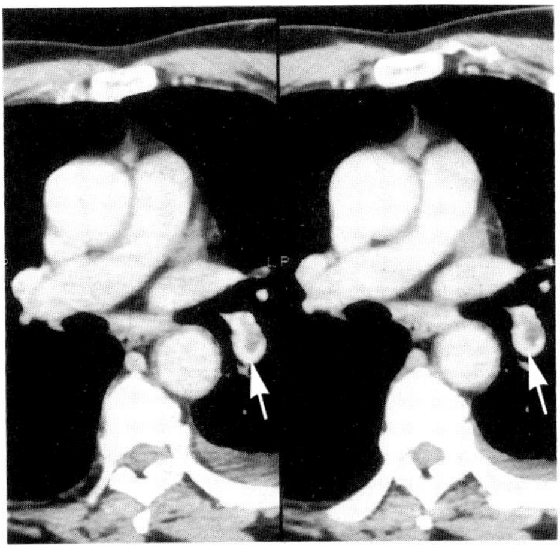

(a) (b)

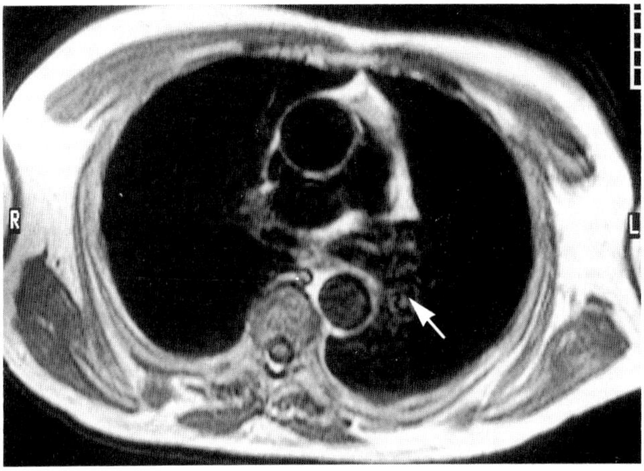

(c)

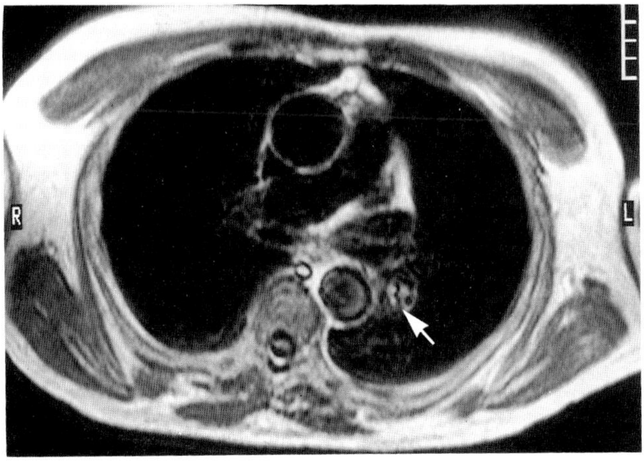

(d)

that pulmonary emboli labelled with non-magnetic barium threads could be identified with MRI in 12 of 19 sites (63 %) documented to have emboli by corresponding CT scans [99]. On spin-echo images, central pulmonary emboli appear as areas of bright signal within corresponding pulmonary arteries; peripherally, emboli are identifiable as discrete foci of relatively high signal intensity, usually present on contiguous scans, without evidence of branching [99]. Unfortunately, due to limited spatial resolution and respiratory motion artefacts, unlike central thrombi, peripheral emboli, clinically are difficult to identify.

As an alternative to routine spin-echo sequences, the pulmonary arteries may be evaluated with cine gradient-refocused images (Fig. 16). In a retrospective study of 11 patients with documented pulmonary emboli, Posteraro et al found cine gradient-images to be more sensitive than routine spin-echo images, identifying thrombi in all cases [28]. Furthermore, using the criteria of low-intensity intraluminal filling defects or abrupt vascular cut-off with high-intensity peripheral flow versus vascular cut-off without high-intensity capping or intravascular webs, Posteraro et al have postulated that it may be possible to differentiate between acute and chronic emboli, respectively [28]. This observation will require further prospective evaluation.

Despite initial enthusiasm, the role of MRI in the evaluation of pulmonary thrombo-embolism is limited. Non-invasive diagnosis of peripheral emboli, in particular, remains elusive. MRI is of value, however, in patients for whom angiography is contra-indicated, or as a means for follow-up in patients with known chronic central emboli. It should be emphasized that MRI may also be of value by diagnosing intravascular filling defects resulting from both primary or secondary (metastatic) tumours. Although there is some overlap in the MRI appearance of tumour within pulmonary arteries and otherwise bland thrombus, it has recently been documented that in the rare case of primary pulmonary artery tumours, this diagnosis may be facilitated by use of contrast enhancement using Gd-DTPA [102].

Recent attention also has been directed towards the use of gradient-recalled echo sequences to evaluate hilar vessels. Edelman et al have produced high quality projection angiograms of the hilar and to a lesser degree the intraparenchymal pulmonary arteries from a series of breath-held, two-dimensional, flow-compensated gradient-recalled images [103].

(a)

(b)

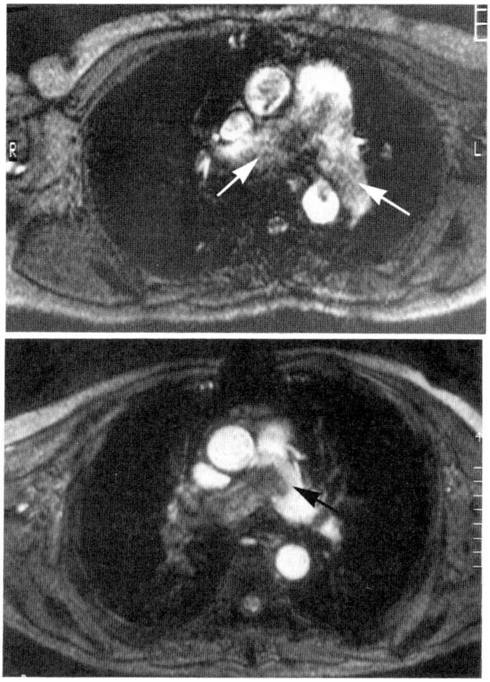

Figure 16. *PULMONARY ARTERIES: EVALUATION WITH GRADIENT-REFOCUSED ECHOES. (a) Gradient-refocused MRI scan shows poorly marginated regions of signal void in both the right and left main pulmonary arteries (arrows) in a patient with documented idiopathic pulmonary artery hypertension. These changes were noted to occur throughout the entire cardiac cycle. (b) Gradient-refocused MRI scan at the same level as shown in (a), in a different patient. In this case, the region of signal void is sharply demarcated and involves not only the entire right pulmonary artery but extends into the proximal portion of the left main pulmonary artery as well (arrow) (compare with a). In this case, signal void is due to the presence of a surgically-confirmed pulmonary artery sarcoma originating in the right main pulmonary artery. Despite differences, it is apparent that changes within the pulmonary arteries on gradient-recalled scans need to be interpreted cautiously.*

SUMMARY

In our experience, MRI primarily serves as a problem-solving device, especially in those cases in which CT has proven equivocal. In patients with thoracic malignancies, MRI has proven more accurate than CT for identifying and delineating the extent both of mediastinal and hilar tumours. MRI has proven especially helpful in assessing chest wall and mediastinal invasion, although this diagnosis still remains problematic in a significant percentage of cases. Additionally, MRI can make an unique contribution to patients both with Hodgkin's and non-Hodgkin's lymphomas by sequentially monitoring their response to therapy. MRI can also be of value in assessing patients with signs of venous obstruction, especially when there is a contra-indication to the use of i.v. contrast media.

MRI is equally as accurate as CT in assessing most benign mediastinal pathology. MRI can easily differentiate aortic aneurysms from enlarged lymph nodes or masses, frequently obviating the need for a more invasive study. MRI is equally efficacious in evaluating patients with cystic lesions, especially patients with complex cysts that are not clearly of water density on CT.

In the hilum, MRI reliably can differentiate between prominent hilar vessels and adenopathy or masses. MRI should be considered the imaging procedure of choice to evaluate suspicious hila identified on plain chest radiographs, especially in patients for whom there is a contra-indication to the use of intravenous contrast. In addition to detecting enlarged nodes and masses, MRI can also be used to differentiate central obstructing hilar tumours and peripheral, collapsed lung. In select cases these findings may be significant in assessing resectability in patients with lung cancer by demonstrating encasement of hilar and mediastinal vessels as well as the central airways.

References

1. Gamsu G, Gostman D. Magnetic resonance imaging of the thorax. *Am Rev Resp Dis* 1989;**139**:254-74.
2. Axel L, Kressel HV, Thickman D, Epstein DM, Edelstein W, Bottomley P, Redington R, Baum S. NMR imaging of the chest at 0.12 T: initial clinical experience with a resistive magnet. *AJR* 1983;**141**:1157-62.

3. Berquist TH, Brown LR, May GR, Jett JR, Bernatz PE. Magnetic resonance imaging of the chest: a diagnostic comparison with computed tomography and hilar tomography. *Magnetic Resonance Imaging* 1984;**2**:3:5-27.
4. Levitt RG, Glazer HS, Roper CL, Lee JKT, Murphy WA. Magnetic resonance imaging of mediastinal and hilar masses: comparison with CT. *AJR* 1985;**145**:9-14.
5. von Schulthess GK, NcMurdo K, Tscholakopff, de Geer G, Gamsu G, Higgins CB. Mediastinal masses: MR imaging. *Radiology* 1986;**158**:289-96.
6. Barakos JA, Brown JJ, Brescia RJ, Higgins CB. High signal intensity lesions of the chest in MR imaging. *J Comput Assist Tomogr* 1987;**13**:797-802.
7. Webb WR, Gamsu G, Stark DD, Moore EH. Magnetic resonance imaging of the normal and abnormal pulmonary hila. *Radiology* 1984;**152**:89-94.
8. Bradly WG, Waluch V. Blood flow magnetic resonance imaging. *Radiology* 1985;**154**:443-50.
9. Dooms GC, Higgins CB. The potential of magnetic resonance imaging for the evaluation of thoracic arterial disease. *J Thorac Cardiovasc Surg* 1986;**92**:1088-95.
10. Glazer HS, Gutierrez FR, Levitt RG, Lee JKT, Murphy WA. The thoracic aorta studied by MR imaging. *Radiology* 1985;**157**:149-55.
11. White RD, Dooms GC, Higgins CB. Advances in imaging thoracic aortic disease. *Invest Radiol* 1986;**21**:761-78.
12. McMurdo KK, de Geer G, Webb WR, Gamsu G. Normal and occluded mediastinal veins. MR imaging. *Radiology* 1986;**159**:33-8.
13. Weinreb JC, Mootz A, Cohen JM. MRI evaluation of mediastinal and thoracic inlet venous obstruction. *AJR* 1986;**146**:679-84.
14. Katz ME, Glazer HS, Siegel MJ, Gutierrez F, Levitt RG, Lee JKT. Mediastinal vessels: postoperative evaluation with MR imaging. *Radiology* 1986;**161**:647-51.
15. White RD, Ullyot DJ, Higgins CB. MR imaging on the aorta after surgery for aortic dissection. *AJR* 1988;**150**:87-92.
16. Batra P, Brown K, Steckel RJ, Collins JD, Ovenfors CO, Aberie D. MR imaging of the thorax: a comparison of axial, coronal, and sagittal imaging planes. *J Comput Assist Tomogr* 1988;**12**:76-81.
17. Webb WR, Gamsu G, Crooks LE. Multisection sagittal and coronal magnetic resonance imaging of the mediastiun and hila. Work in progress. *Radiology* 1984;**150**:475-78.
18. Webb WR, Jensen BG, Gamsu G, Sollitto R, Moore EH. Sagittal MR imaging of the chest: normal and abnormal. *J Comput Assist Tomogr* 1985;**9**:471-9.
19. Gamsu G, Stark DD, Webb WR, Moore EH, Sheldon PE. Magnetic resonance imaging of benign mediastinal masses. *Radiology* 1984;**151**:709-13.
20. Naidich DP, Rumancik WM, Ettenger NA, Feiner HD, Harnaz-Schulman M, Spatz EM, et al. Congenital anomalies of the lungs in adults: MR diagnosis. *AJR* 1988;**151**:13-9.
21. Dooms GC, Hricak H, Sollihotto RA, Higgins CB. Lipomatous tumours and tumours with fatty component. MR imaging potential and comparison of MR and CT results. *Radiology* 1985;**157**:479-83.
22. Glazer HS, Lee JKT, Levitt RJ, Heiken JP, Ling D, Totty WG, Balf DM, Emani B, Wasseman TH, Murphy WA. Radiation fibrosis: Differentiation from recurrent tumour by MR imaging. *Radiology* 1985;**156**:721-6.
23. Zerhouni EA, Fishman EK, Jones R, Siegelman SS, Soulen RL. (Abstr) MR imaging of steralized lymphoma. *Radiology* 1986;**161(P)**:207.
24. Rahmoum AD, Zerhouni EA. Role of MRI in the management of thoracic lymphoma. In: Zerhouni EA (ed.) *CT and MRI of the Thorax*, pp. 23-35. Edinburgh: Churchill Livingstone, 1990.

25. Naidich DP, Zerhouni EA, Siegelman SS. *CT/MR of the Thorax*, 2nd Edition. Raven: New York, 1991.
26. Weinreb JC, Naidich DP. Thoracic MR: clinical applications. In *Imaging Strategies in Pulmonary Disease. Clinics of Chest Medicine.* Philadelphia: Saunders, 1991.
27. Templeton PA, Yang A, Tempany CMC, Zerhouni EA. MR imaging of mediastinal venous obstruction with gradient-echo and spin-echo pulse sequences. *Radiology* 1989;**173(P)**:210.
28. Posteraro RH, Sostman HD, Spritzer CE, Herfkens RJ. Cine-gradient-refocused MR imaging of central pulmonary emboli. *AJR* 1989;**152**:466-8.
29. Hansen ME, Spritzer CE, Sostman HD. Assessing the patency of mediastinal and thoracic inlet veins: value of MR imaging. *AJR* 1990;**155**:1177-82.
30. Shuman WP, Baron RL, Peters MJ, Taziolo PK. Comparison of STIR and spin-echo MR imaging at 1.5T in 90 lesions of the chest, liver and pelvis. *AJR* 1987;**152**:653-9.
31. Bittner RJ, Schoerner W, Schoenfeld N, Schmeizer J, Boeck J, Lodenkemper R et al. Value of contrast-enhanced MR imaging in throracic pathologies. *Radiology* 1990;**177(P)**:97.
32. Konjo M, Adachi S, Tanaka K, Kusumoto M, Sakai E. Gd-DTPA enhanced MR imaging: dynamic study in lung cancer patients. *Radiology* 1990;**177(P)**:97.
33. Dinsmore RE, Liberthson RR, Wismer GL, Miller SW, Liu P, Thompson R, et al. Magnetic resonance imgang of thoracic aortic aneurysms: comparison with other imaging modalities. *AJR* 1986;**145**:309-14.
34. Fletcher BD, Jacobstein MD. MRI of congenital abnormalities of the great arteries. *AJR* 1986;**146**:941-8.
35. Gomes AS, Lois JF, George B, Alpan G, Williams RG. Congenital abnormalities of the aoritic arch: MR imaging. *Radiology* 1987;**165**:691-5.
36. Kersting-Sommerhoff BA, Sechten UP, Fischer MR, Higgins CB. MR imaging of congenital anomalies of the aortic arch. *AJR* 1987;**149**:9-13.
37. Kersting-Sommerhoff BA, Sechtem UP, Schiller NB, Lipton MJ, Higgins CB. MR imaging of the thoracic aorta in Marfan patients. *J Comput Assist Tomogr* 1987;**11**:633-9.
38. von Schulthess GK, Higashino SM, Higgins SS, Didier D, Fisher MR, Higgins CB. Coarctation of the aorta: MR imaging. *Radiology* 1986;**158**:469-74.
39. Amparo EG, Higgins CB, Hricak H, Sollitto R. Aortic dissection: Magnetic resonance imaging. *Radiology* 1985;**155**:399-406.
40. Dinsmore RE, Wedeen VJ, Miller SW, Rosen BR, Fifer M, Vlahakes GJ, Edelman RR, Brady TJ. MRI of dissection of the aorta: recognition of the intimal tear and differential flow velocities. *AJR* 1986;**146**:128.
41. Kersting-Sommerhoff BA, Higgins CB, White RD, Sommerhoff CP, Lipton MJ. Aortic dissection: sensitivity and specificity of MR imaging. *Radiology* 1988;**166**:651-5.
42. Pernes JM, Grenier P, Desbleds MT, de Brix JL. MR evaluation of chronic aortic dissectiion. *J Comput Assist Tomogr* 1987;**11**:975-81.
43. Heelan RT, Martini N, Westcott JW, Bains MS, Watson RC, Caravelli JF, et al. Carcinomatous involvement of the hilum and mediastum: computed tomographic and magnetic resonance evaluation. *Radiology* 1985:**156**:111-5.
44. Musset D, Grenier P, Carette MF, Frija G, Hauuy MP, Desbleds MT, Girard P, Bigot JM, Lallemand D. Primary lung cancer staging: prospective comparative study of MR imaging with CT. *Radiology* 1986;**160**:607-11.
45. Webb WR, Jensen BG, Sollitto R, de Geer G, McCowin M, Gamsu G, Moore E. Bronchogenic carcinoma: staging with MR compared with staging with CT and surgery. *Radiology* 1985;**156**:117-24.

46. Glaze GM, Gross BH, Aisen AM, Quint LE, Francis IR, Orringer MB. Imaging of the pulmonary hilum: a prospective comparative study in patients with lung cancer. *AJR* 1985;**145**:245-8.
47. Cohen AM, Creiston S, LiPuma JP, Bryan PJ, Haaga JR, Alfidi RJ. NMR Evaluation of hilar and medistinal lymphadenopathy. *Radiology* 1983;**148**:739-42.
48. Dooms GC, Hricak H, Crooks LE, Higgins CB. Magnetic resonance imaging of the lymph nodes: comparison with CT. *Radiology* 1984:**153**:719-28.
49. Dooms GC, Hricak H, Moseley ME, Bottles K, Fisher M, Higgins CB. Characterization of lymphadenopathy by magnetic resonance relaxation times: Preliminary results. *Radiology* 1985;**155**:691-7.
50. Glazer GM, Orringer MB, Chenevert TL, Borrello JA, Penner MW, Quint LE, Li KC, Aisen AM. Mediastinal lymph nodes: relaxation time/pathologic correlation and implications in staging of lung cancer with MR imaging. *Radiology* 1988;**168**:428-31.
51. Farmer DW, Moore E, Amparo E, Webb WR, Gamsu G, Higgins CB. Calcific fibrosing mediastinitis: Demonstration of pulmonary vascular obstruction by magnetic resonance imaging. *AJR* 1984;**143**:1189-91.
52. Rholl KS, Levitt RG, Glazer HS. Magnetic resonance imaging of fibrosing mediastinitis. *AJR* 1985;**145**:255-9.
53. Libsnitz HJ, Jing BS, Walace S, Logothethis CJ. Sterilized metastases: a diagnostic and therapeutic dilemma. *AJR* 1983;**140**:14-19.
54. Jochelson M, Mauch P, Balikian J, Rosenthal D, Cancellos G. The significance of the residual mediastinal mass in treated Hodgkin's disease. *J Clin Oncol* 1988;**3**:627-40.
55. Nyman RS, Rehn SM, Glimelius BLG, Hagber ME, Hemmingsson AL, Sundström CJ. Residual mediastinal masses in Hodgkin disease: prediction of size with MR imaging. *Radiology* 1989;**170**:435-40.
56. Rhen SM, Nyman RS, Glimelius BLG, Hagberg HE, Sundström JC. Non-Hodgkin lymphoma: predicting prognostic grade with MR imaging. *Radiology* 1990;**176**:249-53.
57. Nyman R, Rehn S, Glimelius G, Hagberg H, Hemmingsom A, Jung B. Magnetic resonance imaging for assessement of treatment effects in mediastinal Hodgkin's disease. *Acta Radiologica* 1987;**28**:145-51.
58. Negendank WG, Al-Katio AM, Karanes C, Smith MR. Lymphomas: MR imaging contrast characteristics with clinical-pathologic correlations. *Radiology* 1990;**177**:209-16.
59. Lae JKT, Glazer HS. Controversy in the MR appearance of fibrosis. *Radiology* 1990;**177**:21-2.
60. London J, Kim EE, Wallace S, Shirkhoda A, Coan J, Evans H. MR imaging of liposarcomas: correlation of MR features and histology. *J Comput Assist Tomogr* 1989;**13**:832-5.
61. Siegel MJ, Glazer HS, Wiener JL, Molina PL, Normal and abnormal thymus in childhood: MR imaging. *Radiology* 1987;**172**:367-71.
62. DeGeer G, Webb WR, Gamsu G. Normal thymus. Assessement with MR and CT. *Radiology* 1986;**158**:313-7.
63. Rollins NK, Currarino G. MR imaging of posterior mediastinal thymus. *J Comput Assist Tomogr* 1988;**12**:518-20.
64. Shiarkhoda A, Chasen MH, Eftekhari F, Goldman AM, Decaro L. MR imaging of mediastinal thymolipoma. *J Comput Assist Tomogr* 1987;**11**:364-5.
65. Batra P, Herrmann C Jr, Mulder D. Mediastinal imaging in myastheia gravis: correlation of chest radiology, CT, MR and surgical findings. *AJR* 1987;**148**:515-9.
66. Molina PL, Siegel MJ, Glazer HS. Pictorial essay. Thymic masses on MR imaging. *AJR* 1990;**155**:495-500.

67. Stark DD, Moss AA, Gamsu G, Clark OH, Gooding GAW, Webb WR. Magnetic resonance imaging of the neck, part 1. Normal anatomy. *Radiology* 1984;**150**:447-54.
68. Stark DD, Moss AA, Gamsu G, Clark OH, Gooding GAW, Webb WR. Magnetic resonance imaging of the neck, part 2. Pathologic findings. *Radiology* 1984;**150**:455-61.
69. Stark DD, Clark OH, Moss AA. Magnetic resonance imaging of the thyroid, thymus and parathyroid glands. *Surgery* 1984;**96**:1083-91.
70. Higgins CB, McNamara MT, Fisher MR, Clark OH. MR imaging of the thyroid. *AJR* 1986;**147**:1255-61.
71. Mountz JM, Glazer GM, Dmuchowski C, Sisson JC. MR imaging of the thyroid: comparison with scintigraphy in the normal and diseased gland. *J Comput Assist Tomogr* 1987;**11**:612-9.
72. Gefter WB, Spritzer CE. Eisenberg B, LiVolsi VA, Axel L, Velchik M, et al. Thyroid imaging with high-field strength surface-coil MR. *Radiology* 1987;**164**:483-90.
73. Noma S, Nishimura K, Togashi K, Itok K, Fujisawa I, Nakano V. et al. Thyroid gland: MR imaging. *Radiology* 1987;**164**:495-9.
74. Noma S, Kanaoka M, Minami S, Sagoh T, Vamashita K, Nishimura K, et al. Thyroid masses: MR imaging and pathologic correlation. *Radiology* 1988;**168**:759-64.
75. Higgins CB, Auffermann W. MR imaging of thyroid and parathyroid glands: a review of current status. *AJR* 1988;**151**:1095-106.
76. Auffermann W, Clark OH, Thurnher S, Galante M, Higgins CB. Recurrent thyroid carcinoma: characteristics on MR images. *Radiology* 1988;**168**:753-7.
77. Barakos JA, DeMarco RJ, Higgins CB. MR imaging of recurrent medullary thyroid carcinoma. *Radiology* 1989;**173(P)**:252.
78. Holliday RA, Weinreb J. Utility of MR imaging in post-thyroidectomy patients. *Radiology* 1987;**173(P)**:253.
79. Miller DL, Doppmann JL, Shawker TH, Krudy AG, Norton JA, Vucich JJ, et al. Localization of parathyroid adenomas in patients who have undergone surgery. Part 1. Non-invasive imaging methods. *Radiology* 1987;**162**:133-7.
80. Kneeland JB, Krubsack AJ, Lawson TL, Wilson SD, Collier BD, Froncisz W, Jesmanowicz A, Hyde JS. Enlarged parathyroid glands: high-resolution local coil MR imaging. *Radiology* 1987;**162**:143-6.
81. Peck WW, Higgins CB, Fisher MR, Ling M, Okerlund MD, Clark OH. Hyperparathyroidism: comparison of MR imaging with radionuclide scanning. *Radiology* 1987;**163**:415-20.
82. Spritizer CE, Gefter WB, Hamilton R, Greenberg BM, Axel L, Kressel HV. Abnormal parathyroid glands: high-resolution MR imaging. *Radiology* 1987;**162**:487-91.
83. Auffermann W, Gooding GAW, Okerlund MD, Clark OH, Thrurnher S, Levin KE, Higgins CB. Diagnosis of recurrent hyperparathyroidism: comparison of MR imaging and other imaging techniques. *AJR* 1988;**150**:1027-33.
84. Burk DK. Brundberg JA, Kanal E, Latchaw RE, Wolf GL. Spinal and paraspinal neurofibromatosis: surface coil MR imaging at 1.5 T. *Radiology* 1987;**162**:797-801.
85. Dietrich RB, Kangarloo H, Lenarsky C, Feig SA. Neuroblastoma: the role of MR imaging. *AJR* 1987;**148**:927-42.
86. Siegel MJ, Jamroz GA, Glazer HS, Abramson CL. MR imaging of intraspinal extension of neuroblastoma. *J Comput Assist Tomogr* 1986;**10**:593-5.
87. Levine E, Huntrakoon M, Wetzel LH. Malignant nerve-sheath neoplasms in neurofibromatosis: distinction from benign tumours by using imaging techniques. *AJR* 1987;**149**:1059-64.
88. Webb WR. RDOG data.

89. Mayr R, Heywang SH, Ingrisch H, Huber RM, Haussinger K, Lissner J. Comparison of CT with MR imaging of endobronchial tumours. *J Comput Assist Tomogr* 1987;**11**:43-8.
90. Huber DJ, Kobzik L, Malanson G, Adams DF. The detection of inflammation in collapsed lung by alterations in proton nuclear magnetic relaxation times. *Invest Radiol* 1985;**20**:460-4.
91. Shioya S, Haida M, Ono Y, Fukuzaki M, Yamabayashi H. Lung cancer differentation of tumour, necrosis, and atelectasis by means of T1 and T2 values measured in vitro. *Radiology* 1988;**167**:105-9.
92. Tobler J, Levitt RG, Glazer HS, Moran J, Crouch E, Evens RG. Differentiation of proximal bronchogenic carcinoma from postobstructive lobar collapse by magnetic resonance imaging. Comparison with computed tomography. *Invest Radiol* 1987;**22**:538-43.
93. Herold CJ, Kuhlman JE, Zwrhouni EA. Pulmonary atelectasis: signal patterns with MR imaging. *Radiology* 1990;**177(P)**:140.
94. Burke M, Fraser R. Obstructive pneumonitis: a pathologic and pathogenetic reappraisal. *Radiology* 1988;**166**:699-704.
95. Bouchard A, Higgins CB, Byrd B, Amparo EG, Osaki L, Axelrod R. Magnetic resonance imaging in pulmonary artery hypertension. *Am J Cardiol* 1985;**56**:938-42.
96. von Schulthess GD, Fisher MR, Higgins CB. Pathologic blood flow in pulmonary vascular disease as shown by gated magnetic resonance imaging. *Ann Intern Med* 1985;**103**:317-23.
97. White RD, Winkler ML, Higgins CB. MR imaging of pulmonary arterial hypertension and pulmonary emboli. *AJR* 1987;**149**:15-21.
98. Fisher MR, Higgins CB. Central thrombi in pulmonary arterial hypertension detected by MR imaging. *Radiology* 1986;**158**:223-6.
99. Gamsu G, Hirjii M, Moore EH, Webb WR, Brito A. Experimental pulmonary emboli detected using magnetic resonance. *Radiology* 1984;**153**:467-70.
100. Moore EH, Gamsu G, Webb WR, Stulbarg MS. Pulmonary embolus: detection and follow-up using magnetic resonance. *Radiology* 1984;**153**:471-2.
101. Pope CF, Sostman D, Carbo P, Gore JC, Holcomb W. The detection of pulmonary emboli by magnetic resonance imaging. Evaluation of imaging parameters. *Invest Radiol* 1987;**22**:937-46.
102. Weinreb JC, Davis SD, Berkmen YM, Isom W, Naidich DP. Case report. Pulmonary artery sarcoma: evaluation using Gd-DTPA. *J Comput Assist Tomogr* 1990;**14**:647-9.
103. Edelman RR, Wentz KU, Mattle H, Zhao B, Liu C, Kim D, Laub G. Projection arteriography and venography: initial clinical results with MR. *Radiology* 1989;**172**:351-7.

Magnetic resonance imaging and computed tomography of the chest wall.

Peter Vock
Department of Diagnostic Radiology, University Hospital, Bern, Switzerland

---

Imaging Methods for the Chest Wall

With the clear exception of mammography for breast disease, conventional chest radiography is in most cases a prerequisite for any evaluation of chest wall disorders. Some lesions, e.g. displaced rib fractures or soft tissue emphysema, are easily discovered; other pathological changes, such as localized bony destruction and most soft tissue lesions, will be better demonstrated with low-kilovoltage radiography or one of the modern tomographic techniques [1-3]. Before we discuss the specific pathological entities we shall mention some of the general principles that guide the use of imaging methods for the chest wall.

The strength of nuclear bone scanning is that it offers a sensitive overview of thoracic bone turnover similar to the morphological overview of chest radiography. Computed tomography (CT) and magnetic resonance imaging (MRI) afford the complete overview of one plane at one time, whereas ultrasound (US) is limited by a relatively small field of view with more difficulties in anatomical orientation (Table 1). Among the tomographic techniques, only US and MRI offer a true

Table 1. *MRI and CT of the chest wall: advantages as compared to other imaging procedures*

Method	Overview	Multiplanar tomography	Real-time (function)	Bone	Bone marrow	Soft tissues	Simultaneous imaging of the lungs
Radiography	+	-	+ (fluoro)	+	-	-(breast ++)	(+)
Nuclear scanning	++	-	-	++ (functional)	+	-(+monoclonal antibodies)	-
US	-	+	+	-	-	+	-
CT	+	-	-(+*)	++ (morpho-logical)	(+)	+	+
MRI	+	+	-(+*)	+	++	++	(+)

*Technical development areas: new hardware design will improve the performance of the method multiplanar approach, whereas CT and single photon emission computed tomography (SPECT) (the tomographic version of nuclear scanning) are essentially limited to the axial plane. Fluoroscopy and US allow real time analysis and, therefore, functional imaging of the chest wall. Ultrafast CT and MRI are likely to approach real time imaging.

Plain radiography, the functional overview of nuclear bone scans and the detailed morphological information of CT are the preferred imaging methods for cortical bone. With involvement of bone marrow, MRI becomes the most sensitive and, in many cases, the most specific imaging method, whereas CT relies on an increase of bone marrow density due to replacement of marrow fat by any pathological process of soft tissue density. In the soft tissues, US, CT and MRI play the predominant role, with MRI being more and more preferred because of its wide range of contrast and overview. The fact that disease may involve the lung and the chest wall simultaneously may sometimes favour CT instead of MRI, even though the two methods are equivalent for the specific chest wall disorder.

On the other hand, several disadvantages should always be kept in mind when deciding on the appropriate imaging method for the chest wall (Table 2). With the exception of US and MRI, all procedures use ionizing radiation. Angiography and many CT studies require injection of a contrast agent containing iodine with its inherent risks for susceptible patients and in cases of reduced renal function. MRI is absolutely contra-indicated for patients with pacemakers or metallic magnetic foreign bodies. Arrhythmia, such as most often seen with atrial fibrillation, is a relative contra-indication since cardiac gating will not be successful and image quality will suffer. This introduces the problem of motion artefacts caused by any muscle but, above all, respiration and cardiovascular activity. With the most modern scanners, CT will hardly be affected by this problem, and similarly, ultafast MRI sequences are being developed. This is an important problem, since currently the better contrast resolution of MRI is often neutralized by motion artefacts.

In the near future, the cost factor will remain important and will favour US, CT and nuclear scanning instead of MRI. Faster sequences that increase the throughput will hopefully reduce the cost of this important imaging tool.

Table 2. *MRI and CT of the chest wall: disadvantages as compared to other imaging procedures*

Method	Ionizing radiation	Risk of contrast agent (iodine)	Contra-indication	Cardio-respiratory artefacts	Cost
Radiography	+	-/+	-	-	-
Nuclear scanning	+	-	-	-	(+)
US	-	-	-	-	-
CT	+	-/+	-	-(+)	(+)
MRI	-	-	+ pacemaker, magnetic foreign bodies, (arrhythmias)	+(-*)	+

*Technical development areas: new hardware design is likely to overcome this disadvantage.

Thoracic Inlet and Shoulder Girdle

This most superior portion of the chest wall connects the upper extremity to the trunk of the body. Muscles, tendons, the clavicules, the scapulae and the articulations between them and the humerus or the sternum and rib cage respectively guarantee an extraordinary range of motion. In a small cross-sectional area, the thoracic inlet contains a number of important connections from the mediastinum to the neck and the upper extremity, such as the oesophagus and trachea, blood vessels, lymphatics and nerves [4]. The narrow space between the sternum, the clavicules, the uppermost ribs and the vertebral column causes space-occupying lesions to threaten these functionally-important connections. Similarly, the axillae contain delicate soft-tissue structures, such as the vascular supply of the upper extremity, the branches of the brachial plexus and an important group of lymph nodes.

Non-neoplastic Disease

Rib-modelling variations, cervical ribs (one of the causes of the thoracic outlet syndrome) [5-7] and defective or absent clavicles (whether isolated or as part of a generalized syndrome such as cleidocranial dysostosis) are some of the congenital anomalies of this area. Traumatic fractures or dislocations at birth or later in life are likewise mostly evaluated by radiography. However, they may be accompanied by soft tissue lesions of the nearby vessels and nerves. Since radiographic signs of thoracic soft tissue injury such as the apical cap [8], localized swelling or soft-tissue emphysema are neither specific nor sensitive signs CT, MRI or sometimes even angiography may be necessary to detect haematomas and to visualize lacerated vessels or nerves. Using local surface coils, MRI is the only non-invasive imaging procedure that may hclp show traumatic transections of the brachial plexus or the nerve roots. The ultimate goal will be to replace myelographic CT; currently, even using the best equipment available, visualization of the normal brachial plexus remains difficult.

Degenerative disease may also result in a thoracic outlet syndrome [5-7]. Angiography, CT or MRI show the vascular or neural impingement by ligaments and other lesions that are not detected on plain radiographs. Diffuse idiopathic skeletal hyperostosis (DISH) may similarly cause an impingement and, in the case of the oesophagus, may cause dysphagia and imitate an extramucosal tumour.

Rotator cuff tears are often detected on radiographs by an elevated position of the humeral head and soft tissue calcifications. High-resolution US [9-10] and MRI [11] are more and more replacing conventional arthrography: instead of showing the joint and its capsule, they directly demonstrate degeneration and tears of the muscle tendons (Fig. 1). Lesions of the chondral limbus are best studied by CT arthrography or by MRI.

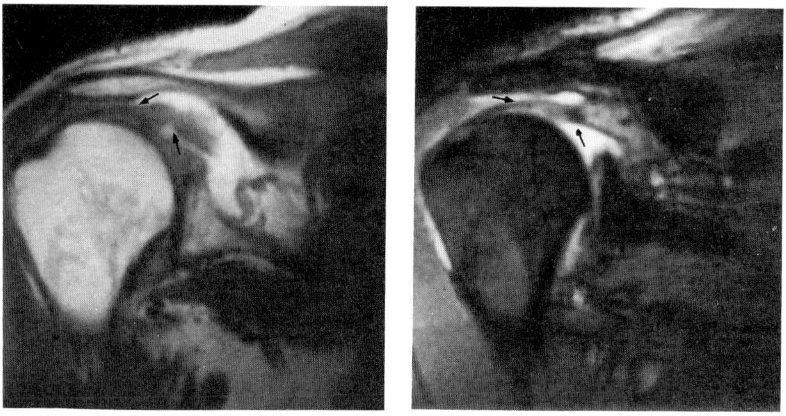

(a) (b)

Figure 1. *MRI OF ROTATOR CUFF TEAR. Degeneration and tear of the supraspinatus muscle is detected in an oblique coronal plane by thinning and a localized interruption of the tendon (arrows) on T1-weighted images (a). On T2-weighted images (b) intra-articular fluid and fluid in the subacromial bursa are bright and highlight the findings of (a). Note the elevated position of the humeral head, a sign that is also detected by conventional radiographs.*

Early infections of the bones and joints, especially in the case of multiple lesions, are best detected by an increased local activity on nuclear bone scans. To differentiate the specific pathology, better morphological imaging is often needed. Both CT and MRI demonstrate the bony and the contiguous soft tissue components of osteomyelitis or arthritis [12,13] as well as soft tissue infections (Fig. 2a).

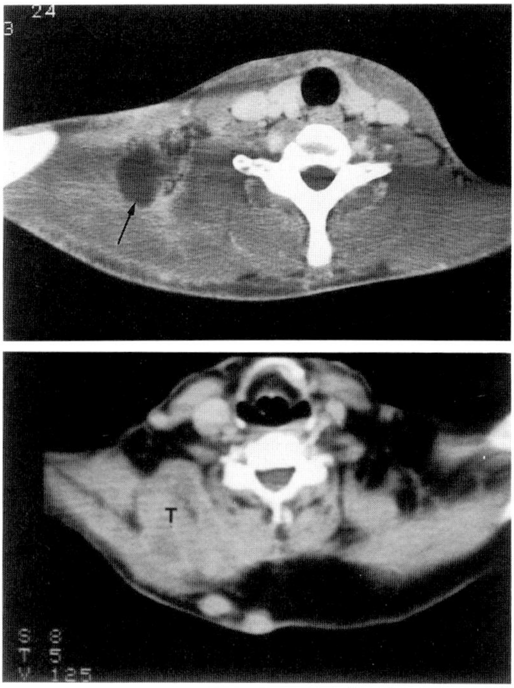

(a)

(b)

Figure 2. *CT COMPARISON OF RIGHT SUPRACLAVICULAR ABSCESS (a) AND MALIGNANT FIBROUS HISTIOCYTOMA (MFH) (b). (a) The acute abscess (arrow) is characterized by a hypo-dense collection of pus surrounded by an enhancing rim of an inflammatory capsule. (b) MFH involves the neck muscles, forming a major mass lesion of soft tissue density (T). There is mild peripheral enhancement and central hypodensity, and two other tumour nodes are seen posteriorly.*

Neoplasms (Table 3)

Localized benign space-occupying lesions of the thoracic inlet and the shoulder girdle, such as nodular goitres and parathyroid adenomas, are detected and characterized by US. However, not all locations are accessible by US and as soon as a lesion becomes large, it is important to see the entire extent of the lesion on one tomographic section. Therefore, CT and MRI are preferred in evaluating most neoplasms of this area [3,14,15]. Lipomas are diagnosed specifically due to their tissue characteristics identical to subcutaneous fat tissue (Fig. 3) [16], whereas most other benign neoplasms require a biopsy unless they have specific morphological features, such as osteochondroma (Table 3).

Table 3. *Common neoplasms of the thoracic inlet and the shoulder girdle.*

Origin	Benign neoplasms	Malignant neoplasms
Parathyroid and thyroid gland	Adenoma, goitre	Carcinoma, haemangioendothelioma
Trachea, oesophagus, soft tissues	Adenoma, leiomyoma, lipoma, neurogenic tumours, haemangioma, lymphangioma	Sarcoma, malignant fibrous histiocytoma,
Lymph nodes		Malignant lymphoma, metastases
Neighbourhood		Superior sulcus tumours
Bone	Osteochondroma, aneurysmal bone cyst, mesenchymomas	Ewing's sarcoma, myeloma, osteosarcoma, chondrosarcoma, fibrosarcoma, malignant fibrous histiocytoma, malignant lymphoma, metastases

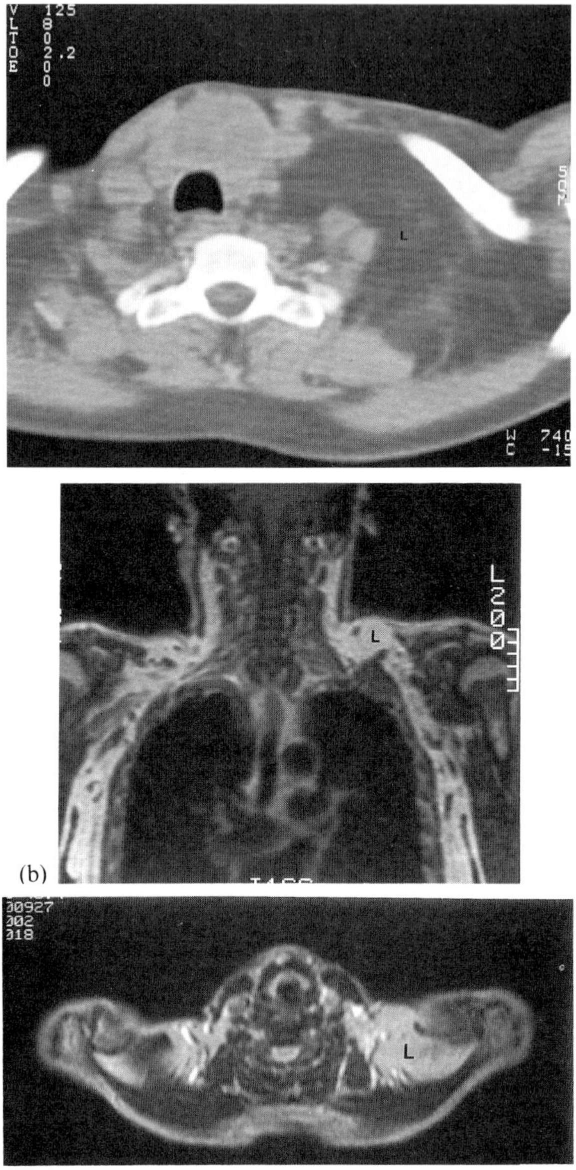

(a) (b) (c)

Figure 3. *LEFT SUPRACLAVICULAR LIPOMA BY CT (a) AND, IN ANOTHER PATIENT, BY MRI (b and c). Lipoma is characterized by a density of around -100 to -180 HU (L), identical to subcutaneous fat on CT scans. Similarly, signal intensity on MR images equals other fatty layers, no matter whether the sequence is T2-weighted (axial image, b), or T1-weighted (coronal image, c).*

Malignant neoplasms are more frequent in the upper thorax than benign neoplasms, and among them haematogenous or lymphatic metastases and tumours infiltrating from the neighbourhood outnumber the primary lesions [3,14,15]. Any organ within the thoracic inlet may give rise to malignancies, most often the oesophagus, the thyroid gland and the trachea. More laterally, primary bone neoplasms such as Ewing's sarcoma, multiple myeloma, osteosarcoma and chondrosarcoma are seen as well as soft tissue sarcoma, malignant lymphoma [17-19] and malignant fibrous histiocytoma (Fig. 2b).

Since the bones of the upper chest wall contain mostly red marrow, they are frequent sites of haematogenous metastases. Metastatic lymphadenopathy to the thoracic inlet, supraclavicular or axillary stations is most often caused by malignant lymphoma, breast cancer, malignant melanoma or lung cancer (Fig. 4). Since the lymph

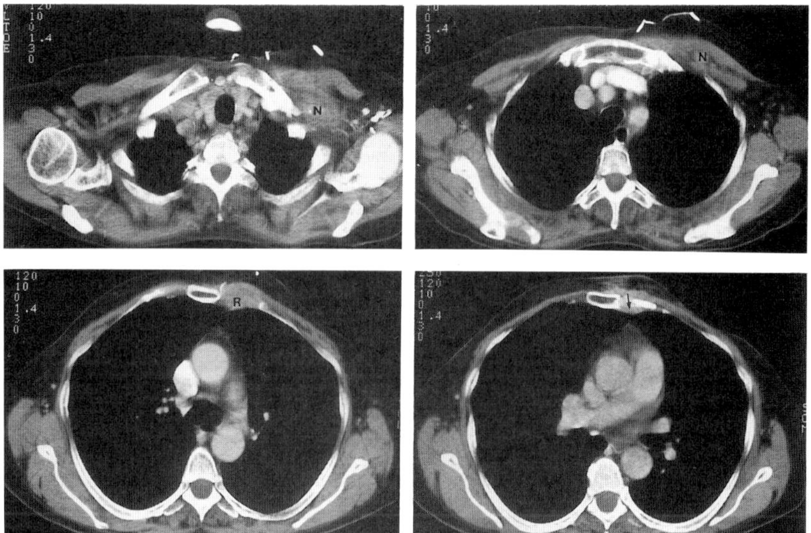

(a) (b) (c) (d)

Figure 4. *FOUR SLICES OF A CT STUDY IN RECURRENT BREAST CANCER. (a) Left axillary lymph node metastases (N) with obstruction of the axillary vein and small subcutaneous collaterals. (b) Left interpectoral lymph node metastasis (N), a significant finding in case of surgical treatment of breast cancer. (c) Local relapse (R) in the left parasternal chest wall and the insertion of the pectoralis major muscle. A mass lesion continues to the inner side of the chest wall where internal mammary lymph node metastases (arrow in d) are found.*

drainage of the entire body eventually reaches the venous angle in the thoracic inlet, lymph node metastases from the neck, the chest and, above all, the abdomen are also seen here. Biopsy guided by US or CT is often helpful in case of an unknown primary tumour. Superior sulcus tumour (Fig. 5) causes Pancoast's syndrome (Horner's syndrome due to involvement of the sympathetic trunk, ulnar pain and wasting of small hand muscles due to brachial plexus infiltration, infiltration of the bone and the subclavian vessels). Apical lung cancer is the most frequent aetiology of Pancoast's syndrome, but other tumours, such as breast cancer, may give rise to identical findings. CT shows the cross-sectional extent of the lesion [20]. Higher soft tissue contrast, the possibility of demonstrating the coronal and other planes and the relative lack of motion in the thoracic inlet favour MRI over CT in this specific situation [2].

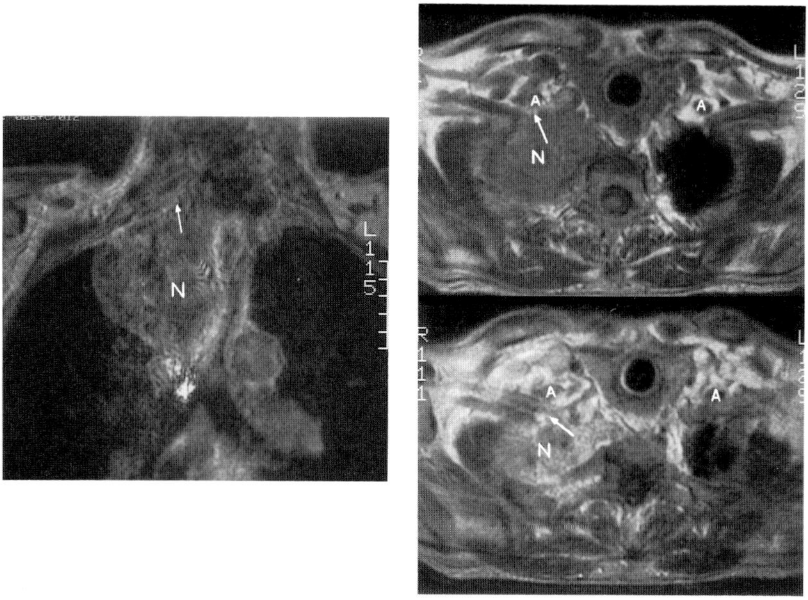

(a) (b) (c)

Figure 5. *APICAL LUNG CANCER WITH INFILTRATION OF THE THORACIC INLET, CAUSING PANCOAST'S SYNDROME. Because of the use of the coronal plane (a), MRI demonstrates the exact extent of the neoplasm (N) in the direction of the brachial plexus, the subclavian vessels (arrows) and the spine as well as the ribs. T1-weighted images; before contrast medium (b) and after Gadolinium-DTPA (a,c), there is a significant, irregular enhancement. Anterior scalene muscle (A).*

Examination of the Anteromedial and Lateral Chest Wall

The breast is the single most important organ in this section of the chest wall and is primarily evaluated by mammography and US. The ribs and the anterior and posterior surface of the sternum are generally well displayed on radiographs, whereas the lateral contours of the sternum, sternocostal articulations, costal cartilage and all other soft tissues require tomographic imaging to show morphological details [21].

Non-neoplastic Disease

Asymmetric or supernumerary breast glands and nipples, or the congenital absence of the pectoralis major muscle (Poland syndrome) generally are meaningless but may rarely cause diagnostic problems. The same is true for hyperplastic, splayed, bifid and fused ribs or a sternal notch [22]. The funnel chest (pectus excavatum), in contrast to the pigeon chest (chicken chest, pectus carinatum), includes a depression of the lower part of the anterior chest wall toward the spinal column with consecutive rotation of the heart to the left. Cardiomegaly and right middle lobe disease are often simulated; chronic bronchitis and bronchiectasis in the underlying lung are serious complications in severe cases. In Tietze's syndrome, unilateral painful swelling of one or more sternocostal chondral junctions is often combined with soft-tissue inflammation [23]; the entity is mostly self-limiting and must be differentiated from more serious aetiologies of chest pain. CT and/or MRI are rarely indicated to evaluate this condition. Metabolic diseases, bone marrow disorders (e.g. thalassaemia) or primary osteopathy (e.g. achondroplasia, osteogenesis imperfecta) tend to affect the ribs more diffusely, distorting both shape and the trabecular structure.

In aortic obstruction, subclavian arterial obstruction or pulmonary oligaemia, arterial collaterals cause inferior rib notching that is most often detected in the posterolateral part of the third to eighth ribs [24,25]. Other causes are venous collaterals in chronic superior vena caval obstruction, arteriovenous malformations or neurofibromatosis. Superior rib notching is mostly acquired and much less common [26].

Trauma to the chest wall is often combined with serious pleural, pulmonary and mediastinal disease. Soft-tissue emphysema is an obvious sign. In contrast to non-traumatic disease, its presence in trauma is of minimal importance. On the other hand, anterior rib fractures, sternal fractures and soft-tissue trauma are hardly detected and may require one of the tomographic imaging methods [27]. Aside from trauma, osteomalacia, osteoporosis, cough, alcohol abuse, multiple myeloma and bony metastases are prone to cause multiple rib fractures and must be excluded in case of inadequate trauma. Postoperative rib changes are mostly detected on chest radiographs, whereas after coronary bypass surgery, retroparasternal haematomas arising from the internal thoracic (mammary) artery may cause diagnostic problems and even require further surgical intervention. CT is generally faster than MRI in demonstrating the exact extent and in differentiating more serious disease of the mediastinum, such as pericardial effusion or lesions of the big vessels.

Among inflammatory disorders, rheumatoid arthritis often involves the manubriosternal and sternoclavicular joints [28]; heroin addicts may develop septic arthritis of the sternochondral and sternoclavicular joints. Again, nuclear bone scans are sensitive but non-specific whereas CT and MRI demonstrate the entire extent of the infectious process [29] both in the bone and in the soft tissues. Image-guided fluid aspiration may be essential in identifying the aetiology. The same imaging tools are used for soft-tissue infections, whether they arise within the chest wall, the skin or from the pleura (e.g. actinomycosis). CT and MRI are likely to show the entire extent of the inflammatory process, but contrast injection into a sinus under fluoroscopic control may rarely be required to show the communication to deeper structures.

Neoplasms (Table 4)

In the sternum and the ribs, enchondroma and osteochondroma are particularly frequent at the costochondral junctions [14,15]. Osteochondroma is similarly well identified by the continuity of trabecular bone between its base and the contiguous bone as well as the cartilaginous cap. More posteriorly, fibrous dysplasia, eosinophilic granuloma and aneurysmal bone cysts are the most frequent tumours and tumour-like lesions. Most other osseous neoplasms of this area are malignant. Metastasis and multiple myeloma are most often characterized by sharply demarcated osteolytic lesions, multiple myeloma often having a soft-tissue component. Chondrosarcoma is the leading primary bone neoplasm and typically presents with large

Table 4. *Common neoplasms of the anteromedial and lateral chest wall*

Origin	Benign neoplasms	Malignant neoplasms
Breast	Fibroadenoma, etc	Carcinoma, sarcoma, malignant lymphoma
Soft tissues	Skin tumours, desmoid tumour, angioma, lipoma, neurofibroma	Skin cancer, liposarcoma, fibrosarcoma
Lymph nodes (parasternal, cardiophrenic)		Malignant lymphoma, metastases
Neighbourhood		Lung and skin cancer, malignant mesothelioma, malignant lymphoma
Bone	Enchondroma and osteochondroma, (fibrous dysplasia), aneurysmal cyst, eosinophilic granuloma	Chondrosarcoma, osteosarcoma, Ewing's sarcoma, myeloma, malignant lymphoma, metastases

lobulated masses with bone destruction and scattered calcifications [14,15]. Other malignant lesions are malignant lymphoma, osteosarcoma and round cell tumours. CT or MRI are extraordinarily valuable in preoperative staging [2,3]. As in other areas of the chest, MRI is slightly superior in defining the soft tissue and bone marrow components but may suffer from respiration and cardiac motion, whereas CT is hardly ever affected by motion artefacts and superbly shows the morphology of the calcified tissues.

Extra-osseous neoplasms arise from the skin, subcutaneous, muscular, tendinous and subpleural soft tissues and, above all, the breast. Lipoma, desmoid tumour, haemangioma, neurofibroma and the variety of benign breast neoplasms are all seen and are characterized by expansive lesions with relatively sharp borders that hardly ever infiltrate.

Among malignant soft tissue tumours, breast cancer predominates all other entities (Table 4). Mammography has become the screening tool of choice [30,31]. Supported by US, it is the only imaging method required to verify the diagnosis by guided biopsy, and for local pre-operative staging in lower stages of breast cancer, whereas in advanced stages with local infiltration of muscles and regional lymphatic metastases to the interpectoral, axillary or internal mammary sites, CT and MRI are similarly helpful (Figs. 4 and 6) Recent experience indicates that contrast medium enhancement may be a relatively specific MRI sign to differentiate malignancies from benign lesions of the breast [32]. However, biopsy is still needed before a decision on treatment is taken. Other malignant lesions of the breast include sarcoma, malignant lymphoma and metastasis. Outside the breast, liposarcoma and fibrosarcoma (which may be detected many years after radiotherapy for Hodgkin's disease [33]) are characterized by an irregular border due to local infiltration, liposarcoma also being characterized by its mixed composition of typical fatty tissue and other components of mixed density and intensity on CT and MRI respectively. In suspected infiltration of the chest wall from the pleura (malignant mesothelioma) [34,35] and the lung (peripheral lung cancer) [36-38], the lack of an extrapleural fat layer does not prove extrapleural invasion, according to the recent literature. Destruction of the rib and clear invasion of intercostal muscles are reliable signs, however they are not very sensitive to either CT or MRI. Malignant internal mammary adenopathy [39-43] is seen in malignant lymphoma, metastasis of breast cancer (mainly when arising in the medial

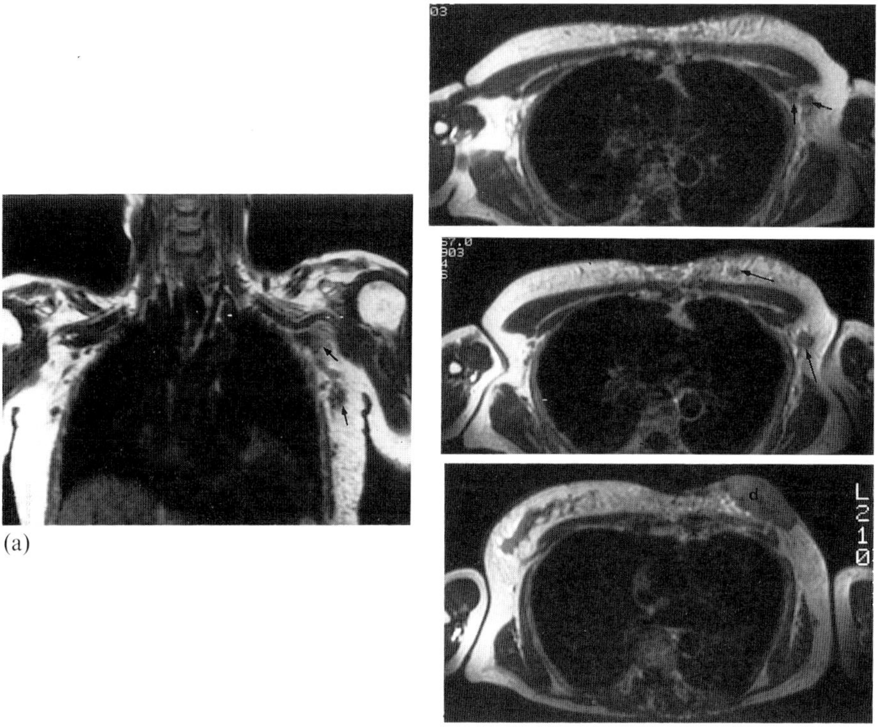

Figure 6. *MRI OF BREAST CARCINOMA WITH LYMPHATIC METASTASES AND LOCAL INFILTRATION. T1-weighted coronal plane before (a) and T1-weighted axial images after injection of gadolinium-DTPA (b - d). Besides the huge primary tumour (d), there are several subcutaneous nodes (arrows, c) as well as a diffuse infiltration of the skin and the subcutaneous fat tissue of the anterior left chest wall. Axillary lymph node metastases (short arrows) are present on the left side, and their topographical relation to the axillary and subclavian vessels and the branches of the brachial plexus is well demonstrated on coronal images (a).*

quadrants) and, less often, following malignant invasion of superior diaphragmatic (cardiophrenic angle) lymph nodes, e.g. in peritoneal malignancies (such as ovarian cancer) (Fig. 7). Three to five nodes are located bilaterally within 3 cm of the sternal edge, most often in the first three intercostal spaces. In adenopathy, they may rarely be detected on lateral chest radiographs by a local bulge of the anterior pleural reflection. Even on cross-sectional tomographic images, this region must be examined carefully in order to identify these nodes.

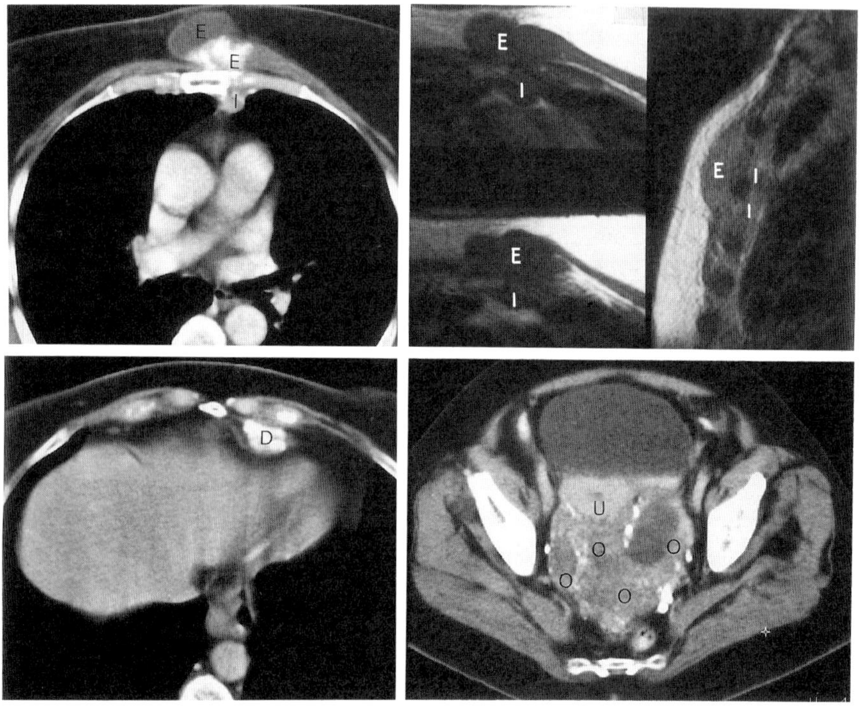

Figure 7. *CT AND MRI OF OVARIAN CANCER WITH CARDIOPHRENIC ANGLE AND INTERNAL MAMMARY LYMPH NODE METASTASES AND LOCAL INFILTRATION OF THE PARASTERNAL AREA. The peristernal tumour (E) has a soft tissue and a calcified component. Calcium is more easily detected on CT scans (upper left) than on MRI (upper right, two axial slices and one sagittal slice). The intrathoracic internal mammary component (I) is equally well demonstrated by both methods. Calcified left superior diaphragmatic (cardiophrenic angle) lymph node metastasis (D, lower left), whereas the right sided station has only lymph nodes of a few millimeters that are in the normal range. Hiatal hernia is an accessory finding. The primary tumour in the pelvis (O, lower right) has calcified, solid and liquid components and pushes the uterus (U) anteriorly. It involves the entire peritoneal space down to the pelvic floor.*

Examination of the Vertebral and Paravertebral Area

Non-neoplastic Disease

Congenital lesions include vertebral anomalies (hemivertebrae, diastematomyelia, dysraphism with or without meningoceles) and kyphoscoliosis. Severe congenital kyphoscoliosis may be responsible for pulmonary arterial hypertension. Besides diffuse deformities of the bones containing red marrow, extra-osseous disease is another manifestation of extramedullary haematopoiesis [44,45]: its rounded extrapulmonary paravertebral soft-tissue mass lesions, quite similar to lymphadenopathy, are typically located at the thoracic level. Another reason for paravertebral, laterally convex soft tissue lesions is an acute vertebral fracture with an accompanying haematoma that displaces the posterior pleural reflection lines bilaterally and helps differentiate acute disease from a pre-existing vertebral compression. Acute vertebral fractures, whether accompanied by a neural deficit or not, require cross-sectional imaging whenever the stability is in question. CT will differentiate a pure fracture of the anterior vertebral body that is stable from an additional involvement of the posterior wall of the vertebral body or the vertebral arch (Fig. 8). MRI, although not as good for demonstrating the osseous lesion, may sometimes be required to estimate the extent of the medullary lesion or the compression by haematoma [46].

Spondylitis, whether tuberculous, fungal or nonspecific bacterial, mostly involves an intervertebral disc and the adjacent vertebral end-plates. CT demonstrates the amount of osseous destruction and paravertebral as well as extradural intraspinal involvement. MRI alone is able to directly show the longitudinal extent without the need for secondary reformation [46-48]. Paravertebral abscesses may descend towards the retroperitoneum. Lymphadenopathy in sarcoidosis is a rare cause of benign paravertebral rounded mass lesions and has to be differentiated from more serious neoplastic disease [49].

Neoplastic Disorders (Table 5)

Neurogenic tumours and meningiomas are responsible for most benign soft tissue neoplasms in the paravertebral area. The dorsal vertebral column gives rise to haemangiomas, osteoblastomas, osteoid osteomas, aneurysmal bone cysts and lipomas [3,14,15].

As in other areas of the chest wall, malignant neoplasms outnumber benign lesions by far. Ewing's sarcoma, osteosarcoma, chondrosarcoma and myeloma are the primary malignancies of the thoracic spine [14,15,50]. Metastatic deposits are seen more frequently and arise mainly from the breast, lung, prostate, kidney, rectum and thyroid gland. In the soft tissues, neurofibromatosis may degenerate

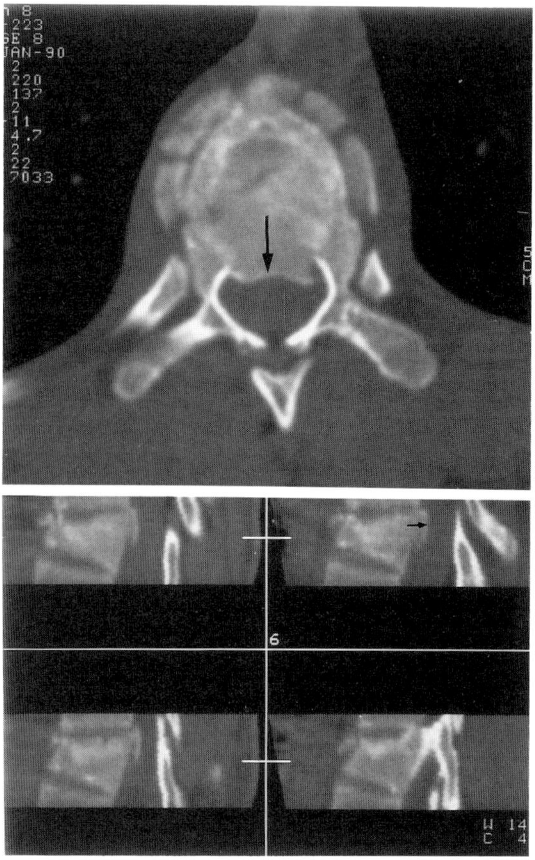

(a)

(b)

Figure 8. *ACUTE UNSTABLE VERTEBRAL FRACTURE IN THE AXIAL PLANE AT THE LEVEL OF THE PEDICLES (a) AND IN SAGITTAL REFORMATIONS (b). The upper posterior wall of the vertebral body is involved and displaced into the spinal canal (arrow).*

and develop neurofibrosarcoma. Again, secondary lesions are more important. They may invade the paravertebral area from the spine, the pleura, the lung or may represent malignant lymphadenopathy in malignant lymphoma (Fig. 9) [17-19] or retroperitoneal tumours. Since in the area of the spine and its neighbourhood motion is less a problem than in the anterior parts of the chest wall, and since the multiplicity of lesions often asks for demonstration of most of the dorsal spine, MRI using a surface coil is mostly preferred to CT in

Table 5. *Neoplasms of the vertebral column and the paravertebral area*

Origin	Benign neoplasms	Malignant neoplasms
Soft tissues	Neurogenic tumours, meningioma (extramedullary haemopoiesis)	Neurogenic sarcoma
Lymph nodes	(Sarcoidosis)	Metastases, malignant lymphoma
Neighbourhood		Lung cancer, malignant mesothelioma
Vertebral column	Haemangioma, osteoblastoma, osteoid osteoma, aneurysmal cyst	Ewing's sarcoma, osteosarcoma, chondrosarcoma, myeloma, malignant lymphoma, metastases

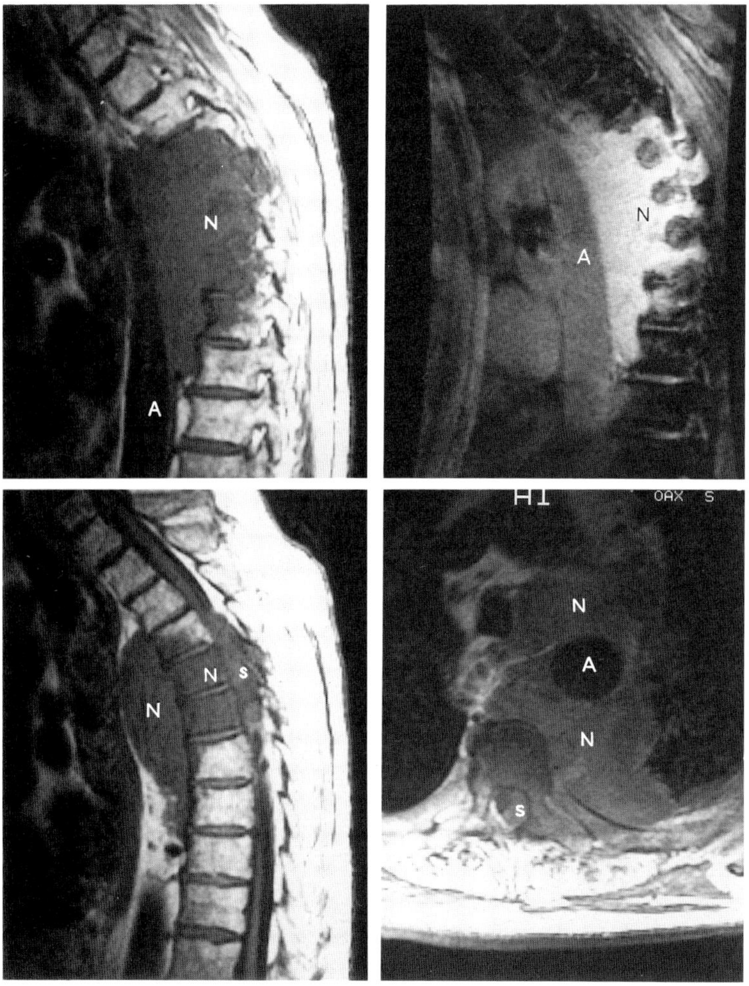

(a) (b) (c) (d)

Figure 9. *MALIGNANT NON-HODGKIN'S LYMPHOMA INVOLVING THE SPINE. Left sided sagittal sections show the voluminous tumour (N) as a mass lesion of low signal intensity on the T1-weighted image (a) and of high intensity on the T2-weighted image (b). The space between the aorta (A) and the spine is completely filled up, and the tumour continues through the intervertebral foramina into the spinal canal. (c) The median sagittal T1-weighted image shows the prevertebral and intravertebral tumour component (N) and the lesion within the spinal canal (S) that is better demonstrated on the oblique axial image (d, after injection of a contrast agent). Note the displacement of the dural sac by the enhanced tumour (S) that correlates with the clinical sign of paraparesis. The aorta (A) is completely surrounded by tumour (N).*

evaluating inflammatory and neoplastic diseases. As soon as the entire cross-section including the lung and the mediastinum is likely to contain lesions (e.g. lung metastases), CT remains the current method of choice.

Aknowledgement

I thank Barbara Le Blanc for her secretarial and administrative assistance in preparing this manuscript.

References

1. Gouliamos AD, Carter BL, Emami B. Computed tomography of the chest wall. *Radiology* 1980;**134**:433-436.
2. Gefter WB. Chest applications of magnetic resonance imaging: an update. *Radiol Clin North Am* 1988;**26**:573-588.
3. Jafri SZH, Roberts JL, Bree RL,Tabor HD. Computed tomography of chest wall masses. *Radiographics* 1989;**9**:51-68.
4. Vock P, Owens A. Computed tomography of the normal and pathological thoracic inlet. *Eur J Radiol* 1982;**2**:187-193.
5. Crawford FA. Thoracic outlet syndrome. *Surg Clin North Am* 1980;**60**:947-956.
6. Stallworth JM, Horne JB. Diagnosis and management of thoracic outlet syndrome. *Arch Surg* 1984;**119**:1149-1151.
7. Bilbey JH, Müller NL, Connell DG, Luoma AA, Nelems B. Thoracic outlet syndrome: evaluation with CT. *Radiology* 1989;**171**:381-384.
8. McLoud TC, Isler RJ, Novelline RA, et al. Review: The apical cap. *AJR* 1981;**137**:299-306.
9. Mack LA, Matsen FA III, Kilcoyne RF, Davies PK, Sickler ME. US evaluation of the rotator cuff. *Radiology* 1985;**157**:205-209.
10. Mack LA, Nyberg DA, Matsen FA. Sonographic evaluation of the rotator cuff. *Radiol Clin North Am* 1988;**26**:161-177.
11. Zlatkin MB, Iannotti JP, Roberts MC, Esterhai JL, Dalinka MK, Kressel HY, Schwartz JS, Lenkinski RE. Rotator cuff tears: diagnostic performance of MR imaging. *Radiology* 1989;**172**:223-229.
12. Destouet J M, Gilula LJA, Murphy WA, Sagel SS. Computed tomography of the sternoclavicular joint and sternum. *Radiology* 1981;**138**:123-128.
13. Dillmann W. *Gelenke-Wirbelverbindungen*, 3rd ed. p 228, New York: Thieme Verlag, 1987.
14. Omell GH, Anderson LS, Bramson RT. Chest wall tumours. *Radiol Clin North Am* 1973;**11**:197-214.
15. Stelzer P, Gay WA Jr. Tumours of the chest wall. *Surg Clin North Am* 1980;**60**:779-791.
16. Buxton RC, Tan CS, Khine NM. Atypical transmural thoracic lipoma. *J Comput Assist Tomogr* 1988;**12**:196-198.

17. Press GA, Glazer HS, Wasserman TH, Aronberg DJ, Lee JKT, Sagel SS. Thoracic wall involvement by Hodgkin disease and non-Hodgkin lymphoma: CT evaluation. *Radiology* 1985;**157**:195-198.
18. Khan A, Herman PG. Intrathoracic manifestations of lymphoma. *Semin US CT MR* 1986;**7**:18.
19. Khoury MB,Godwin JD, Halvorsen RA Jr, Hanun Y, Putman CE. Role of chest CT in non-Hodgkin lymphoma. *Radiology* 1986;**158**:659-662.
20. Webb WR, Jeffrey RB, Godwin JD. Thoracic computed tomography in superior sulcus tumours. *J Comput Assist Tomogr* 1981;**5**:361-365.
21. Hatfield MK, Gross BH, Glazer GM, et al. Computed tomography of the sternum and its articulations. *Skeletal Radiol* 1984;**11**:197-203.
22. Stark P. Midline sternal foramen: CT demonstration. *JCAT* 1985;**9**:489-490.
23. Levey GS, Calabro YY. Tietze's syndrome. Report of two cases and review of literature. *Arthritis Rheum* 1962;**5**:261.
24. Boone ML, Swenson BE, Felson B. Rib notching: Its many causes. *AJR* 1964;**91**:1075-1088.
25. Tadavarthy SM, Klugman J, Castaneda-Zuniga WR, Nath PH, Amplatz K. Systemic-to-pulmonary collaterals in pathological states. A review. *Radiology* 1982;**144**:55-59.
26. Sargent EN, Turner AF, Jacobson G. Superior marginal rib defects. An etiologic classification. *AJR* 1969;**106**:491-505.
27. Feigin DS, Madewell JE. In Teplick JG, Haskin ME (eds). *Disorders of the chest wall*, pp. 1294-1319, Surgical Radiology. Philadelphia, WB Saunders, 1981.
28. Sebes JL, Salazar JE. The manubriosternal joint in rheumatoid disease. *AJR* 1983;**140**:117-121.
29. Webb W. Actinomycosis involving the chest wall: CT findings. *AJR* 1982;**139**:1007-1009.
30. Feig SA. Decreased breast cancer mortality through mammographic screening: Results of clinical trials. *Radiology* 1988;**167**:659-665.
31. Turner DA, Alcorn FS, Shorey WD, Stelling CB, Mategrano VC, Merten CW, Silver B, Economou SG, Straus AK, Witt TR, Norusis MJ. Carcinoma of the breast: detection with MR imaging versus xeromammography. *Radiology* 1988;**168**:49-58.
32. Kaiser WA, Zeitler E. MR imaging of the breast: imaging sequences with and without Gd-DTPA. *Radiology* 1989;**170**:681-686.
33. Souba WW, McKenna RJ Jr, Meis J, et al. Radiation-induced sarcomas of the chest wall. *Cancer* 1986;**57**:610-615.
34. Alexander ES, Clark RA, Coley DP, et al. CT of malignant pleural mesothelioma. *AJR* 1981;**137**:287.
35. Adams VI, Unni KK, Muhm JR, et al Diffuse malignant mesothelioma of pleura. Diagnosis and survival in 92 cases. *Cancer* 1986;**58**:1540-1551.
36. Glazer HS, Duncan-Meyer J, Aronberg DJ, Moran JF, Levitt RG, Sagel SS. Pleural and chest wall invasion in bronchogenic carcinoma: CT evaluation. *Radiology* 1985;**157**:191-194.
37. Pearlberg JL, Sandler MA, Beute GH, et al. Limitations of CT in evaluation of neoplasms involving chest wall. *JCAT* 1987;**11**:290.
38. Haggar AM, Pearlberg JL, Froelich JW, et al. Chest-wall invasion by carcinoma of the lung: Detection by MR imaging. *AJR* 1987;**148**:1075-1078.
39. Cho CS, Blank N, Castellino RA. Computerized tomography evaluation of chest wall involvement in lymphoma. *Cancer* 1985;**55**:1892-1894.
40. Ege GN, Clark RM. Internal mammary lymphoscintigraphy in the conservative management of breast carcinoma: Update and recommendations for the new TNM staging. *Clin Radiol* 1985;**36**:469-472.

41. Meyer JE, Munzenrider JE. Computed tomographic demonstration of internal mammary lymph node metastasis in patients with locally recurrent breast carcinoma. *Radiology* 1981;**139**:661-663.
42. Scatarige JC, Fishman EK, Zinreich ES, Brem RF, Almaraz R: Internal mammary lymphadenopathy in breast carcinoma: CT appraisal of anatomic distribution. *Radiology* 1988;**167**:89-91.
43. Vock P, Hodler J. Cardiophrenic angle adenopathy: Update of causes and significance. *Radiology* 1986;**159**:395-399.
44. Long JA, Doppman JL, Nienhuis AW. Computed tomographic studies of thoracic extramedullary haematopoiesis. *J Comput Assist Tomogr* 1980;**4**:67-70.
45. Savader SJ, Otero RR, Savader BL. MR imaging of intrathoracic extramedullary haematopoiesis. *J Comput Assist Tomogr* 1988;**12**:878-881.
46. Karnaze MG, Godo MH, Sartor KY, et al. Comparison of MR and CT myelography in imaging the cervical and thoracic spine. *AJNR* 1987;**8**:983.
47. Modic MT, Hardy RW, Weinstein MA, et al. Nuclear magnetic resonance of the spine: Clinical and potential limitations. *Neurosurgery* 1984;**15**:583-592.
48. VanLom KY, Kellerhouse LE, Pathria MN, Moreland SI, et al. Infection versus tumour in the spine: Criteria for distinction with CT. *Radiology* 1988;**166**:851.
49. Berkmen YM. Radiologic aspects of intrathoracic sarcoidosis. *Semin Roentgenol* 1985;**20**:356.
50. Hudson TM, Hamlin DJ, Enneking WF, Pettersson H. Magnetic resonance in imaging of bone and soft tissue tumours: Early experience in 31 patients compared with computed tomography. *Skeletal Radiol* 1985;**13**:134-146.

Magnetic resonance imaging of the brachial plexus

Lynne S. Steinbach and Charles Higgins
University of California, San Francisco, California, USA

Introduction

A variety of abnormalities can produce brachial plexopathy and patients with this problem are difficult to evaluate. Trauma, with avulsion of the lower cervical nerve roots, is a leading cause of brachial plexopathy. When non-traumatic, there is the underlying question of whether the plexopathy is a pathological lesion or idiopathic. Idiopathic brachial plexopathy is a self-limiting disorder with symptoms usually resolving within 3 years, whereas plexus mass lesions are usually due to neoplasm, especially metastases [1-7]. The presence of a neoplasm in the lung, breast, or elsewhere in the body raises suspicion for direct or metastatic invasion of the plexus. Brachial plexopathy is often seen in patients following radiation therapy for neoplasms such as lung or breast carcinoma.

The brachial plexus is difficult to examine clinically because the nerves lie deep within the neck and axilla and are not accessible to the palpating hand. Palpable masses in this region signify advanced disease. Neurologic signs and symptoms can be subtle or confusing. Patients frequently complain of pain or numbness in the neck or shoulder, paraesthesias, or upper extremity weakness. It is important to exclude other causes of such symptoms including cervical spondylitis, peripheral nerve entrapment syndromes, rotator cuff tears, vascular insufficiencies, and thoracic outlet syndrome. Even with the aid of electromyography (EMG), a clinician may have difficulty with localization along the length of the brachial plexus [8]. EMGs can be incomplete and misleading and cannot distinguish between a mass and other causes of plexopathy [5,9,10]. These patients require a reliable method for localizing and characterizing a lesion and distinguishing identifiable pathology from idiopathic brachial plexopathy.

Prior to magnetic resonance imaging (MRI), conventional radiographs, myelography, and computed tomography (CT) were utilized for evaluation of the brachial plexus. Conventional radiographs were useful only for demonstrating osseous abnormalities that might be impinging on the nerves, such as cervical osteophytes or fractures, enlarged C7 transverse processes, cervical ribs, or clavicular pathology such as a mass or fracture. Soft tissue masses were not usually seen unless they contained calcification or displaced fat planes. Myelography was invasive and limited to evaluation of the structures within and adjacent to the thecal sac including the cervical spinal cord, the dura, and the nerve roots [8]. CT provided better soft tissue contrast discrimination, allowing for more precise and non-invasive evaluation of the peripheral components of the brachial plexus. Disadvantages included shoulder artefact from beam hardening from the humeral head and scapula as well as difficulty in discriminating vascular structures from nerves and masses, even with the aid of intravenous contrast. The CT was also limited to the axial plane, which was better for demonstrating the more central components of the brachial plexus such as the neural foramina, and not as helpful for evaluating the portion of the plexus that courses in an oblique plane - the nerve trunks and roots [6,7,11-17].

MRI is being increasingly utilized for the evaluation of disease of the brachial plexus. Patients are evaluated for two reasons: (1) symptoms referable to the brachial plexus such as pain or neural deficit; or (2) pathology, usually a mass, suspected to be in the region of the brachial plexus. Advantages of MRI include high soft-tissue contrast, direct multiplanar imaging capability, non-invasiveness, lack of ionizing radiation, and lack of beam hardening artefact. Problems that can exist with MRI include artefacts from respiratory and cardiac motion, but these are not usually significant.

Anatomy

A thorough knowledge of the complex anatomy of this region is required for interpreting images of the brachial plexus (Fig. 1).The brachial plexus supplies nerve fibres primarily to the upper extremity, parallelling the course of the subclavian and axillary arteries into the axilla. It is composed of the anterior rami from nerve roots of C5 to T1, with occasional contributions from C4 and T2. It is usually comprised of five roots, three trunks, six divisions, three cords, and terminal peripheral nerves

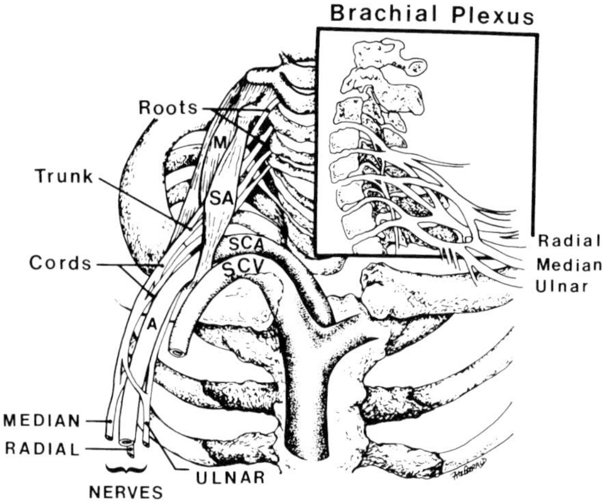

Figure 1. *NORMAL ANATOMY IN THE REGION OF THE BRACHIAL PLEXUS. The roots of the brachial plexus are seen between the anterior and middle scalene muscles and posterosuperior to the subclavian artery. The trunks begin lateral to the scalene muscles and divide into three cords which surround the axillary artery. The cords terminate in peripheral branches that include the median, radial and ulnar nerves. Abbreviations: SA, anterior scalene muscle; M, middle scalene muscle; SCA, subclavian artery; SCV, subclavian vein; A axillary artery.*

Roots

At the level of the seventh cervical and first thoracic vertebra, the brachial plexus roots are formed between the anterior and middle scalene muscles. The intermediate signal intensity roots can be identified on axial and coronal MRI as they exit the intervertebral foramina and course anterolaterally, posterior to the subclavian artery and anterior scalene muscle and anterior to the middle scalene muscle (Figs. 2a and 3). Since the roots course posterior to the vertebral

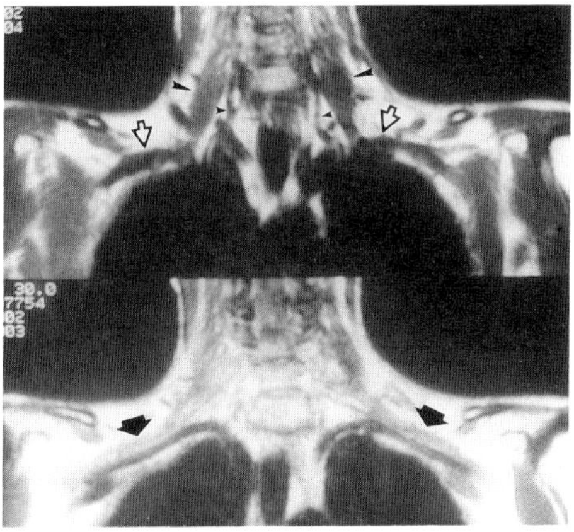

(a)

(b)

Figure 2. *NORMAL BRACHIAL PLEXUS IN THE CORONAL PLANE. (a) (top) On this T1-weighted MR image, the visualization of the anterior scalene muscles large arrowheads indicate a tomographic level just anterior to brachial plexus. The vertebral arteries are also located anterior to the roots of the brachial plexus (small arrowheads). The low signal intensity subclavian veins are seen above the lung apices (open arrows). (b) (bottom) The adjacent slice demonstrates the course of the brachial plexus which travels parallel and cranial to the subclavian arteries (arrows).*

artery and anterior scalene muscle and anterior to the middle scalene muscle, the important coronal MR images for evaluation of the roots are between these structures (Fig. 2). The subclavian vein, which is usually larger in diameter than the corresponding artery, lies anterior to the anterior scalene muscle beneath the clavicle and subclavius muscle. Although they are usually low signal intensity, the vessels may contain higher signal intensity, caused in some cases by flow-related enhancement. The anterior scalene muscle arises from the transverse process of the third through seventh cervical vertebrae and extends infero-laterally to insert on the first rib. The middle scalene muscle is bulkier, longer, and slightly higher in signal intensity than

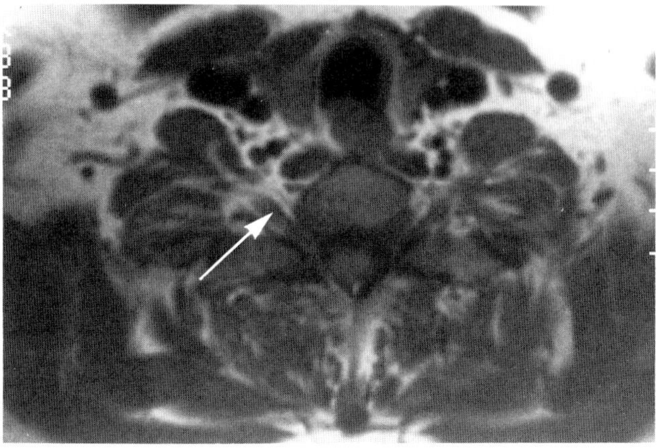

Figure 3. *NORMAL BRACHIAL PLEXUS IN THE AXIAL PLANE (AT THE LEVEL OF THE THYROID). Proximally on this T1-weighted MR image, the intermediate signal intensity nerve roots (arrowhead) lie behind the low signal intensity subclavian artery. Distally, the nerves lie between the anterior and middle scalene muscles (arrow).*

the anterior scalene muscle, and arises from the posterior aspect of the transverse processes of the second to seventh cervical vertebra, with a broad insertion along the first rib. The posterior scalene muscle often merges with the middle scalene muscle, and arises from the transverse processes of the fifth to seventh cervical vertebrae inserting on the outer surface of the second rib. There is a groove in the first rib between the insertions of the anterior and middle scalene muscles which is traversed by the subclavian artery and brachial plexus.

Trunks

At the lateral border of the scalene muscles, three trunks are formed. The C5 and C6 nerve roots unite to form the upper trunk, the roots of C7 supply the middle trunk, and C8 and T1 nerve roots supply the lower trunk. The intermediate signal intensity trunks of the brachial plexus lie in a supraclavicular position parallelling the course of the low signal intensity subclavian artery, well seen on coronal MRI (Fig. 2b).

Divisions and cords

Each of the three trunks of the brachial plexus divides into an anterior and posterior division. The anterior and posterior divisions supply the flexor and extensor muscles of the upper extremity, respectively. The divisions then merge into cords. The relative position of the cords to the axillary artery gives rise to their respective names - lateral, posterior and medial. The divisions and cords lie lateral to the anterior scalene muscle and extend behind the clavicle and pectoralis muscle and inferior to the coracoid process into the axilla. The cords are best seen in cross section on sagittal MRI (Fig. 4). Distal to the pectoralis muscle, the brachial plexus divides into terminal nerve branches that supply the upper extremity. The terminal nerve branches will not be discussed in this chapter.

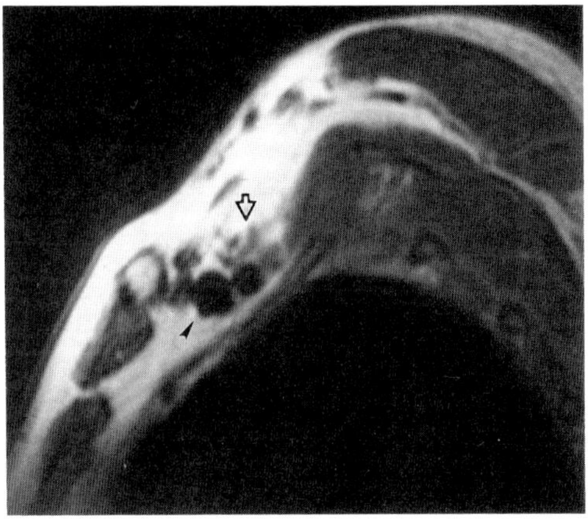

Figure 4. *NORMAL BRACHIAL PLEXUS IN THE SAGITTAL PLANE. On T1-weighted MRI the low signal intensity subclavian vein (arrowhead) lies anterior to the artery. The intermediate signal intensity nerves are located posterior and superior to the subclavian artery, surrounded by high signal intensity fat.*

MRI Technique

Since the brachial plexus takes a long, oblique course from the neck to the upper arm, it is preferable to image in multiple planes. We prefer to image both sides of the brachial plexus, utilizing T1-weighted pulse sequences for depicting the anatomy in the region. T2-weighted or similar sequences are then obtained for further characterization of pathology such as a mass, haemorrhage, fibrosis, or inflammation. Gradient-echo sequences tend to image the brachial plexus with decreased signal-to-noise and spatial resolution, and we do not use them routinely.

Most patients examined for brachial plexopathy at our institution are imaged using a spin-echo technique based upon diagnostic effectiveness and economy of imaging times (Table). The study begins with T1-weighted images of both sides of the brachial plexus in the coronal plane with the body coil or a transverse rectangular coil placed posteriorly in the interscapular region. This acquisition is usually electrocardiogram (ECG) gated (TR = RR interval of the ECG). The field of view varies between 32 and 38 cm. This is followed by proton density and T2-weighted spin-echo images of both sides of the brachial plexus in the axial plane using a neck coil with a field of view of (FOV) 28 - 34 cm. On all sequences the matrix is 256 × 192 with 2 number of exitations (NEX) and a 5 mm slice thickness. The entire study takes approximately 20 minutes of scan time.

Table. *Routine MRI protocol for imaging the brachial plexus*

Plane	Pulse sequence (TR:TE)	Slice thickness (mm)	Skip (mm)	Matrix	FOV (cm)	NEX
Coronal[a]	SE 600; 25	5	0	192	38	2
Axial[b]	SE 2000; 25/60	5	2	192	32	2

a. Body coil or transverse rectangular coil.
b. Neck coil.

Further study of an area of interest can be done with surface coil images [18-20]. Surface coil images can be obtained in the axial plane to evaluate nerve roots or in the coronal or sagittal planes to look at the trunks or cords, respectively. One can use a shoulder coil or two five inch receive-only surface coils placed in a Helmholtz configuration anterior and posterior to the apex of the lung and supraclavicular fossa. With surface coil imaging, we use a slice thickness of 3 mm and a FOV of 20 - 24 cm. In general, respiratory gating is not needed. It is helpful to reduce motion artefact (ghosting) by placing the frequency-encoded axis in the plane of respiratory motion. One investigator has recommended the use of additional T1-weighted sequences following intravenous administration of gadolinium-DTPA for further characterization of lesions such as scar or tumour [21]. We have found the use of contrast media advantageous in the evaluation of the brachial plexus after operation in order to distinguish scar from chronic inflammation. With further experience it may also prove useful for the assessment of tumours.

Pathology

MRI is useful for demonstrating pathology in the region of the brachial plexus. The high soft tissue contrast allows for accurate assessment of posttraumatic and postoperative lesions, metastases, primary tumours, inflammation and scarring (including that produced by radiation), and anatomical impingement of the plexus. Lack of visualization of an abnormality suggests an intact brachial plexus, although the patient may be experiencing symptoms caused by an idiopathic brachial plexopathy. It is assumed that stretch injuries of the nerves can be missed by all imaging studies including MRI.

Trauma

Trauma to the brachial plexus is sometimes seen after a patient has been involved in a motorcycle, traffic, or sports accident. A common mechanism in these patients is direct traction on the plexus caused by shoulder compression or dislocation with fixation of the brachial plexus between the clavicle and first rib. Brachial plexus injuries may be divided into supraclavicular and infraclavicular lesions. In general, supraclavicular injuries are more damaging than infraclavicular injuries [22].

Supraclavicular injuries may be divided into pre- and post-ganglionic types. If the lesion is between the spinal ganglion and the medulla, it is preganglionic. These patients can have meningoceles, which are well seen on MRI extending from the involved neural foramina with signal characteristics similar to cerebrospinal fluid.

Horner's syndrome, which is associated with anhidrosis, miosis, enophthalmos, ptosis, and paralysis of several muscles including the levators and rhomboids, is seen with avulsions of the T1 nerve root.

Postganglionic lesions occur when the spinal nerve is ruptured and the nerve roots are intact. These patients are prone to proximal stump and neuroma formation, and do not have meningoceles. The eighth cervical and first thoracic nerve roots are more susceptible to preganglionic or avulsion injuries, due to the fact that these nerves do not have musculo-tendinous attachments to the transverse processes and vertebral artery. We have observed a characteristic 'hammocking' of the trunks and cords of the brachial plexus on MRI following traumatic avulsion of the nerve roots from the spinal cord (Fig. 5). The fifth to seventh cervical nerve roots are more firmly attached centrally and they are therefore more vulnerable to postganglionic injury. Spinal nerve injury can result in oedematous infiltration of the tissue surrounding the nerves resulting in increased signal intensity on T2-weighting [18].

Patients involved in accidents may also receive fractures of the lower cervical transverse processes, first rib, or clavicle. Fresh clavicular fractures usually cause extensive supraclavicular traction injuries to the brachial plexus, since they permit increased mobility of the tissues between the head and shoulder [22,23]. The fracture fragments can compress the brachial plexus. These injuries are often accompanied by vascular damage and resulting haematoma. In patients with signs and symptoms of brachial plexopathy several months following fracture, MRI is useful for demonstrating external compression upon the brachial plexus caused by mal-union or non-union of the fracture fragments or due to scarring and callus formation (Fig. 6). Such patients may require correction or resection of the bone and soft tissue responsible for compression.

Stabbing or gunshot wounds to the area may be associated with nerve transection. A haematoma associated with rupture of the surrounding vessels can compress the brachial plexus (Fig. 7). Haemorrhage will have different characteristics on MRI, depending upon its stage of evolution [24-29]. Acute haemorrhage is usually low signal intensity on T1-weighted images due to the presence of deoxyhaemoglobin in intact red blood cells. On T2-weighting, the more central portion of an area of haemorrhage or haematoma contains more deoxyhaemoglobin and may remain low signal intensity, particularly at higher field strengths, due to magnetic suscepti-

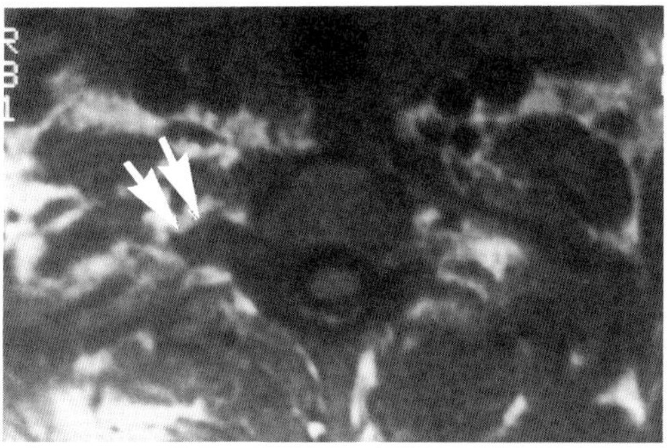

(a)

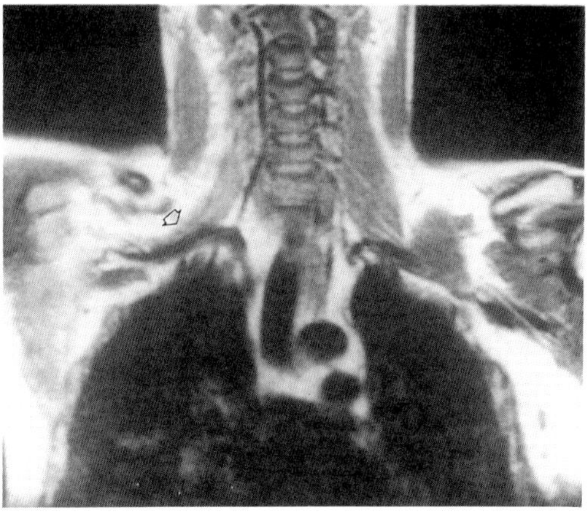

(b)

Figure 5. *THIS PATIENT HAD RIGHT ARM PARALYSIS FOLLOWING A TRAUMATIC AVULSION OF THE C8 NERVE ROOT DURING A MOTOR VEHICLE ACCIDENT. An MRI was obtained 4 months following the injury. (a) Axial T1-weighted MRI demonstrates a low signal intensity mass in the right neural foramina (arrows), later found to be a neuroma. (b) There is thickening and loss of definition of the nerve trunks on the right on coronal proton density MRI (open arrow). There is also a characteristic 'hammocking' of the nerve trunks, occasionally seen in patients with cervical nerve root avulsion.*

bility of the deoxyhaemoglobin, while the periphery oxidizes more rapidly to methaemoglobin, displaying a higher signal intensity. Subacute and chronic haemorrhage are characterized by methaemoglobin, resulting in a shortening of T1 relaxation time and a lengthening of T2 relaxation time which causes high signal intensity on T1- and T2-weighted spin-echo sequences. With time, haeme iron is converted by macrophages into haemosiderin, which lines the margin of the

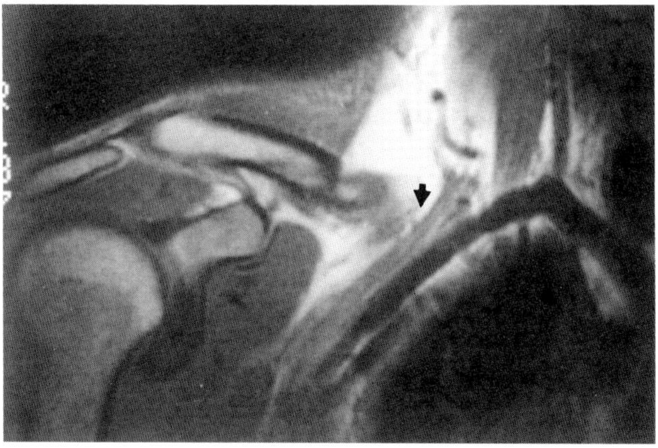

Figure 6. *THE CLAVICLE OF THIS MAN WAS FRACTURED DURING A MOTORCYCLE INJURY SEVERAL MONTHS PRIOR TO THIS MRI. There is exuberant callus formation and scarring around the fracture, causing compression of the superior aspect of the brachial plexus (arrow).*

haematoma and produces a low signal intensity rim that has magnetic susceptibility and is most evident on higher field strength images, and those obtained with T2-weighting or gradient echo technique.

Other patients may experience trauma to the brachial plexus following anaesthesia or axillary arteriography, with resultant symptoms from nerve transection, haematoma, or ischaemia [30-34]. Post-anaesthetic palsy results from injury to the brachial plexus following a surgical procedure unrelated to the brachial plexus. Patients usually have an excellent recovery from this disorder. Posttraumatic neuromas may be seen following trauma or surgery and are characterized on MRI as well-defined masses in the region of the brachial plexus that are of intermediate signal intensity on T1-weighting and increased signal intensity on T2-weighting (Fig. 8). There may be multiple neuromas in the region of the brachial plexus, since many nerves are involved.

Tumours

It is important to identify the presence of a mass or infiltration along the course of the brachial plexus. The distinction must be made between a mass that is adjacent to the plexus but not displacing or

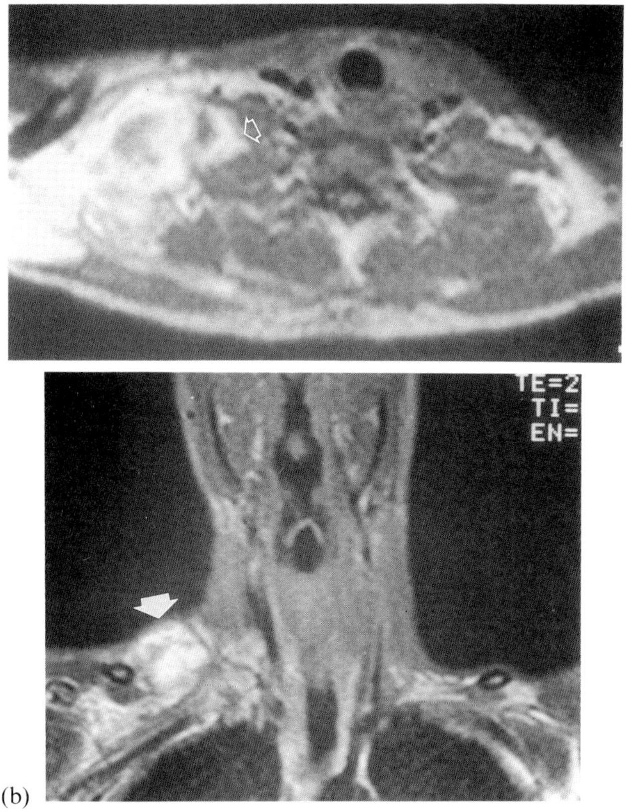

(a)

(b)

Figure 7. *A HAEMATOMA DEVELOPED IN THE SUPRACLAVICULAR AREA AT THE SITE OF A RECENT GUNSHOT WOUND. (a) Axial T1-weighted MRI shows an extensive haematoma infiltrating into the area of the brachial plexus, between the anterior and middle scalene muscles (open white arrow). The haematoma is characteristically high signal intensity in the periphery and low signal intensity centrally. (b) The haematoma lies just above the brachial plexus on T2-weighted coronal MRI (arrow).*

compressing it, and one that actually compresses or invades the brachial plexus or subclavian artery. Such a mass is more likely to be malignant; however the diagnosis cannot be certain. It should be remembered that benign tumours such as aggressive fibromatosis and invasive lipomas can simulate malignant tumours on MRI due to their invasive tendencies. MRI can be utilized to demonstrate the degree of invasion of a tumour in relation to the structures surrounding the

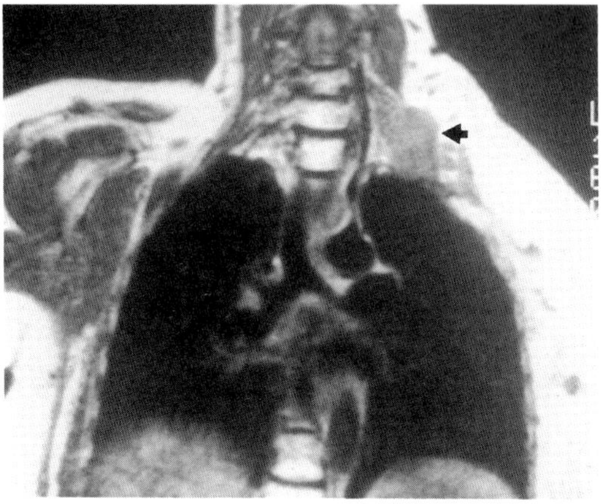

Figure 8. *THIS WOMAN HAD AN AMPUTATION OF HER ARM AND SHOULDER GIRDLE 22 YEARS PRIOR TO THIS MRI. In the interim, she formed multiple neuromas in the region of the brachial plexus. Coronal T1-weighted MRI demonstrates a homogeneous, fusiform, intermediate signal intensity mass in the region of the brachial plexus consistent with a postamputation neuroma (arrow).*

brachial plexus, including the subclavian vessels, oesophagus, trachea, and chest wall.

Secondary Tumours

Metastasis to the brachial plexus is the most common aetiology of brachial plexopathy [35]. The brachial plexus is commonly affected by metastatic spread from primary tumours in the lung, breast, stomach, oesophagus, kidney, and head and neck. Metastases to the region of the brachial plexus can produce loss of the normal landmarks due to infiltration of the surrounding fat by tumour or a mass. Because of high soft tissue contrast on the T2-weighted image, MRI is particularly useful in identifying infiltrative metastases that may not be detected by CT (Fig. 9), and alteration in signal intensity in the muscles adjacent to the brachial plexus may be a sign of tumour invasion. Occasionally, metastases will not be detected with MRI [19].

The brachial plexus can also be involved through direct spread from a Pancoast tumour of the lung [17]. This is better seen with MRI than CT [11]. It is important to determine if there is preservation of the thin rim of adipose tissue (and fat or fat pad) that sepa-

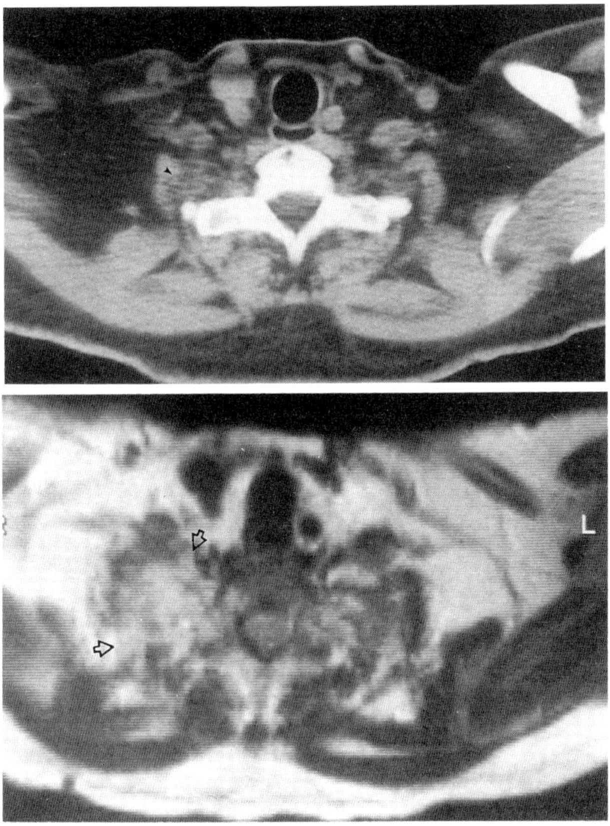

(a)

(b)

Figure 9. *THIS PATIENT HAD KNOWN BREAST CANCER AND SYMPTOMS OF BRACHIAL PLEXOPATHY. (a) CT shows a subtle low attenuation mass on the right in the region of the brachial plexus, infiltrating the middle scalene muscle (arrow). (b) T2-weighted MRI further delineates the extent of the high signal intensity metastasis which invades the scalene muscles, altering their signal intensity (open arrow).*

rates the apex of the lung from other structures above the lung apex, including blood vessels and the brachial plexus. When the tumour extends beyond the lung apex superiorly, the normally intact apical fat pad above the lung is invaded. This is easily visualized on sagittal and coronal T1-weighted MRI (Fig. 10). Most Pancoast tumours are inhomogeneous with predominantly low signal intensity on T1-weighted images and high signal intensity on T2-weighted images. Besides demonstrating involvement of the brachial plexus, knowledge

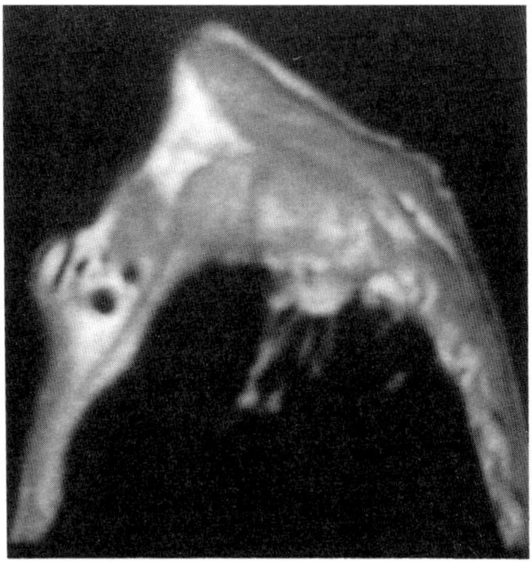

Figure 10. *PROTON DENSITY SAGITTAL MRI DEMONSTRATES A PANCOAST TUMOUR THAT EXTENDS THROUGH THE APICAL FAT INTO THE SOFT TISSUES SUPERIOR AND ANTERIOR TO THE LUNG. The tumour is surrounding the nerves of the brachial plexus, just above the subclavian artery.*

of invasion of a Pancoast tumour beyond the lung is important information for use in therapeutic decision-making. When a Pancoast tumour extends beyond the lung parenchyma superiorly into the chest wall, surgery is usually deferred in favour of radiation therapy [11].

Lymphoma can involve the lymph nodes in the region of the brachial plexus [36], compressing the nerves with resultant symptoms of brachial plexopathy (Fig. 11). Other secondary tumours that we have seen on MRI in the region of the brachial plexus include aggressive fibromatosis and haemangiomatosis. These benign tumours were extensive with indistinct margins and produced compression of the neighbouring brachial plexus.

Primary Neurogenic Tumours

The primary tumours of the brachial plexus include benign and malignant neurogenic tumours [3]. These are most commonly benign neuromas, schwannomas (also referred to as neurilemmomas) and neurofibromas. Benign neural tumours are slow-growing, and produce symptoms of pain, tenderness, paraesthesias, or functional impairment in the distribution of the brachial plexus. They are usually too deep in the soft tissues to be palpable.

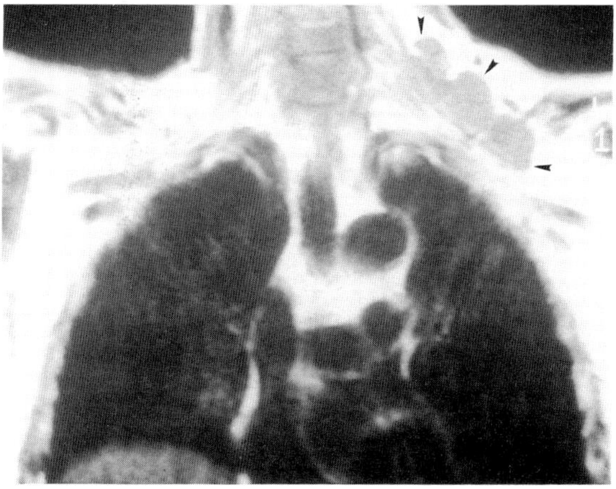

Figure 11. *T1-WEIGHTED CORONAL MRI FROM A PATIENT WITH LYMPHOMA, shows multiple enlarged intermediate signal intensity lymph nodes compressing the roots and trunks of the brachial plexus on the left (arrowheads).*

Neuromas are non-neoplastic proliferations of neural tissue created in the proximal stump of a severed nerve and are seen following trauma or surgery. They are usually homogeneous and well-defined and are seen along the course of the brachial plexus (Fig. 8).

The schwannoma arises from Schwann cells and is eccentric, but intraneural. It can usually be removed surgically without disruption of nerve function. Recurrence or malignant transformation is rare [37].

Neurofibromas are not encapsulated and infiltrate the surrounding nerve fascicles, making it more difficult to remove without impairing nerve function. Neurofibromas can be solitary and unrelated to neurofibromatosis (von Recklinghausen's disease) or they can be multiple and related to the disease which is an autosomal dominant disorder. There is a 15 - 30% chance of malignant degeneration in neurofibromatosis [22].

Neurogenic tumours are characterized on MRI as wellcircum-scribed round or cylindrical lesions. A mass in the region of the brachial plexus in a patient without a known carcinoma suggests the diagnosis of primary neural tumour. On MRI, neural tumours are usually low or intermediate signal intensity on T1-weighted images and intermediate to high signal intensity on T2-weighted images (Fig. 12). The more collagenous, hypocellular lesions can present with low

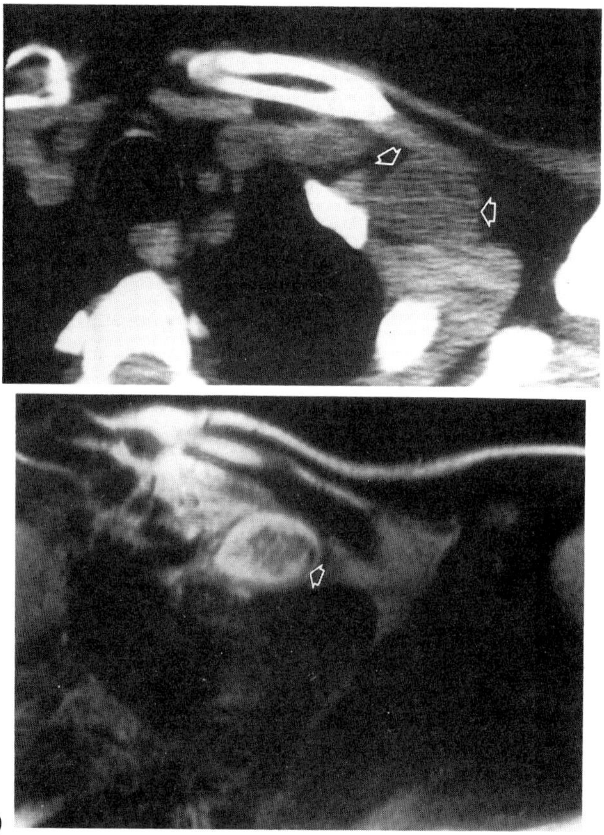

(a)

(b)

Figure 12. *THIS PATIENT HAD A BRACHIAL PLEXUS SCHWANNOMA. (a) CT shows a round, homogeneous low attenuation mass in the region of the brachial plexus on the left side (open white arrows). (b) The schwannoma is better delineated on a T2-weighted axial MRI as an inhomogeneous high signal intensity mass in this region (open white arrow).*

signal intensity on T2-weighted images [38]. Neural tumours can be inhomogeneous and may contain central areas of low signal intensity. It is difficult to distinguish benign from malignant neural tumours, and a tissue diagnosis is required in suspected cases of malignancy.

Other causes of Brachial Plexopathy

Radiation injury to the brachial plexus represents another cause of brachial plexopathy in patients with cancer. These patients are frequently irradiated in the supraclavicular fossa for primary treatment of lymphoma, head-and-neck, breast, or lung tumours. Radiation therapy may also be indicated for patients with recurrent or metastatic carcinoma. Involvement of the brachial plexus following radiation therapy is unusual at doses less than 6 000 rads but has been reported at doses as low as 4800 rads. The onset of brachial plexopathy following radiation therapy can range from 18 months to 10 years [39].

MRI can demonstrate abnormalities associated with radiation injury; however it is non-specific. Infiltration of the tissue surrounding the brachial plexus with abnormal signal intensity can be seen at all stages following radiation therapy. The time required for fibrotic repair is variable [40]. Early stages will usually display an infiltrative pattern on MRI with signal intensity characteristics consistent with oedema, necrosis, or granulation tissue, demonstrating increased signal on T2-weighted images. The problem here is that infiltrative tumour may also have this appearance and cannot be distinguished from radiation change. With maturation of the granulation tissue to fibrous tissue, the MRI will display low signal intensity infiltration of the soft tissues surrounding the brachial plexus on all imaging sequences (Fig. 13). This finding is non-specific, however, and we have seen one patient with a recurrent scirrhous breast carcinoma in this region who displayed such signal characteristics.

Inflammation of the nerves of the brachial plexus (neuritis) can have a variety of aetiologies or may be idiopathic [4,9]. In some patients, it is believed to be caused by an infection or a hypersensitivity reaction and has been seen in patients who have received sera or vaccines. It can also be seen in patients with primary malignancies without evidence of metastatic involvement of the brachial plexus [5]. In these patients, the disorder is usually self-limiting. We have observed such a patient with MRI who had renal cell carcinoma. The nerves of the brachial plexus were indistinct and demonstrated high signal intensity on T2-weighting, consistent with inflammation (Fig. 14).

Thoracic outlet syndrome represents a symptomatic disorder related to anatomic impingement upon the brachial plexus in the region of

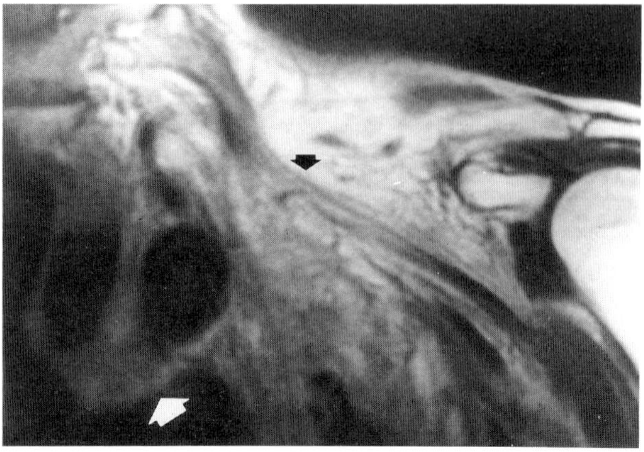

Figure 13. *THIS PATIENT HAD IRRADIATION OF THE LUNG AND SUPRACLAVICULAR REGION FOR TREATMENT OF BREAST CARCINOMA MANY YEARS PRIOR TO THIS MRI EXAMINATION, AND WAS NOW SYMPTOMATIC. T1-weighted coronal MRI obtained with a surface coil demonstrates the indistinct nature of the nerves of the brachial plexus and infiltration of the surrounding fat by low signal intensity scar tissue (black arrow). There is also extensive scarring and bullae in the left lung apex (white arrow).*

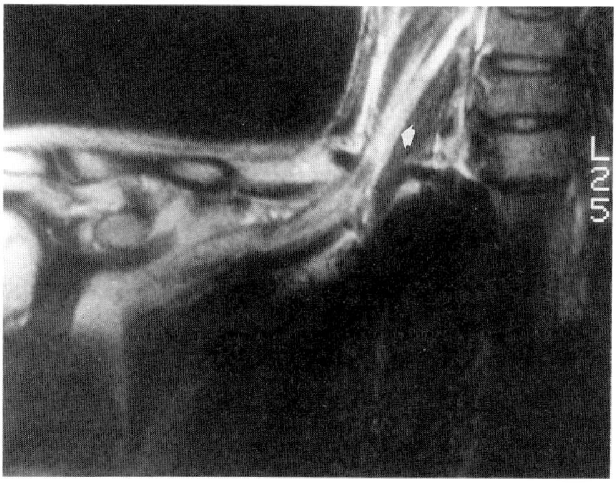

Figure 14. *THIS 31-YEAR-OLD WOMAN HAD A HISTORY OF RENAL CELL CARCINOMA AND NEW ARM PAIN. There is abnormally high signal intensity in the roots and trunks of the brachial plexus on T2-weighted coronal MRI, consistent with neuritis (white arrow).*

the thoracic outlet [41,42]. MRI can be utilized to demonstrate impingement upon the brachial plexus by these normal anatomic variants. Soft tissue structures that can predispose to brachial plexus impingement include anomalous soft tissue bands and an anomalous relationship of the scalene muscles to the transverse processes [43]. Osseous impingement may be caused by cervical ribs, or abnormally long, drooping transverse processes at the C7 level. The symptoms of thoracic outlet syndrome are intermittent and are often positional. It may occur or intensify when an arm is raised, which causes anatomic crowding. It is suggested that an additional T1-weighted MRI sequence be obtained in patients with thoracic outlet syndrome with the arm raised above the head in an attempt to demonstrate an impingement that could be missed with conventional MRI.

Conclusion

MRI is the procedure of choice for imaging patients with brachial plexopathy. In contrast to CT, where vessels and nerves must be differentiated using intravenous contrast, these structures have differing signal intensity on MRI. CT is limited to the axial plane, while MRI can image directly in multiple planes, allowing for better evaluation of the brachial plexus. The coronal and sagittal planes are particularly helpful for imaging the brachial plexus beyond the roots. Beam-hardening artefacts produced by cortical bone in the shoulders on CT is not present with MRI. Abnormalities that can be well seen include secondary tumours such as Pancoast tumours, where a sagittal MR image is helpful for determining involvement of the chest wall and brachial plexus. Alteration in signal intensity in adjacent muscle may be a sign of tumour spread, not well appreciated on CT. Primary neurogenic tumours are identified with MRI in the path of the brachial plexus. Posttraumatic problems such as impingement of the plexus by fracture callus, the presence of neuromas following nerve laceration, haematoma, and nerve root avulsion are demonstrated with MRI. Inflammation of the nerve can present with thickened nerve roots, trunks, and cords while radiation fibrosis can be seen within the supraclavicular fossa surrounding the nerves, but the MRI appearance is non-specific. MRI can also be used to show osseous and soft tissue compression of the brachial plexus in thoracic outlet syndrome.

References

1. Thomas J, Colby M. Radiation-induced or metastatic brachial plexopathy? *JAMA* 1972;**222**:1392-5.
2. Handler S, Canalis R, Jenkins Weiss A. Management of brachial plexus tumors. *Arch Otolaryngol* 1977;**103**:653-7.
3. Dart LH, MacCarty CS, Love JG, Dockerty M. Neoplasms of the brachial plexus. *Minn Med* 1970;**53**:959-64.
4. Tsairis P, Dyck P, Mulder D. Natural history of brachial plexus neuropathy. *Arch Neurol* 1972;**27**:109-17.
5. Kori S, Foley K, Posner J. Brachial plexus lesions in patients with cancer: 100 cases. *Neurology* 1981;**31**:45-50.
6. Usselman JA, Vint VC, Waltz TA. CT demonstration of a brachial plexus neuroma. *AJNR* 1980;**1**:346-7.
7. Webb WR, Jeffrey RB, Godwin JD. Thoracic computed tomography in superior sulcus tumors. *J Comput Assist Tomogr* 1981;**5**:361-5.
8. Armington WG, Harnsberger HR, Osborn AG, Seay AR. Radiographic evaluation of brachial plexopathy. *AJNR* 1987;**8**:361-7.
9. Pezzimenti JF, Bruckner HW, DeConti RC. Paralytic brachial neuritis in Hodgkin's disease. *Cancer* 1973;**31**:626-9.
10. Synek VM, Cowan JC. Somatosensory evoked potentials in patients with metastatic involvement of the brachial plexus. *Electromygr Clin Neurophysiol* 1983;**23**:545-51.
11. Heelan RT, Demas BE, Caravelli JF, Martini N, Bains MS, McCormack PM, Burt M, Panicek DM, Mitzner A. Superior sulcus tumors: CT and MR imaging. *Radiology* 1989;**170**:637-41.
12. Gebarski KS, Glazer GM, Gebarski SS. Brachial plexus: anatomic, radiologic, and pathologic correlation using computed tomography. *J Comput Assist Tomogr* 1982;**6**:1058-63.
13. Cascino TL, Kori S, Krol G, Foley KM. CT of the brachial plexus in patients with cancer. *Neurology* 1983;**33**:1553-1557.
14. Stewart JD, Schmidt B, Wee R. Computed tomography in the evaluation of plexopathies and proximal neuropathies. *Can J Neurol Sci* 1983;**10**:244-7.
15. Takasugi JE, Godwin JD, Halvorsen RE, Williford ME, Silverman PM, Putman CE. Computed tomographic evaluation of lesions in the thoracic apex. *Invest Radiol* 1985;**33**:1553-7.
16. Powers SK, Norman D, Edwards MSB. Computerized tomography of peripheral nerve lesions. *J Neurosurg* 1983;**59**:131-6.
17. Vock P, Owens A. Computed tomography of the normal and pathological thoracic inlet. *Europ J Radiol* 1982;**2**:187-93.
18. Rapoport S, Blair DN, McCarthy SM, Desser TS, Hammers LW, Sostman HD. Brachial plexus: correlation of MR imaging with CT and pathologic findings. *Radiology* 1988;**167**:161-5.
19. Kneeland JB, Kellman GM, Middleton WD, Cates JD, Jesmanowicz A, Wojciech F, Hyde JS. Diagnosis of diseases of the supraclavicular region by use of MR imaging. *AJR* 1987;**148**:1149-51.
20. Castagno AA, Shuman WP. MR imaging in clinically suspected brachial plexus tumor. *AJR* 1987;**149**:1219-22.
21. Nelson MC, Stull MA, Freedman MT. MR evaluation of the brachial plexus: pre- and post-gadolinium. *Invest Radiol* 1990;**25**:1368.
22. Green D. *Operative Hand Surgery* 2nd Ed. New York: Churchill Livingstone, 1988.
23. Alnot JX. Traumatic brachial plexus palsy in the adult. *Clin Orth* 1988;**237**:9-16.

24. Cohen MD, McGuire W, Cory DA, Smith JA. MR appearance of blood and blood products: an in vitro study. *AJR* 1986;**146**:1293-7.
25. Gomori J, Grossman Rl, Goldberg HI, Zimmerman RA, Bilaniuk LT. Intracranial hematomas: imaging by high-field MR. *Radiology* 1985;**157**:87-93.
26. Edelman RR, Johnson K, Buxton R, Shoukimas G, Rosen BR, Davis KR, Brady TJ. MR of hemorrhage: a new approach. *AJNR* 1986;**7**:751-6.
27. Bradley WGJr, Schmidt PG. Effect of methemoglobin formation on the MR appearance of subarachnoid hemorrhage. *Radiology* 1985;**156**:99-103.
28. Swensen SJ, Keller PL, Berquist TH, McLeod RA, Stephens DH. Magnetic resonance imaging of hemorrhage. *AJR* 1985;**145**:921-7.
29. Unger EC, Glazer HS, Lee JKT, Ling D. MRI of extracranial hematomas: preliminary observations. *AJR* 1986;**146**:403-7.
30. Orkin FK, Cooperman LH. *Complications of anesthesia*, pp 648-54. Philadelphia: J.B. Lippincott, 1983.
31. Jackson L, Keats AS. Mechanisms of brachial plexus palsy following anesthesia. *Anesthesiology* 1965;**26**:190-4.
32. O'Keefe DM. Brachial plexus injury following axillary arteriography. *J Neurosurg* 1980;**53**:853-7.
33. Molnar W, Paul DJ. Complications of axillary arteriotomies. An analysis of 1,762 consecutive studies. *Radiology* ;**104**:269-76.
34. Lyon BB, Hansen BA, Mygind T. Peripheral nerve injury as a complication of axillary arteriography. *Acta Neurol Scand* 1975;**51**:29-36.
35. Posner JB. Neurological complications of systemic cancer. *Med Clin North Am* 1979;**63**:783-800.
36. Wechsler RJ, Rao VM, Newman LM. The subclavian triangle: CT analysis. *AJR* 1989;**152**:313-7.
37. Carstens H, Schrodt G. Malignant transformation of a benign encapsulated neurilemmoma. *Am J Clin Pathol* 1969;**51**:144.
38. Sundaram M, McGuire MH, Schajowicz F. Soft tissue masses: histologic basis for decreased signal (short T2) on T2-weighted MR images. *AJR* 1987;**148**:1247-50 .
39. Cascino TL, Kori S, Krol G, Foley KM. CT of the brachial plexus in patients with cancer. *Neurology* 1983;**33**:1553-7.
40. Match RM. Radiation-induced brachial plexus paralysis. *Arch Surg* 1975:**110**:384-6.
41. Lord JW, Rosati LM. Thoracic outlet syndromes. *Ciba Clin Symp* 1971;**23**:1-32.
42. McCormick CC, Gubbay SS, Lekias JS. Upward dislocation of the first rib: a rare cause of nerve entrapment, producing brachialgia. *Br J Radiol* 1981;**54**:140-2.
43. Bilbey JH, Muller NL, Connell DG, Luoma AA, Nelems B. Thoracic outlet syndrome: evaluation with CT. *Radiology* 1989;**171**:381-4.

Magnetic resonance imaging of breast disease

Sylvia H. Heywang-Köbrunner
Department of Radiology, Klinikum Großhadern, University of Munich, Munich, Germany

Introduction

Since large studies proved the significant impact of mammographic screening on both early detection of malignancy and survival rates [1,2], breast imaging has attracted more and more attention. Owing to its easy, fast and reproducible application to its excellent accuracy in the detection of microcalcifications and of even tiny malignancies in fatty breasts, mammography is and remains the primary method for screening and problem solving. Ultrasound (US) has proven a valuable adjunct for demonstration of palpable malignancy within mammographically dense tissue and for demonstration of cysts.

In spite of the very good results obtained by these imaging techniques combined which clinical examination further improvement of diagnostic accuracy remains desirable. In dense breasts sensitivity of mammography is limited [3,4]. Sonography cannot for certain exclude non-palpable malignancy of less than 1 cm [5,6]. Furthermore, specificity of all methods is limited, especially since small and early malignancies may present with quite uncharacteristic appearance.

Plain magnetic resonance imaging (MRI) initially appeared quite promising for breast imaging because of its well-known high soft-tissue contrast [7-9]. Furthermore tissue-specific information was expected from calculated T1 and T2 values. However, the calculated T1 and T2 values of benign and malignant tissue overlapped significantly and have therefore not yet been diagnostically useful [10-14]. Unfortunately, interpretation of the varying contrast of lesions and tissues with different pulse sequences has also turned out to be more difficult than expected [11,12,14-16]. Therefore the diagnostic value of plain MRI so far has been quite limited. Only in a few cases (diagnosis of fibrous fibroadenoma, demonstration of cysts or the internal structure of some lesions) was interesting information provided by plain MRI. It was primarily based on the close correlation of the signal intensity on the T2-weighted image and the macroscopic content of fibrosis, cells or water within the examined tissue: Fibrosis displays very low signal intensity, whereas a higher amount of cells and water within the tissue causes intermediate to strong signal intensity.

For the large majority of lesions, however, neither this information nor the information gained by evaluation of further pulse sequences has so far allowed a reliable distinction between benign and malignant aetiology. Thus investigations concerning the use of Gd-DTPA for MRI enhancement in breast carcinoma were undertaken [17,18].

Meanwhile, contrast-enhanced MRI is proving more and more valuable as an additional tool in diagnostically difficult cases [19-26]. Since all carcinomas thus far examined were enhanced, absence of enhancement quite reliably excludes malignancy larger than the slice thickness. This information has been most helpful for detection or exclusion of malignancy within mammographically very dense and/or irregularly shaped tissue (e.g. differential diagnosis of indeterminate mass, ill-defined asymmetric tissue, extensive scarring versus malignancy). Due to its tomographic technique contrast-enhanced MRI is especially suited for evaluation of patients with silicon implants. Considering its inherent limitations, (high costs, necessary interpretation of about 100 images per breast, influence of partial volume effect, lack of specificity in cases with diffuse enhancement) contrast-enhanced MRI is not suitable for screening. Furthermore, it is not recommended for evaluation of lesions smaller than the slice thickness and for diseases where diffuse enhancement is to be expected (known proliferative dysplasia, inflammation), since in these cases MRI cannot exclude malignancy.

Imaging Technique

To obtain a sufficient signal-to-noise ratio (S/N), which allows slice thicknesses below 5 mm and a resolution below 1 mm within an acceptable imaging time, the use of special surface coils is necessary. Breast coils are designed to examine the patient in the prone position with the breast pending. Thus artefacts caused by respiratory motion of the anterior chest wall are minimized. Furthermore it is very important that the amplification within the coil volume is as homogeneous as possible to avoid misinterpretation caused by local differences in reception [27].

Most experience presently concerns single breast coils. Among the double breast coils we only recommend those types which allow separate imaging of each breast [22]. The possibility of using a small field of view (FOV) and off-centre zoom means that these coils allow the same resolution and image quality as single breast coils. Finally motion artefacts caused by the heart need to be optimally eliminated. With standard equipment they can be removed from the breast by switching phase and frequency encoding gradients. With the latest equipment these artefacts can optimally be avoided by local pre-saturation of the heart region.

For plain MRI a multitude of pulse sequences exists. Even though the optimum combination of pulse sequences is not yet known, a plain MRI study should at least include a T1-weighted pulse sequence, such as a short TR - short TE spin-echo or Inversion Recovery (IR) or Short T1 Inversion Recovery (STIR), and a T2- and proton density-weighted pulse sequence, such as double or multiple echo (long TR spin-echo). Further possible pulse sequences include gradient echo sequences such as Fast Low Angle Shot (FLASH), Fast Imaging with steady State free Precession (FISP), Gradient Recalled Acquisition at Steady State (GRASS) or fat-water separating sequences such as Dixon, PEACH, CHEmical Shift Selective (CHESS) etc.

For contrast studies with Gd-DTPA the same T1-weighted pulse sequence is applied before and usually twice after the administration of Gd-DTPA. It is injected intravenously through an existing infusion tube. We recommend a dose of 0.16 mmol/kg body weight for FLASH imaging.

Fast gradient echo imaging (FLASH with a flip angle of 50-90°, TR < 40 ms, TE < 14 ms) has proven optimum. Owing to the excellent sensitivity of FLASH to Gd-DTPA enhancing lesions are quite obvious by their significant increase of signal intensity. In general, fat even displays a lower signal intensity than enhancing lesions. Furthermore, when three-dimensional imaging is used, the complete breast can be imaged at slice thicknesses below 3 - 4 mm within less than 5 minutes. Dynamic imaging, which has so far been possible in preselected slices only, and, if used for the complete breast would produce extreme numbers of images, is not recommended as a routine procedure by us.

Normal Breast

On T1-weighted images all breast tissues except fat display low signal intensity. Fat shows high signal intensity. Thus T1-weighted MRI compares well with mammographic or computed tomography (CT) images of the breast. Normal skin itself is visualized as a very thin, barely visible, low signal intensity line. The nipple also displays low signal intensity. Vessels mostly show low signal intensity, sometimes high signal intensity, depending on the velocity and direction of the flowing blood.

On T2-weighted images the signal intensity of fat is only intermediate. The signal intensity of ductal, glandular and connective tissue depends on its contents of fibrosis, cells and water and thus usually varies from low to intermediate. High signal intensity may be seen in dilated ducts or within cysts. Considering the wide variations of morphology and signal intensity within normal breast tissue no reliable definition of the 'normal appearance' can be given for plain MRI.

When Gd-DTPA is applied, normal breast tissue usually enhances insignificantly and in a delayed manner. Diffuse enhancement has only rarely been encountered, e.g. at the end of the menstrual cycle, during hormone treatment or during lactation. Therefore contrast-enhanced MRI, like mammography, should be performed within the first 10 days after menstruation.

Since all carcinomas thus far examined were shown to enhance significantly, absence of enhancement quite reliably excludes malignancy. This information, which is provided by contrast-enhanced MRI, appears to be unique and has proven most helpful in those cases with indeterminate findings because of mammographically asymmetric or irregularly shaped tissue or because of mammographically dense tissue with a questionable palpable abnormality (Fig. 1).

Benign Conditions of the Breast

Dysplasia

Whereas normal breast tissue consists of varying amounts of fat, ductal, glandular, loose and dense connective tissue, dysplasia describes a qualitative or quantitative alteration of one or more of these components.

Simple or non-proliferative dysplasia is not associated with an increased risk of malignancy.

Proliferative dysplasias are characterized by increased intraductal (papillomatous, solid or adenomatous) or extraductal (adenotic) growth. Whereas the association of moderate proliferative dysplasia with an increased risk of malignancy is controversial, high-grade proliferative dysplasia is generally considered a risk factor [6,9].

Mammographically and clinically dysplasia may pose diagnostic problems due to its increased nodularity and roentgen-density. Furthermore, proliferative dysplasia may contain microcalcifications, which usually are scattered but which may appear suspicious if they are clustered or asymmetric. On T2-weighted plain MRI, again the signal intensity of dysplasia correlates well with its macroscopic content of fibrosis, cells and water. Therefore the same wide variations of appearance are seen in dysplasias as in normal breast tissue. On T1-weighted images all dysplasias display low signal intensity like normal breast tissue.

After the administration of Gd-DTPA non-proliferative dysplasia usually does not enhance - like normal breast tissue. With increasing proliferation moderate to even strong usually diffuse enhancement may be encountered (Figs. 2 and 3). On dynamic studies most proliferative dysplasias exhibit delayed enhancement, some, however, enhance early and strongly. Focal enhancement is seen infrequently in cases of focal proliferative dysplasia. Thus malignancy larger than slice thickness can quite reliably be excluded in all cases with absent or little enhancement. Since few carcinomas with delayed and/or diffuse enhancement exist, neither diffuse nor delayed enhancement can reliably exclude malignancy, even though proliferative dysplasia

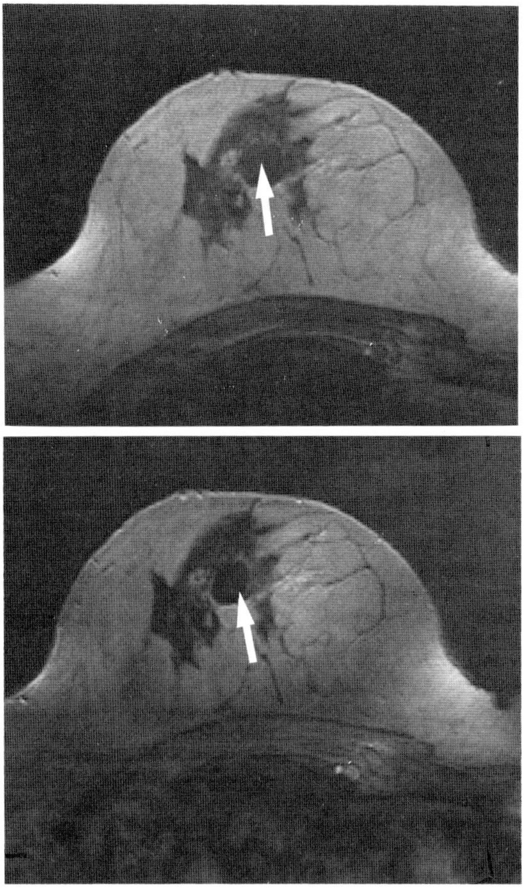

(a)

(b)

Figure 1. *NORMAL BREAST TISSUE WITH A CYST. (a) On the T1-weighted precontrast image (one of 32 images of a FLASH-3D pulse sequence: TR = 40 ms, TE = 14 ms, FA = 50°, acquisition time: 5 min) the complete breast tissue displays low signal intensity. It contains a well-circumscribed cyst (arrow) with very low signal intensity. The surrounding and interposed fat displays strong signal intensity. (b) With postcontrast MRI (same slice, same pulse sequence) no change of signal intensity is noted within breast tissue, fat or cyst.*

or inflammatory changes are the most probable causes of diffuse and delayed enhancement.

In case of focal enhancement further work-up (usually biopsy) is necessary.

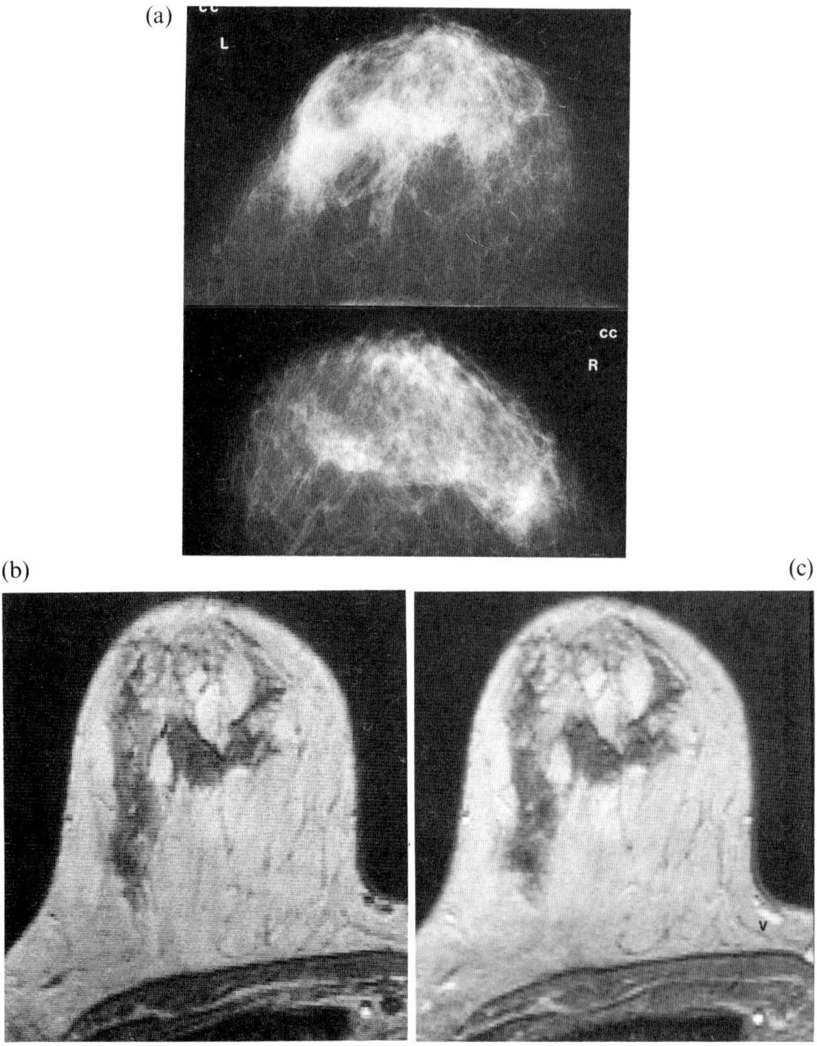

Figure 2. *PATIENT WITH PALPABLE AND MAMMOGRAPHIC ASYMMETRY. (a) Due to the palpable and mammographic asymmetry, as shown here on the craniocaudad views of this patient's first mammogram, MRI was recommended to exclude a mass. (b) Representative precontrast transverse MRI (one of 32 slices of a FLASH-3D study: TR = 40 ms, TE = 14 ms, FA = 50°). (c) On the postcontrast study (same slice, same pulse sequence) no significant enhancement was shown within the complete breast tissue. Significant increase of signal intensity is only noted within some vessels (v), which can be followed through the slices. These findings are compatible with asymmetric dysplasia and exclude malignancy larger than the slice thickness (4 mm). This diagnosis was confirmed by 2-year follow-up.*

(a)

(b)

(c)

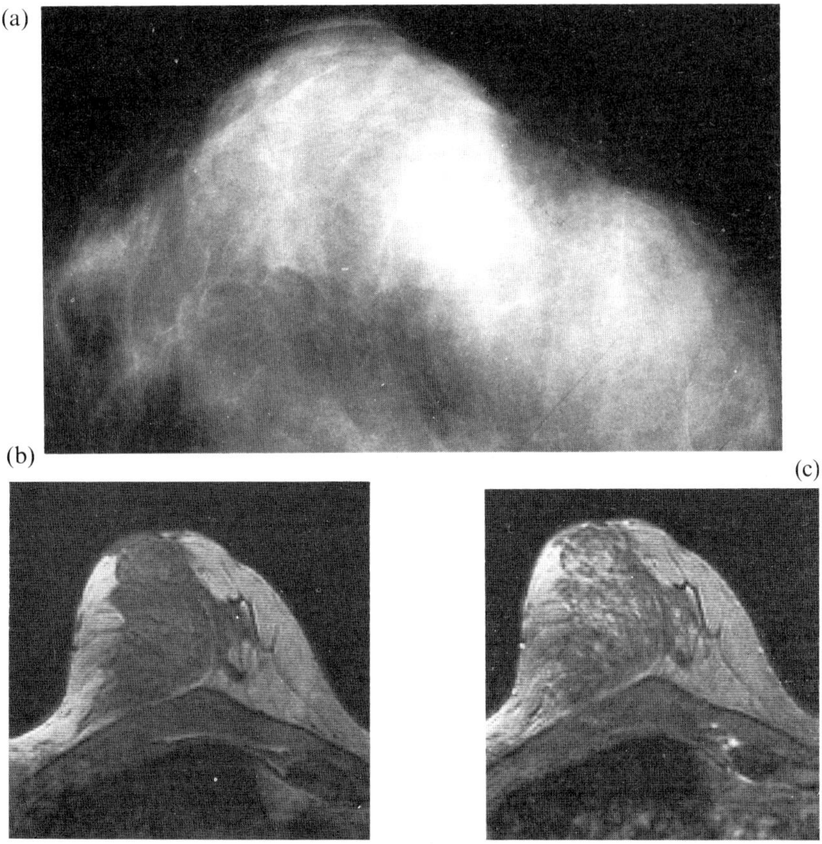

Figure 3. *PATIENT WITH A DENSE MAMMOGRAM AND SUSPICIOUS PALPABLE FINDINGS IN THE OUTER QUADRANT OF THE BREAST. (a) Mammography (craniocaudad view) exhibits very dense tissue and therefore cannot exclude malignancy in the presence of the palpable abnormality. (b) T1-weighted precontrast MRI (FLASH-3D: TR = 440 ms, TE = 14 ms, FA = 50°) displays the dense breast tissue. (c) Postcontrast MRI (same slice, same pulse sequence) shows patchy diffuse enhancement within the complete breast tissue. Even though this finding is highly compatible, e.g., with proliferative dysplasia, malignancy cannot be excluded by MRI due to the underlying enhancement and biopsy had to be performed. Histology proved proliferative dysplasia with atypias.*

Cysts

Cysts are a frequent and harmless finding in the female breast. Due to the excellent sonographic sensitivity and specificity for cysts MRI is usually not necessary for this diagnosis. On plain MRI simple cysts are characterized by a very low signal intensity on T1-weighted images (lower than or similar to normal breast tissue) and by a homogeneous and very strong signal intensity on T2-weighted images.

With higher protein contents (e.g. in complicated cysts) the signal intensity on T2-weighted images is less high. In the case of contents tinged with blood very high signal intensity may be encountered on T1-weighted images.

After the application of Gd-DTPA neither the contents nor the wall of a simple cyst enhance (see Fig. 1).

Fibroadenomas

The fibroadenoma is the most common benign tumour of the breast. It may present with round, oval or lobulated shape and typically has well-defined outlines. Only if mammography shows the typical popcorn-like coarse calcifications, can it for certain be distinguished from a rare well-circumscribed malignancy. Histologically older fibroadenomas are fibrous and sometimes calcified (sclerosing fibroadenomas). The younger fibroadenomas usually contain larger amounts of cells and loose interstitium (adenomatous, myxoid, juvenile fibroadenoma).

On T1-weighted MRI fibroadenomas show low signal intensity, which is as low or lower than the signal intensity of normal breast tissue.

On T2-weighted MRI fibrous or calcified fibroadenomas display very low signal intensity, adenomatous, myxoid and juvenile fibroadenomas display intermediate to high signal intensity. Since the fibrous fibroadenoma is the only well-circumscribed lesion which is composed of dense fibrosis, it can easily be distinguished from the other well-circumscribed tumours on the T2-weighted image, since they all contain higher amounts of cells and water and therefore display intermediate to high signal intensity (e.g. medullary, papillary or mucinous carcinomas, metastases, lymphoma, intramammary lymph node, cystosarcoma, non-fibrous fibroadenomas).

On contrast-enhanced MRI fibrous fibroadenomas usually exhibit little (and delayed) enhancement. Adenomatous and myxoid fibroadenomas enhance strongly, mostly delayed, but sometimes also early. Because of their enhancement, MRI detects more fibroadenomas than mammography and sonography within dense tissue. Unfortunately, however, a definite diagnosis of benignity is only possible in the case of absent or non-significant enhancement. Delayed but strong enhancement cannot for certain exclude a medullary, papillary or other well-circumscribed carcinoma (Fig. 4).

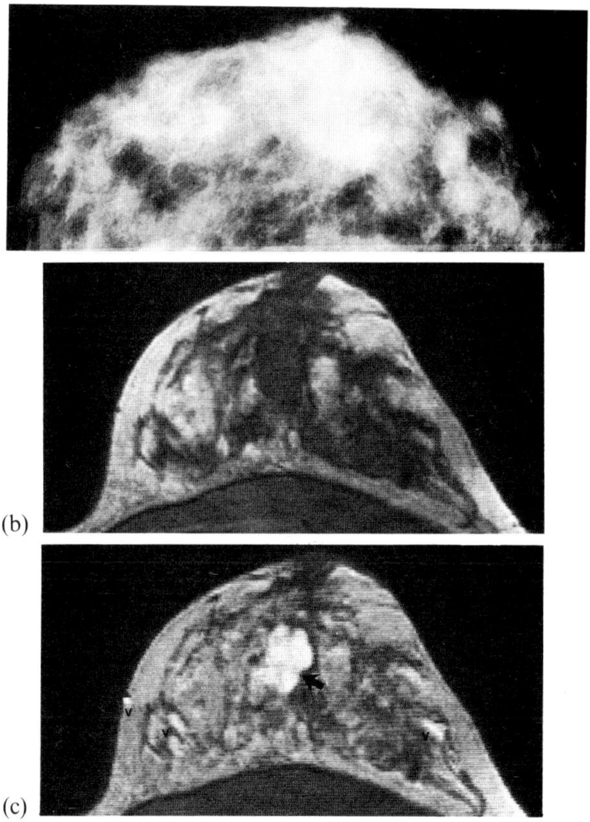

Figure 4. *PATIENT WITH A QUESTIONABLE PALPABLE ABNORMALITY CENTRALLY WITHIN THE BREAST. (a) The dense mammogram (craniocaudad view) cannot exclude malignancy in the presence of the palpable abnormality. Therefore MRI was recommended. (b) Precontrast transverse MRI at the level of the palpable abnormality (FLASH-3D: TR = 40 ms, TE = 14 ms, FA = 50°). (c) On the postcontrast image (same slice, same pulse sequence) a strongly enhancing lobulated mass (arrow) is visualized surrounded by dysplasia with no significant enhancement. Several enhancing vessels (v) can be followed through the adjacent slices. Since MRI could not further distinguish between a strongly enhancing fibroadenoma or a lobulated malignancy (e.g. mucinous carcinoma) biopsy was recommended. Histology revealed an adenomatous fibroadenoma.*

Other Benign Masses

Other common benign breast masses include papilloma, hamartoma, lipoma and intramammary lymph node.

The majority of papillomas are small or very small. Larger papillomas have an appearance similar to fibroadenomas on mammography and MRI. Even though most papillomas (except those, which are completely sclerosed) enhance, contrast-enhanced MRI is not the method of choice to evaluate them. Firstly, tiny papillomas may be smaller than the slice-thickness. Secondly, due to the accompanying nipple discharge and inflammatory reaction, they are frequently surrounded by enhancing tissue. Thirdly and most importantly, MRI cannot further distinguish between enhancing papilloma or early enhancing papillary carcinoma. Therefore mammography and galactography are the methods of choice for their detection. For further differentiation biopsy is necessary.

Hamartomas and lipomas can usually be diagnosed by mammography. The same is true for intramammary lymph nodes, if they are partially replaced by fat and/or situated in the axillary tail. In this regard, MRI is usually not helpful since both benign and infiltrated lymph nodes enhance like other breast tumours and no specific signal behaviour of lymph nodes on MRI is known.

Cystosarcoma Phylloides

The cystosarcoma is a semimalignant tumour, which is usually quite well-circumscribed, oval or lobulated, and presents with fast growth. In large tumours inhomogeneous internal structure is demonstrated on T2-weighted images or on postcontrast T1-weighted images. Whether small cystosarcomas can be distinguished from other enhancing tumours is not yet known.

Carcinoma

Breast cancer is the most common carcinoma in women and the leading cause of death. Its imaging characteristics vary with the wide spectrum of histological types, their morphology and growth pattern. Mammographically most common presentations include spiculated or ill-defined (or rarely smooth) mass, microcalcifications, increased density due to diffuse infiltration, distorted architecture, asymmetric prominent duct, retraction and skin thickening.

As already mentioned, mammographic sensitivity is excellent in fatty breasts. Furthermore mammography has the unique capability to detect microcalcifications, which may be an early sign of malignancy. Its diagnostic accuracy, however, depends on both the surrounding tissue and the size of the lesion in question. Thus, the uncharacteristic mammographic presentation of many small masses necessitates numerous biopsies. Furthermore, dense tissue may obscure lesions without microcalcifications.

Sonography frequently aids in demonstrating palpable malignancy within dense tissue. It is not able to exclude small or *in-situ* carcinomas since they may be invisible sonographically. Even though most carcinomas can be visualized by non-enhanced MRI, it has not been able to provide significant information. On T1-weighted images all carcinomas display low signal intensity - as low as or sometimes lower than normal breast tissue or dysplasias. The signal intensity of carcinomas on T2-weighted images ranges from very low (in scirrhous carcinomas) to very high (in mucinous or oedematous carcinomas), and thus is predominantly determined by the gross composition of each tumour (Fig. 5). Since the same variations have been encountered in benign disease and with other pulse sequences as well, no signal behaviour specific for malignancy has yet been found for non-enhanced MRI [11-16].

After the i.v. application of Gd-DTPA all malignancies thus far examined including *in-situ* carcinomas, enhanced significantly. Most carcinomas in fact exhibit focal and fast enhancement. However diffuse enhancement or delayed enhancement cannot exclude malignancy. In spite of the fact that all malignancies enhanced, MRI is not recommended for evaluation of mammographically detected indeterminate microcalcifications for the following reasons:

1. microcalcifications themselves are not visualized since they are beyond the resolution of MRI;
2. enhancement around a tiny group of microcalcifications or within a duct might be mistaken for an enhancing vessel or vice versa: - furthermore, partial volume effect has to be considered in case of tiny lesions;

(a)

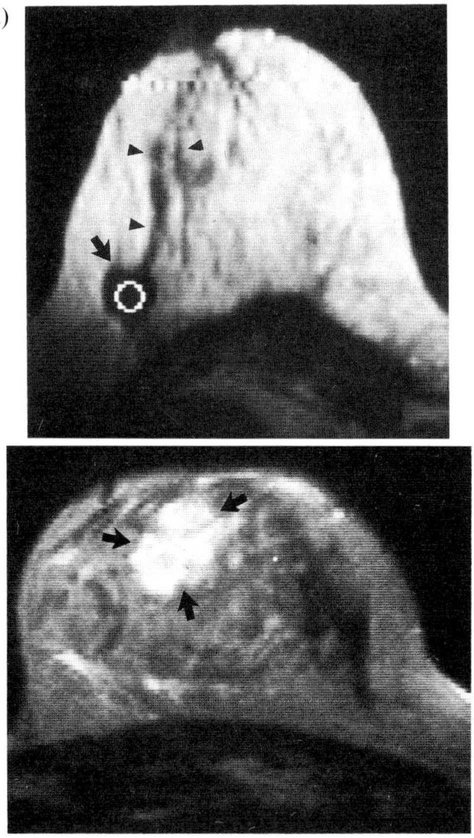

(b)

Figure 5. *VARIABLE PRESENTATIONS OF CARCINOMAS ON T2-WEIGHTED PLAIN MRI. (a) This scirrhous carcinoma (arrow), which is surrounded by fat, displays low signal intensity on a T2-weighted spin-echo sequence. Based on its signal intensity it cannot be distinguished from remaining strands of fibrous dysplasia (arrowheads) nearby. (b) This mucinous carcinoma (arrow) , which is surrounded by fibrous dysplasia, in contrast displays very high signal intensity on a T2 weighted spin-echo sequence.*

3. since microcalcifications are mostly surrounded by either carcinoma or some type of proliferative dysplasia, enhancement has to be expected anyway.

Contrast-enhanced MRI has been shown to provide valuable information for both exclusion and detection of malignancy within mammographically dense tissue. Based on its excellent sensitivity and

Table 1. *Accuracy data in biopsy proven (**a**) and in diagnostically difficult cases (**b**) (from ref. 22).*

	Pre-MRI	Post-MRI
a		
Sensitivity	90%	100%
Specificity	15%	22%
Neg. pred. value	58%	100%
Pos. pred. value	55%	60%
Prevalence of carcinomas: 52%		
b		
Sensitivity	74%	100%
Specificity	32%	53%
Neg. pred. value	85%	100%
Pos. pred. value	19%	31%
Prevalence of carcinomas: 18%		

a. Accuracy in 250 biopsy proven diagnoses: The pre-MRI diagnoses, based on mammography, clinical examination and sonography (if necessary) are compared with the post-MRI diagnoses, based on the above mentioned methods and MRI; all diagnoses were established preoperatively.

b. Accuracy in 192 diagnostically difficult cases: (Cases where a decision between biopsy or follow-up appeared problematic based on mammography, clinical examination, history and sonography were considered 'difficult' and referred to MRI; the diagnoses are meanwhile confirmed by biopsy or at least 2-year follow-up). The pre-MRI diagnoses, based on mammography, clinical examination and sonography (if necessary) are compared with the post-MRI diagnoses, based on the above mentioned methods and MRI; all diagnoses were established preoperatively.

(a)

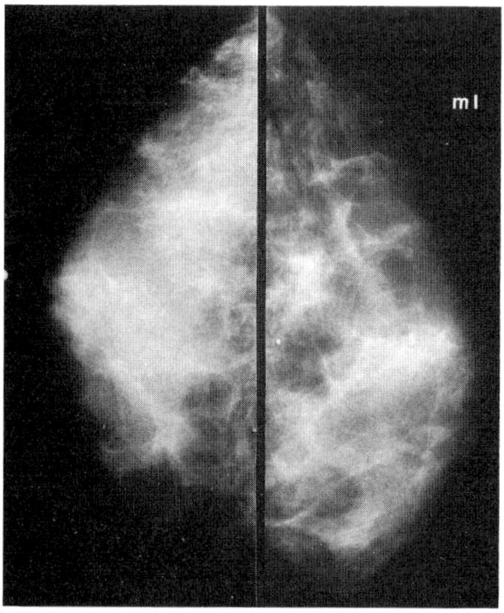

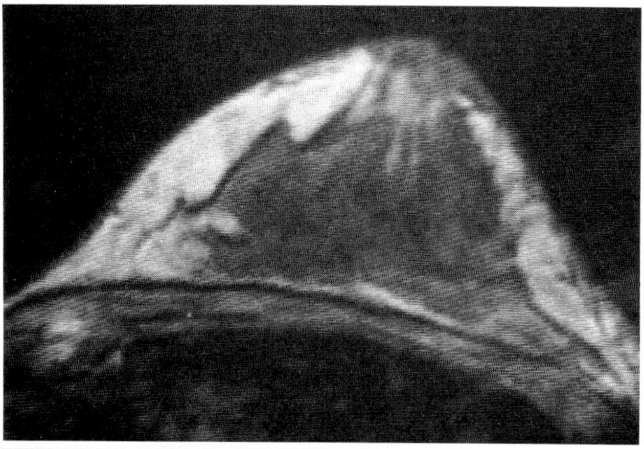

(b)

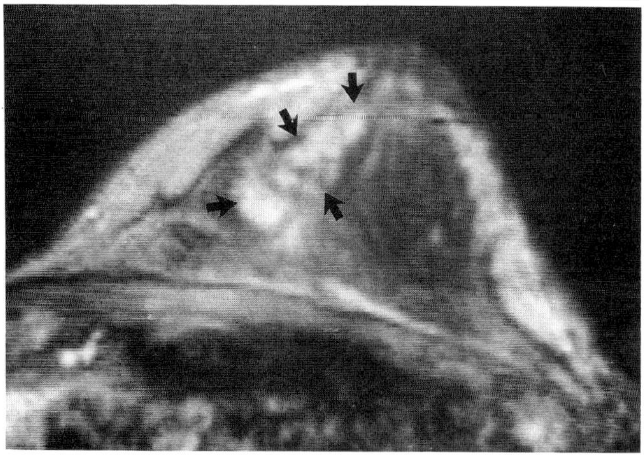

(c)

negative predictive value (Table 1) it allows exclusion of malignancy larger than the slice thickness in cases of absent or little enhancement. Furthermore, focal enhancement, when detected within mammographically dense tissue may be the only hint of malignancy, and is not visible by other modalities (Fig. 6). These observations are supported by the accuracy data of several authors [22-26].

Inflammatory changes

Inflammatory changes predominantly include acute and chronic mastitis, as well as abscess. Even though both T2-weighted non-enhanced MRI and contrast-enhanced MRI may nicely demonstrate the internal structure of an abscess, no specific information can be contributed by plain or contrast-enhanced MRI in most cases with inflammatory change. This is due to the fact that both the signal behaviour on non-enhanced MRI and the usually encountered enhancement of inflammatory changes are non-specific findings. Therefore in cases of insufficient response to treatment, biopsy remains necessary for the clinically relevant distinction between abscess and necrotic carcinoma or between mastitis and inflammatory carcinoma.

Status Postsurgery and/or Radiation Therapy

Extensive scarring after surgery or after surgery and radiation therapy may cause diagnostic problems, since it may obscure or mimic malignancy mammographically and clinically. On non-enhanced MRI no definite distinction between scarring or malignancy has been possible. After the application of Gd-DTPA, significant enhancement is usually encountered during the first 6 months after surgery and up

---

Figure 6. *PATIENT REFERRED TO MRI FOR SEARCH FOR A PRIMARY TUMOUR. (a) Mammographically (craniocaudad and mediolateral views) no malignancy could be detected within the dense breast tissue. MRI was recommended, since sonography and clinical examination also showed no abnormality. (b) Precontrast MRI at the centre of the breast (one of 32 slices of a FLASH-3D study: TR = 40 ms, TE = 14 ms, FA = 50°). (c) Postcontrast MRI (same slice, same pulse sequence) exhibits a strongly enhancing area medially in the breast (arrows). Since this abnormality was not palpable, even in retrospect and since it was only visible by MRI, MR-guided biopsy had to be performed. Histologically an intraductal carcinoma corresponding to the extension of the enhancing area was found. It contained a tiny area of invasive carcinoma of 4 mm. (from ref. 32).*

to about 18 months after radiation therapy. Significant enhancement also occurs in acute fat necrosis. Because of the described enhancement distinction between carcinoma and these early inflammatory changes is not possible. However, mature fibrosis which occurs later does not show significant enhancement. At this stage (usually later

(a)

(b)

(c)

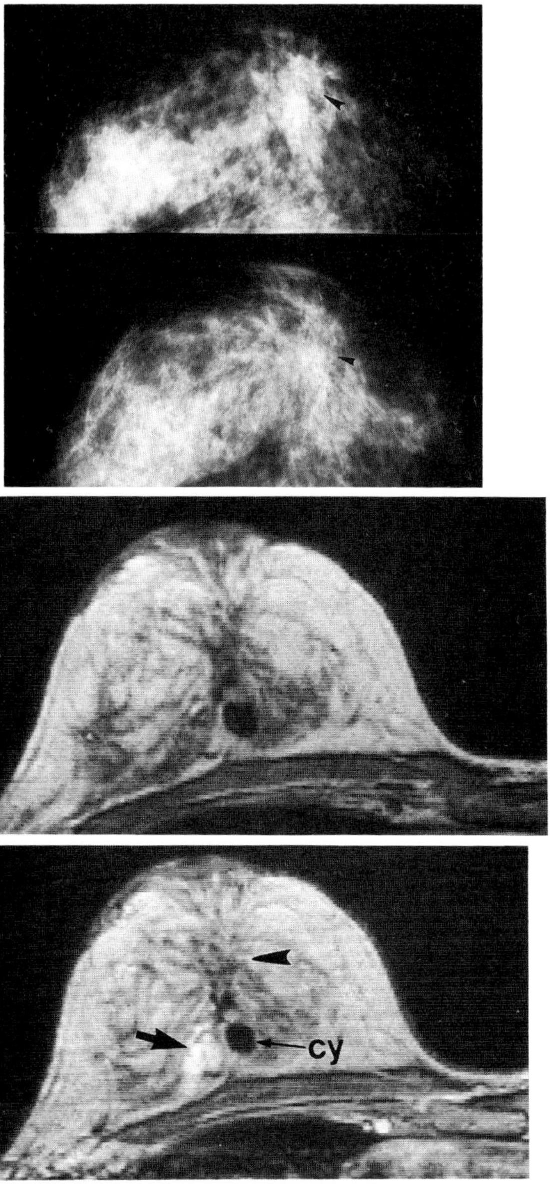

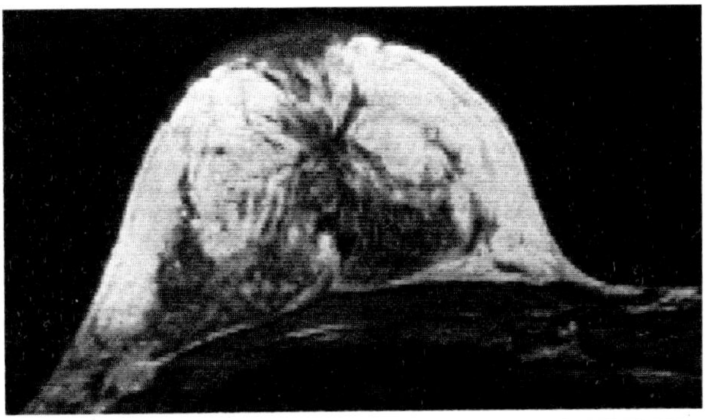

(d)

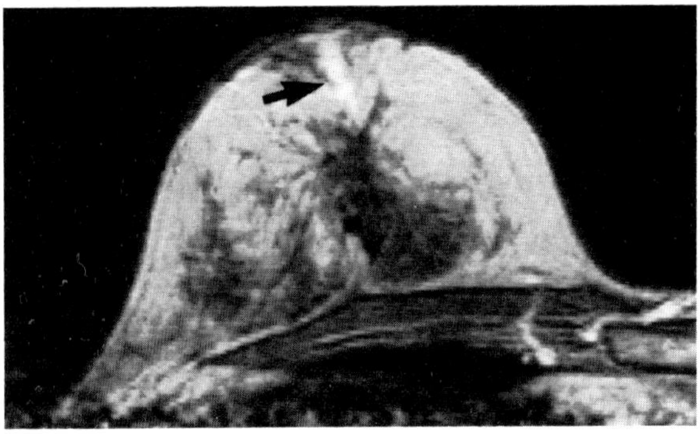

(e)

Figure 7. *RECURRENCE DETECTED BY MRI ALONE. This patient was examined by MRI 26 months after radiation therapy in a study in which all patients with dense tissue after tumourectomy and irradiation were offered an additional MR examination. No palpable abnormality and no expressible nipple discharge were detected. (a) The mammograms [craniocaudad views 1 year previously (top) and before MR examination (bottom)] display moderately dense breast tissue and regressing star-like scarring (arrowhead). (b) Precontrast MRI at the level of the scar (one of 32 slices of a FLASH-3D study: TR = 40 ms, TE = 14 ms, FA = 50°). (c) The post-contrast MRI (same slice, same pulse sequence) demonstrates the star-like scar (arrowhead), which does not enhance. Behind the scar close to the chest wall and adjacent to a non-enhancing cyst (cy), however, a strongly enhancing highly suspicious lesion (arrow) is visualized. (d) Neighbouring precontrast slice through the nipple (same pulse sequence). (e) The post-contrast image of this neighbouring slice shows another independent suspicious enhancement within the retro-areolar ducts (arrow). MR-guided biopsy of the two lesions confirmed a 1.1 cm mucinous invasive recurrent tumour close to the chest wall (b) and (c) and a second intraductal carcinoma independent of the first within the retro-areolar ducts (d) and (e). (from ref. 32).*

than 6 months after surgery or 18 months after radiation therapy) distinction between malignancy, which always enhances, and scarring is excellent. Therefore, MRI has proven valuable as an additional tool in cases with diagnostic problems (Fig. 7).

In patients with silicon implants MRI allows tomographic evaluation of the complete tissue around the implant. This is especially advantageous, since dense silicon implants may obscure significant parts of the surrounding tissue on mammography.

Conclusion

Since 1982 MRI of the breast has developed continuously to become a diagnostically interesting tool for breast imaging. Present technique allows imaging of the breast within acceptable imaging time.

Non-enhanced MRI has not proved as valuable as expected. Due to significant overlap in the appearance of many benign and malignant conditions it does not yet appear suitable for routine clinical application. Research in this field is, continuing with evaluation of new pulse sequences, computer-assisted tissue analysis and evaluation of the potentials of spectroscopy [28-31].

Contrast-enhanced MRI, however, is proving more and more valuable in diagnostically difficult cases. Since evaluation of the enhancement provides physiological information about vascularity and interstitial space (perfusion, permeability of vessels, amount of interstitium), the method adds a new dimension to conventional mammographic and sonographic imaging. In the absence of enhancement, malignancy can reliably be excluded even within dense or irregular tissue. This helps to avoid unnecessary biopsies. Focal enhancement offers the possibility of early detection of otherwise occult lesions, which is particularly helpful in mammographically very dense tissue. Indications, where contrast-enhanced MRI most helpful are listed in Table 2.

Due to its specific limitations (discussed above) contrast-enhanced MRI cannot be used as a screening tool. It should only be used in combination with mammography.

Table 2. *Indications for contrast-enhanced MRI of the breast (to be used in addition to mammography)*

- Diagnostic problems in mammographically dense breasts:
  Questionable palpable abnormality
  Questionable mammographic abnormality
  Exclusion or detection of further foci, when limited surgery of a small malignancy is planned
  Search for a primary tumour
- Distinction between mammographic irregularly-shaped densities:
  Malignancy versus dyplasia
  Malignancy versus superimposition (abnormalities visible on 1 view only)
- Distinction between scarring and malignancy:
  For scarring more than 6 months postoperatively
  For scarring more than 18 months post radiation therapy
- Diagnostic problems in patients with silicon implants

Since Gd-DTPA is still under approval for use in the body and since good breast coils are not yet available with all MRI equipment the optimal method is not widely available. Nevertheless, owing to the increased use of screening mammography and the desire to detect smaller lesions without the use of excess biopsies, this method will gain more and more importance. Present results are being confirmed by an increasing number of investigators.

References

1. Feig SA. Decreased breast cancer mortality through mammographic screening: results of clinical trials. *Radiology* 1988;**2**:659-665.
2. Tabar L, Dean PB. The control of breast cancer through mammography screening; what is the evidence? *Radiol Clin North Am* 1987;**25**:933-1006.
3. Homer MJ. Pitfalls, controversies and some practical thoughts. *Radiol Clin North Am* 1985;**23**:459-472.
4. Page DL, Winfield AC. The dense mammogram. *AJR* 1986;**14**:487-489.
5. Kopans DB. Non-mammographic breast imaging techniques. Current status and future developments. *Radiol Clin North Am* 1986;**25**:961-971.
6. Mc Sweeney MB, Murphy CM. Whole breast sonography. *Radiol Clin North Am* 1985;**23**:157-167.

7. Damadian R, Zaner K, Hor D, Di Maio. Tumors by NMR. *Physiol Chem Phys* 1973;**5**:381-402.
8. El Yousef SJ, Duchesneau RH, Alfidi RJ, et al. Magnetic resonance imaging of the breast. *Radiology* 1984;**150**:761-766.
9. Ross RJ, Thompson JS, Kim K, Bailey RA. Nuclear magnetic resonance imaging and evaluation of human breast tissue: preliminary clinical trials. *Radiology* 1982;**143**:195-205.
10. Alcorn FS, Turner DA, Clark JW. Magnetic resonance imaging in the study of the breast. *Radiographics* 1985;**5**:631-652.
11. Heywang SH, Fenzl G, HahnD, et al. MR of the breast: histopathologic correlation. *Europ J Radiol* 1987;**3**:175-183.
12. Murphy WA, Gohagan JK. In Stark DD, Bradley WG jr. (eds). *Breast. Magnetic Resonance Imaging* ,pp 861-886. St.Louis: C.V. Mosby, 1987.
13. Partain CL, Kulkarni MV, Price RR, et al. Magnetic resonance imaging of the breast: functional T1 and three-dimensional imaging. *Cardiovasc Intervent Radiol* 1986:**8**:292-299.
14. Wiener JI, Chako AC, Merten CW, et al. Breast and axillary tissue MR imaging: correlations of signal intensities and relaxation times with pathologic findings. *Radiology* 1986;**160**:299-305.
15. Stelling CB, Powell DE, Mattingly SS. Fibroadenomas: histopathology and MR imaging features. *Radiology* 1987;**162**:399-407.
16. Kaiser W, Oppelt A. In Lissner J, Margulis AR, (eds). *KST der Mamma mit Schnell-bildverfahren (FISP und FLASH). MR 87,* pp 303-310. Konstanz: Schnetztor Verlag, 1987.
17. Revel D, Brasch RC, Praajanen H, et al. Gd-DTPA contrast enhancement and tissue differentiation in MR imaging of experimental breast carcinoma. *Radiology* 1986;**158**:319-324.
18. Heywang SH, Hahn D, Schmidt H, et al. MR imaging of the breast using Gd-DTPA. *J Comput Assist Tomogr* 1986;**10**:199-204
19. Heywang SH, Wolf A, Pruss E, et al. MRI of the breast with Gd-DTPA - use and limitations. *Radiology* 1989;**171**:95-103.
20. Heywang SH, Hilbertz T, Bauer WM, et al. In Lissner J, Doppman JL, Margulis AR, (eds). *Kontrastmittelkernspintomographie der Mamma bei diagnostisch schwierigen Fällen. MR 1989,* pp 138-142. Köln: Deutscher Ärzteverlag, 1989.
21. Heywang SH, Hilbertz T, Beck R, et al. Contrast-material enhanced MRI of the breast in patients with postoperative scarring and silicon implants. *Comput Assist Tomogr* 1990;**14**:348-356.
22. Heywang SH. In Bydder G, Felix R, Bücheler E (eds). *Contrast-enhanced MRI of the breast. Contrast Media in MRI*, pp 261-266. Berlin: Medicom Europe, 1990.
23. Kaiser WA, Zeitler E. MR imaging of the breast: fast imaging sequences with and without Gd-DTPA. *Radiology* 1989;**170**:681-686.
24. Stack J, Redmond VI, Codd MB, et al. Tissue enhancement profiles with Gd-DTPA in breast carcinoma. *Radiology* 1988;**169**:22.
25. Strigl R, Lukas P. In: *Was leistet die Kernspintomographie im Rahmen der Komple-mentärdiagnostik zur Früherkennung des Mammakarzinoms (Fallberichte)?* Alete wissenschaftlicher Dienst. Proceedings of the 20th Meeting of the Bavarian Assoc. of Obstetrics and Gynecology 1988, pp 155-158. Landshut: Bosch-Druck, 1988.
26. Lewis Jones H, Whitehouse GH, Leinster SJ. In: *Book of Abstracts, 8th Annual Meeting of the Society of Magnetic Resonance in Medicine 1988. Gadolinium enhancement in assessment of recurrent breast carcinoma*,.p. 690 Amsterdam: Excerpta Medica, 1990.

27. Krimmel K, Koebrunner G, Heywang SH. Anpassung einer Mammaspule an klinische Bedürfnisse bei 1 Tesla. *Digitale Bilddiagnostik* 1986;**8**:101-110.
28. König H, Gohagan JK, Laub G, et al. Improved MR breast images by contrast optimization using artificial intelligence. *Radiology* 1986;**161**:27.
29. Gohagan JK, Spitznagel EL, I Murphy WA, et al. Multispectral analysis of MR images of the breast. *Radiology* 1987;**163**:703-707.
30. Heywang SH, Deimling M, Hilbertz T, et al. Improved sequences for T1 and T2 quantification: first applications in breast imaging. *Radiology* 1988;**169**:326.
31. Glaholm J, Colllns D, Leach O, et al. In vivo 31P Magnetic Spectroscopy for monitoring the treatment of human breast carcinoma. *Magn Reson Imag* 1989;**suppl. 1**:1010.
32. Heywang-Köbrunner SH. Contrast-enhanced MRI of the breast. München, Karger publ. 1990.

Tomographic imaging of thoracic aortic disease: emphasis on MRI

Richard D. White
Section of Cardiovascular Imaging, Division of Radiology, Cleveland Clinic Foundation, Cleveland, Ohio, USA

Introduction

Thoracic aortic disease includes a variety of acquired and congenital conditions, some of which may be life threatening. Thus, the suspicion of such disease necessitates the use of an imaging technique capable of its definitive detection or exclusion and, if detected, able to offer a complete description. The optimal technique for this purpose elucidates efficiently, safely, and accurately the pathophysiological elements necessary to establish a diagnostic and prognostic profile for directing proper therapy [1,2].

The traditional approach to the diagnosis of thoracic aortic disease has been contrast aortography [3]. Although aortography has been considered to be the definitive imaging technique, it is somewhat limited in its diagnostic capability; only the intra-aortic regions that become opacified with contrast material are demonstrated in a projective fashion [1]. In addition, aortography may be technically difficult in the setting of tortuous or stenosed vessels, and it carries with it the risk of catheterization and contrast reaction.

In the past two decades, several non-invasive imaging techniques have also been shown to be capable of detecting definitively the presence or absence of thoracic aortic disease, along with providing the essential specific details. These new techniques include two-dimensional (2-D) echocardiography [4], contrast-enhanced computed tomography (CT) [1,2,5], and magnetic resonance imaging (MRI) [1,2,6]. In addition to their relatively risk-free nature and ease of performance, these techniques share the advantages that are common to tomographic techniques, but not characteristic of the standard projection approach used in aortography [1,2]. These advantages include the following: avoidance of superimposition of mediastinal shadows; spatial separation of the various portions of the aorta circumferentially; and demonstration of the intra-aortic space, aortic wall, and peri-aortic regions. Consequently, the overall nature and the extent of thoracic aortic disease can often be more accurately determined by the tomographic techniques. Unfortunately, compared to aortography, they are relatively limited in their ability to evaluate the status of the coronary arteries.

MRI has several attributes that make it especially useful for the evaluation of diseases of the cardiovascular system compared to both echocardiography and CT [2,6,7]. These include the inherent natural contrast between the intracardiac/intravascular spaces and the surrounding walls of the cardiovascular structures; high soft-tissue contrast enabling sharp delineation of the myocardium, vessel walls, pericardium, and adjacent fat; non-interference with imaging of the cardiovascular structures by the surrounding thoracic skeletal or air-filled structures; and the ease of synchronization of imaging to segments of the cardiac cycle. Due to these qualities, and because it does not require either the use of ionizing radiation or injection of contrast materials, MRI is an ideal imaging technique for the evaluation of thoracic aortic disease.

Overview of Pertinent MRI Principles

The signal recorded from resonating protons during MRI is a vector uniquely defined by magnitude (i.e. intensity) and phase (i.e. direction) components [8,9]. The magnitude component can be utilized to produce an anatomy-based image, while the phase component provides the basis for a flow-based image which reflects the movement of proton spins during the time interval between the radio-frequency (RF) excitation pulse and the centre of the signal sampling window (i.e. echo time or TE).

The value of electrocardiographic (ECG) gating in the performance of MRI of the cardiovascular system, including the thoracic aorta, has been described in detail [10]. In ECG-triggered multilevel MRI, the time interval between consecutive RF-excitation pulses (i.e. repetition time or TR) applied at a level is set by the monitored R-waves.

MRI Pulse Sequences

In general, spin-echo sequences have been the foundation of cardiovascular MRI [7]. Varying the TR and/or the TE times will selectively enhance contrast according to T1 (i.e. longitudinal relaxation) or T2 (i.e. transverse relaxation) differences in tissues [11]. Magnitude data from spin-echo sequences produce the standard static images with the intracardiac/intravascular spaces represented by the 'dark blood' appearance (Fig. 1), which is due to a combination of 'time-of-flight' and phase-change effects [9]. In cardiovascular MRI, spin-echo sequences are usually employed in a multilevel format in order to provide a static survey of the thorax and/or abdomen for anatomical abnormalities.

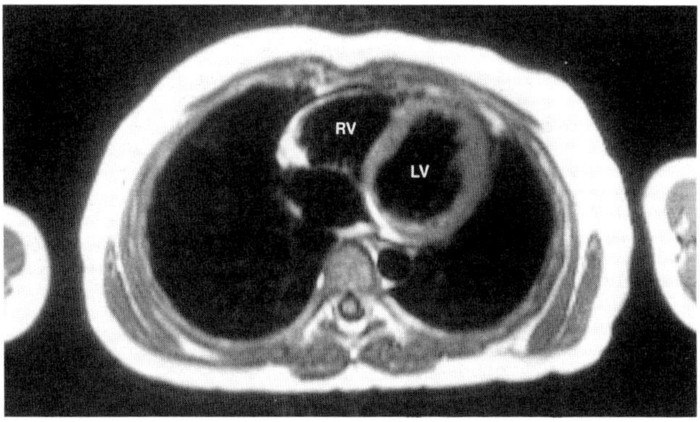

Figure 1. *'DARK BLOOD' APPEARANCE (SPIN-ECHO; TRANSAXIAL).*

Recently, gradient echo sequences (e.g. FLASH) have received greater attention in cardiovascular MRI. They utilize a rapid repetition rate (i.e. short TR), a narrow flip angle (i.e. less than 90°), and a gradient-refocused echo [12]. In gradient echo imaging, a proton spin need only experience one RF pulse to contribute to the echo signal, and short TR values flowing blood to carry a constant influx of fully magnetized protons into the imaging volumes. The net result is flow-related enhancement and a 'bright blood' appearance in the intra-cardiac/intravascular spaces (Fig. 2) [9].

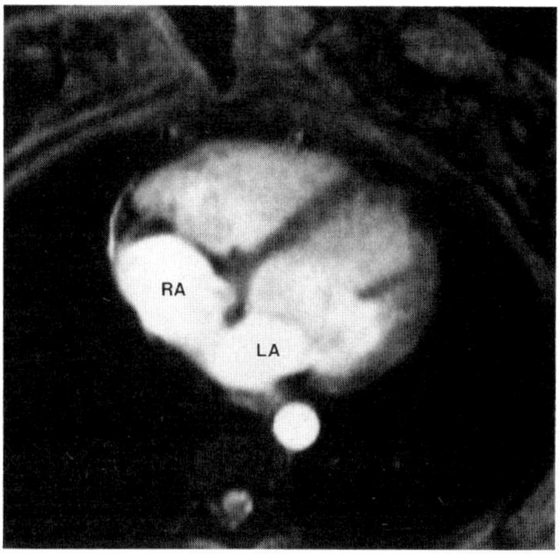

Figure 2. *'BRIGHT BLOOD' APPEARANCE (GRADIENT-ECHO; TRANSAXIAL).*

Dynamic display of gradient echo images acquired repetitively throughout the cardiac cycle is the basis for 'cine MRI' [13]. In cine MRI, the rapid repetition rates allow for one to four anatomical levels of the cardiovascular structures to be imaged at multiple identical segments of the cardiac cycle during a single series. The maximum number of frames in the resulting image loop corresponds to the number of TR intervals which can be applied during the cardiac cycle [14]. Because many anatomical levels may need to be evaluated with cine MRI, simultaneous acquisition of image loops from more than one level is desirable because it reduces total imaging time; this can be accomplished, but at the expense of temporal resolution. Prospective and retrospective gating strategies for cine MRI and their relative advantages and disadvantages have been described in detail [15].

Although qualitative information on blood flow can be derived from spin-echo and cine magnitude data images, quantification is difficult because the signal intensity depends on the flow profile, as well as on proton density and relaxation times [9,16]. On the other hand, the proton spin phase of the signal is more directly related to flow [17]. The spin phase is sensitive to magnetic gradients and varies according to the position of the proton in the gradient fields. As blood protons undergo a change in position due to flow, their spins will incur phase alterations that differ from stationary protons. From either spin-echo or gradient echo series, the phase data can be used to generate several forms of phase reconstructions which correspond to the standard magnitude data images. These phase data images record motion-dependent spin phase changes spatially based on a gray scale [18].

In multiple spin-echo MRI, averaged spin phase can be interpreted on a voxel-by-voxel basis from odd echo data and used to produce a standard phase display image [19]. For protons in stationary structures, the phase change is zero and is, by convention, assigned a shade in the middle of the gray scale (Fig. 3). On the other hand, phase changes for protons in motion (e.g. flowing blood protons) are expressed as positive or negative degree values (i.e. ranging from +180° to -180°). They are represented by increasing degrees of

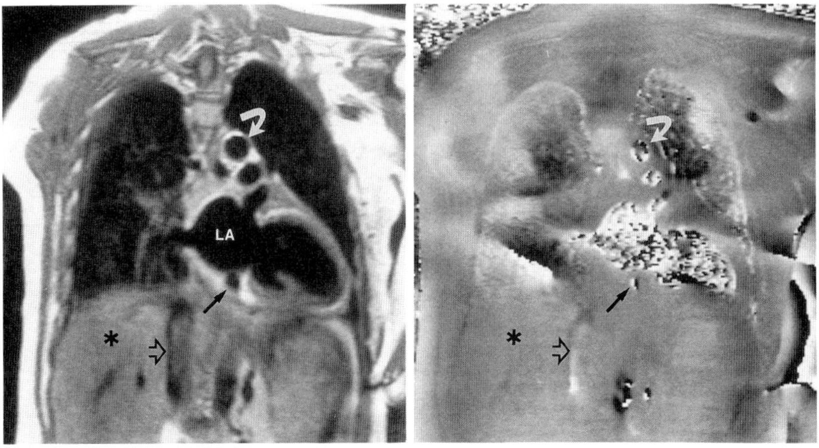

(a) (b)

Figure 3. *PHASE DISPLAY (SPIN-ECHO MAGNITUDE AND PHASE-DISPLAY; TWO-CHAMBER). A first-echo magnitude data image (a), and the corresponding phase-display image (b), are shown. On the latter image, shades of white and black are noted in the same intracardiac/intravascular regions where there is evidence of rapidly flowing blood on the former image. This is evident in the aortic arch (curved arrows) and coronary sinus (straight closed arrows). Inplane slow flow within the inferior vena cava (open arrows) is properly identified because of similar motion dependent phase changes. On the other hand, the liver (asterisks) shows no such phase changes and is represented by a shade in the middle of the gray scale.*

whiteness or blackness, depending on the assignment of the positive and negative values relative to the two ends of the gray scale.

On even-numbered spin-echo images, the net spin phase associated with constant velocity flow is theoretically zero; thus, the phase display appearance of blood protons moving at constant velocity resembles that of stationary blood [9,17]. Such 'even echo rephasing' results in an absolute increase in signal intensity on corresponding magnitude data images [20]. Application of balanced and symmetric gradients for flow compensation will produce the same effect for constant velocity flow in gradient echo MRI. Since the rephasing occurs for a unique timing and amplitude relationship between gradient pulses applied along a given direction, a slight time shift can be introduced into the bipolar gradient to make the velocity insensitive pulse sequence sensitized and the associated signal used for quantitative velocity measurements [21]. This is the basis for the 'velocity mapping' technique, which allows for the calibrated spin phase shifts to be represented spatially based on the phase reconstruction gray scale and ultimately translated into absolute velocity values (cm/sec) [22,23]. A region of interest function then permits direct assessment of the mean flow velocity over an area of multiple voxels. Therefore, the intravascular cross-sectional area (cm^2) of a vessel, such as the ascending aorta, can be measured and multiplied by the derived mean flow velocity in order to calculate mean instantaneous volume flow (ml/s) for that vessel [24].

Imaging Orientations and Acquisition Schemes

The orientations most often used for cardiovascular MRI are the transaxial; coronal, and sagittal planes which are orthogonal to the thorax [7]. However, by electronic axial rotation, orientations related to the inherent axes of the cardiovascular structures, such as the thoracic aorta, can also be obtained [25]. This permits acquisition of important single-oblique images, such as those directed along the long axis of the thoracic aorta (Fig. 4). With further axial rotation, double-oblique imaging can also be performed.

Nevertheless, diseased vasculature is often tortuous and seldom courses in a single plane. Therefore, even obliquely oriented 2-D MRI images may be limited in comparison to conventional angiograms which represent full thickness projections of the blood vessels and are not affected by their courses. Accordingly, MRI angiography methods may be employed to help overcome this limitation [26]. Be

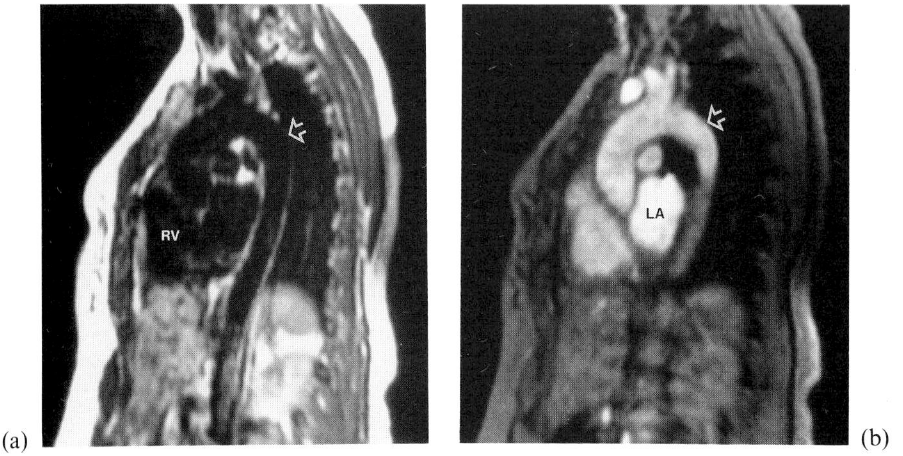

Figure 4. *LONG-AXIS IMAGING OF THE THORACIC AORTA (SPIN-ECHO AND CINE; LONG-AXIS). Both the spin-echo image with its 'dark blood' appearance (a) and the cine image with its 'bright blood' appearance (b) demonstrate the thoracic aorta (open arrows) along its long-axis.*

cause true three-dimensional (3-D) volume MRI angiographic methods may suffer from both motion artefact and loss of intravascular signal due to blood flowing through the thick imaging volume, thin slice, 2-D, flow sensitive acquisition techniques may be better used to obtain projection MRI angiograms of the thoracic aorta [27]. In order to eliminate unwanted signal from adjacent systemic veins, such as the superior vena cava, judiciously placed saturation pulses may be used within a series of such overlapping, flow compensated gradient echo images of the thoracic aorta; the resulting magnitude data may then be postprocessed in several ways. A maximal intensity projection (MIP) technique allows production of projection aortograms in multiple obliqued orientations; the reconstructed images can then be displayed in a dynamic image loop. If the MIP reconstruction artefactually displays discontinuity of the vessels, it is often helpful to view the original series of thin-slice, 2-D tomographic images in the form of a dynamic loop to appreciate vessel continuity. Finally, a multiplanar reconstruction (MPR) through the same stacked series allows indirect production of additional tomographic images oriented through the area of interest.

Anatomical Evaluation of Thoracic Aortic Disease with MRI

Normal haemodynamics are such that little to no signal is usually received from the intra-aortic blood pools on standard static magnitude data images from spin-echo MRI [9,16]. However, under circumstances of blood flowing below a critical velocity, whether physiological or pathophysiological in nature, intra-aortic signal may be noted [28]. When blood flow is exceptionally sluggish or stagnant due to disease of the thoracic aorta, such abnormal signal is frequently observed even on systolic spin-echo images due to the reduction of time-of-flight and phase change effects.

A characteristic of slower flowing blood on intensity images from multiple spin-echo sequences with balanced and symmetric gradient structures is even-echo rephasing [9,20]. It represents enhancement of phase coherence and reduction of signal cancelling effects of proton spins in regions of non-turbulent, slow, constant velocity blood flow with the even numbered 180° RF-refocusing pulses [9,17]. This phenomenon is manifested as an increase in flow signal intensity, both in absolute values and relative to other tissues, from an odd echo image to the subsequent even echo image. Since this signal variation is true only of proton spins moving at constant velocity, slow flow can often be differentiated from fixed, solid, intra-aortic material (e.g. thrombus) which also causes abnormal signal but does not demonstrate even echo rephasing.

Slow blood flow can also be differentiated qualitatively from stationary intra-aortic material using reconstructions of the phase-data from spin-echo MRI sequences [6,19]. Because of its fixed nature, an intra-aortic mass appears with the same gray shade on phase display as other immobile structures [29]. On the other hand, slowly flowing blood has an appearance which is quite different because of its moving protons. Unfortunately, any structure that is moving during the application of the gradients, such as a mobile intra-aortic mass, may produce an observable phase change which may lead to improper identification. In addition, physical factors (e.g. magnetic susceptibility) can alter local phase progression, which then may be misinterpreted as phase change due to motion [9,17].

Physiological Evaluation of Thoracic Aortic Disease with MRI

The pursuit of the evaluation of physiological aspects of cardiovascular disease by MRI has resulted in the development and implementation of a number of interesting techniques [9,30]. Some emphasize the production from magnitude data of anatomically accurate images representing the different segments of the cardiac cycle and others demonstrate physical changes within the acquired phase data that reflect motion (e.g. blood flow).

Cine MRI has assumed an important role in physiological evaluation of cardiovascular disease [9,13]. Normal and abnormal patterns of intra-aortic blood flow are reflected by variations in gradient echo signal intensity. Normally, the intra-aortic blood pool shows almost uniformly increased signal intensity during most of the cardiac cycle, although normal increases in flow rates in systole are represented by increased signal intensity (Fig. 5) [9].

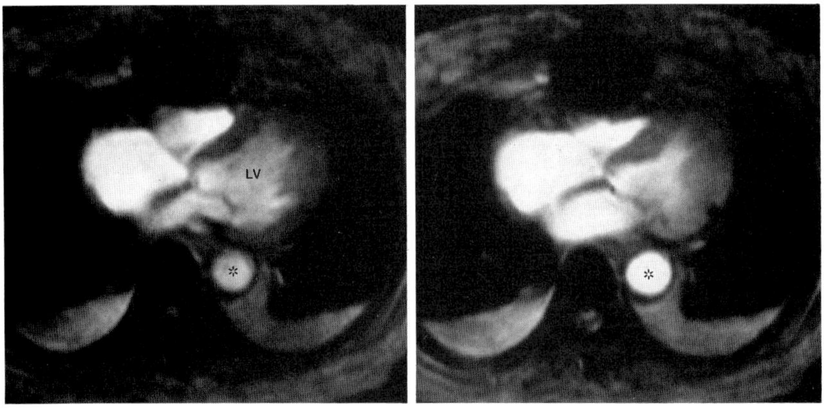

(a) (b)

Figure 5. *NORMAL VARIATION IN INTRA-AORTIC BLOOD FLOW SIGNAL DURING THE CARDIAC CYCLE (CINE; TRANSAXIAL). Compared to the diastolic image (a), the systolic image (b) demonstrates markedly increased signal intensity of blood within the descending thoracic aorta (asterisks) related to higher flow rates. Reprinted from White RD, van Rossum AC. Introduction to the use of magnetic resonance imaging. In: Elliott LP, (ed), The Fundamentals of Cardiac Imaging in Children and Adults, J.B. Lippincott, Philadelphia - 1991;206-220).*

From basic phantom work with cine MRI it is now recognized that signal intensity increases on such images with increasing flow velocity up to a point (i.e. 60 cm/sec), because partially saturated protons are washed out of the imaging plane and completely replaced by fully magnetized protons at a very rapid rate [31]. Beyond this point, there is signal loss primarily due to spin dephasing effects which increase with increasing TE [32]. Phase cancellation, exaggerated by turbulent flow, is a common cause of signal void on cine MRI [33]. A combination of these effects accounts for the characteristic focal pronounced 'signal void jet' found with thoracic aortic disease causing complex flow with high non-uniform velocity distribution, acceleration, and turbulence (Fig. 6) [9,34]. On the other hand, a more diffuse

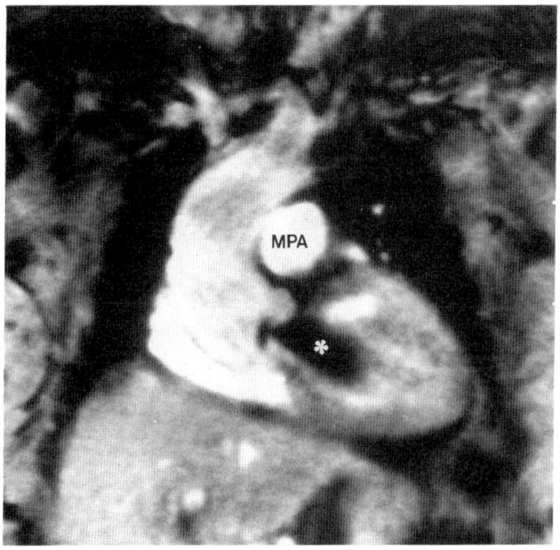

Figure 6. *'SIGNAL-VOID JET' (CINE; CORONAL). A discrete area of pronounced signal void, representing a jet of complex regurgitant flow (asterisk) in diastole, is noted passing into the left ventricle.*

intermediate 'signal void cloud' in regions of slow flow appears to, for the most part, result from saturation effects as these slowly moving proton spins remain in the imaging volume over a longer period of time and, hence, experience a greater number of RF excitation pulses (Fig. 7) [9].

Velocity mapping performed in combination with cine MRI allows a plot of mean instantaneous volume-flow to be made over a cardiac cycle represented on the image loop (Fig. 8) [23,35]. This allows

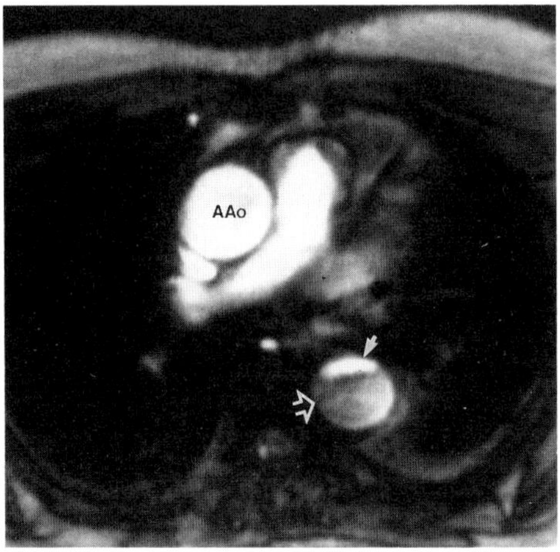

Figure 7. *'SIGNAL-VOID CLOUD' (CINE; TRANSAXIAL). Diffuse intermediate signal loss, representing a cloud of slowly flowing blood (open arrow), is noted within the false lumen of an aortic dissection of the descending thoracic aorta. Evidence of more rapidly flowly blood is noted in the true lumen (closed arrow). Reprinted from White RD, van Rossum AC. Introduction to the use of magnetic resonance imaging. In: Elliott LP (ed), The Fundamentals of Cardiac Imaging in Children and Adults, J.B. Lippincott, Philadelphia - 1991;206-220.*

quantitative characterization of total flow through any segment of diseased thoracic aorta over a complete cardiac cycle and/or calculation of stroke volume of the left ventricle if the volume flow curve from the ascending aorta is integrated.

MRI of Acquired Thoracic Aortic Disease

Aortic Dissection

Definitive diagnosis of aortic dissection rests upon the demonstration of an intimal flap, and current therapeutic management is largely predicated upon the proximal extent of the flap [36,37]. Thus, the evaluation of thoracic aortic disease requires unequivocal detection or exclusion of an intimal flap and, if present, the determination as to whether there is involvement of the ascending aorta [1]. Documentation of aortic dissection involving the ascending aorta (i.e. type A)

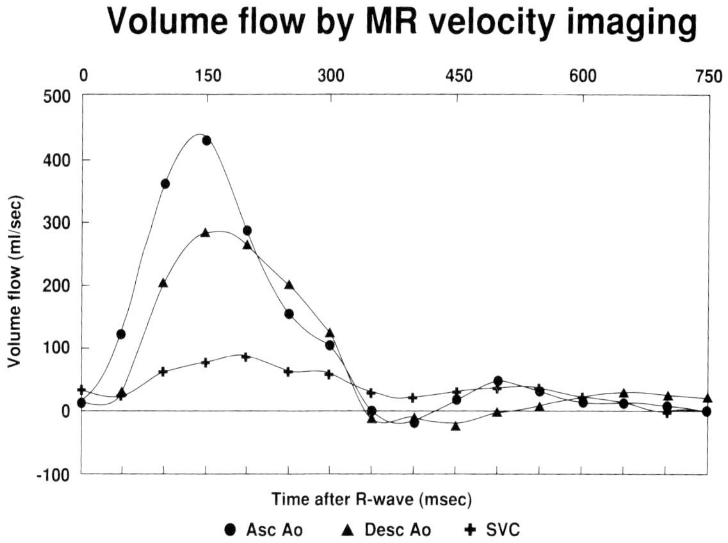

Figure 8. *VOLUME-FLOW OVER A CARDIAC CYCLE (VELOCITY MAPPING; TRANSAXIAL). This figure represents the volume-flow (ml/sec) averaged over the transaxial cross-section of the thoracic great vessels during a complete cardiac cycle. The volume-flow wave form of the superior vena cava is noted to be biphasic. Total flow in each vessel per cardiac cycle is obtained by integrating the area under the respective volume-flow curve. The difference between ascending aortic and descending aortic volume-flow represents flow to the head and upper extremities (courtesy of A.C. van Rossum, M.D., Free University Hospital, Amsterdam).*

generally warrants immediate surgical repair, whereas establishing that a dissection is limited to the descending portion of the aorta (i.e. type B) generally indicates the need for only medical therapy.

A valuable application of MRI, identified early in its development, has been the non-invasive evaluation of suspected aortic dissection [1,2,6]. An intimal flap of aortic dissection is usually well visualized on MRI. On static spin-echo MRI images, an intimal flap is readily identified when there is rapidly flowing blood in both the true and false lumina; the flap appears as a linear structure located within the intra-aortic space and surrounded by signal void of rapidly flowing blood within both channels (Fig. 9) [1,2,6] Intimal flap detection on spin-echo MRI has been reported in 58% up to 100% of cases of aortic dissection [38,40]. The appearance of an intimal flap in a similar haemodynamic setting can be quite dramatic on cine MRI; the flap is outlined by the bright blood appearance of the rapidly flowing blood within two lumina (Fig. 10) [6,41-44]. In addition, mobility of the intimal flap during the cardiac cycle can be appreciated with cine MRI.

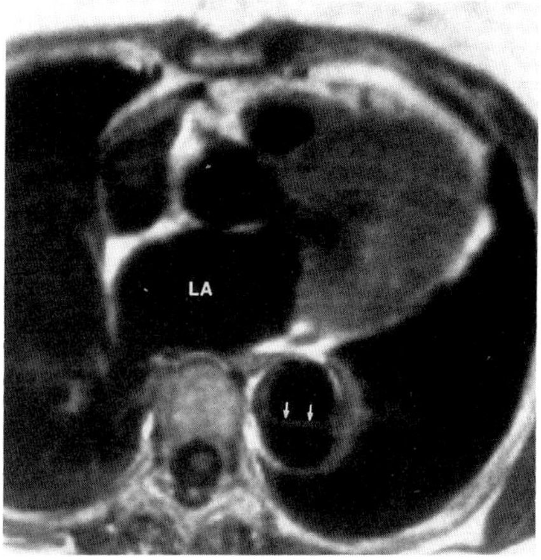

Figure 9. *INTIMAL FLAP OF AORTIC DISSECTION (SPIN-ECHO; TRANSAXIAL). The intimal flap (arrows) of the dissected descending thoracic aorta is surrounded by signal void of rapidly flowing blood in the true and false lumina.*

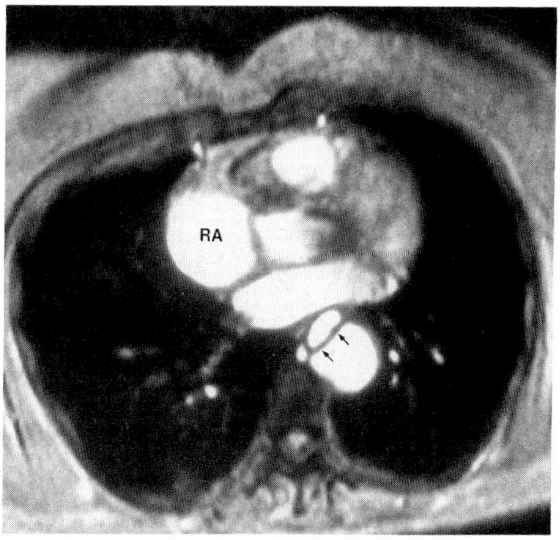

Figure 10. *INTIMAL FLAP OF AORTIC DISSECTION (CINE; TRANSAXIAL). The intimal flap (arrows) is clearly delineated by high signal intensity of rapidly flowing blood in the true and false lumina.*

Identifying the presence or absence of flow in the false lumen of an aortic dissection has therapeutic and prognostic significance [45]. Cases with false channel flow have been shown to have a worse prognosis than those in whom the channel appeared to be fully thrombosed. Flow in the false lumen indicates the presence of a re-entry point back into the true lumen [46].

Abnormal intravascular signal is often identified on MRI within the false lumen of an aortic dissection; this signal may be due to slow blood flow and/or thrombus [1,2,6]. On spin-echo MRI, increased intra-aortic signal due to slow flow may be properly identified and distinguished from that due to thrombus by detecting even echo rephasing or motion dependent phase changes (Fig. 11) [6,44,47,48].

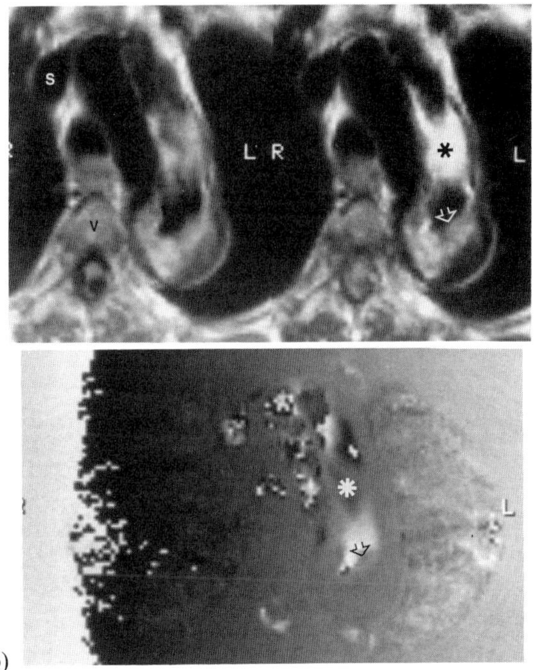

(a)

(b)

Figure 11. *DIFFERENTIATION BETWEEN CAUSES OF ABNORMAL SIGNAL IN THE FALSE LUMEN (SPIN ECHO MAGNITUDE AND PHASE-DISPLAY; TRANSAXIAL). Abnormal intra-aortic signal due to slow blood flow (asterisks) is easily differentiated from that due to thrombus (open arrows) because it demonstrates both even-echo rephasing from first-echo (left) to second-echo (right) magnitude images (a) and evidence of motion dependent phase changes on the corresponding first-echo phase-display image (b) (reprinted from permission from Ref. 2 and 6).*

Cine MRI provides increased capabilities for identifying and differentiating patterns of abnormal signal within the false lumen [6,9,41-44,47]. On cine MRI, the false lumen is typically characterized by delayed systolic signal enhancement relative to the true lumen. In addition, a fluctuating signal void cloud of slow flow is often seen within the false lumen, and this can be differentiated from a more fixed appearing and darker thrombotic mass (Fig. 12). Finally, the

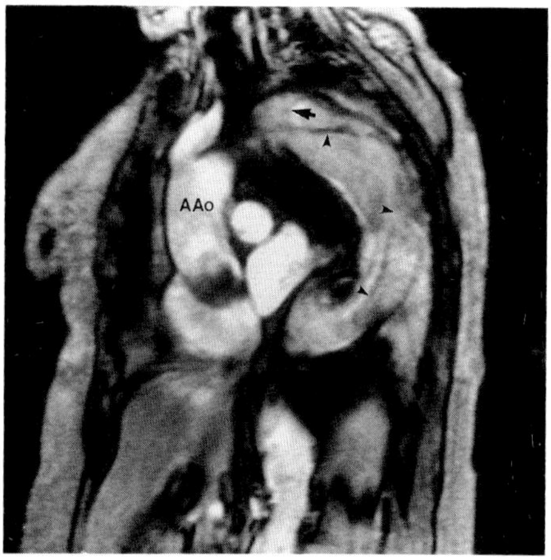

Figure 12. *THROMBUS WITHIN THE FALSE LUMEN (CINE; LONG-AXIS). Within the false lumen of a type B dissection there is a fixed appearing mass representing thrombus (arrow). The intimal flap (arrowheads) is delineated by signal-void cloud of slow flow within the true and false lumina of the dissected segment.*

detection of a signal void jet of complex flow can be used to identify an entry site for blood flowing from the true lumen into the false lumen (Fig. 13) [42].

Velocity mapping has also been used in the evaluation of aortic dissection [35,49,50]. It has been useful both in confirming the presence of flow within the false lumen and in describing the pattern of perfusion of branches to vital organs. Plots of flow velocity versus time has shown decreased antegrade velocity in the false lumen compared to the true lumen during systole and sometimes retrograde flow in the false lumen during diastole (Fig. 14). This reversal of flow in the false channel suggests intimal tears both proximally and distally [46].

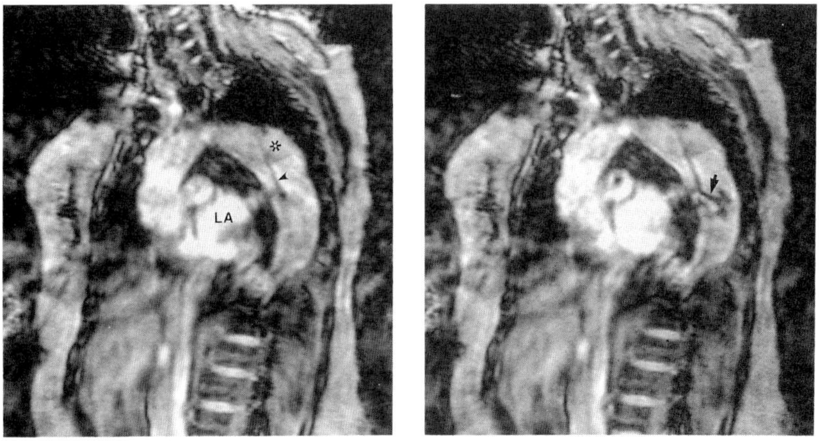

Figure 13. *DEMONSTRATION OF ENTRY SITE (CINE; LONG-AXIS). On the diastolic image (a), the intimal flap (arrowhead) is noted. Thrombus (asterisk) is seen in the most superior aspect of the false lumen. On the systolic image (b), a signal-void jet of complex flow reveals the site of communication at the entry site (arrow).*

However, the differentiation between aortic dissection with a completely thrombosed false lumen and a thoracic aortic aneurysm with mural thrombus can be problematic even for MRI [6]. However, for this differentiation, MRI has distinct advantages over other imaging techniques. These advantages include the non-reliance on contrast administration, and the availability of multiple schemes for detection of even minimal flow in a false lumen. Unfortunately, inwardly displaced intimal calcification, which is easily seen on CT, is not well shown on MRI [1,2]. However, this is not a reliable diagnostic characteristic even for CT, due to partial volume errors associated with a tortuous aorta which may create the appearance of intra-aortic calcification.

If flowing blood within the false lumen cannot be demonstrated, the morphological method of differentiation of an aortic dissection with false channel thrombosis from a thoracic aortic aneurysm with adherent mural thrombus is the same as with CT [1,2,5,6]. With such an aortic dissection, the residual intra-aortic space (i.e. true lumen) typically becomes asymmetrically narrowed due to compression by the thrombus-filled crescentic or oval-shaped false lumen, the outline of which is relatively rounded by the enveloping layers of the

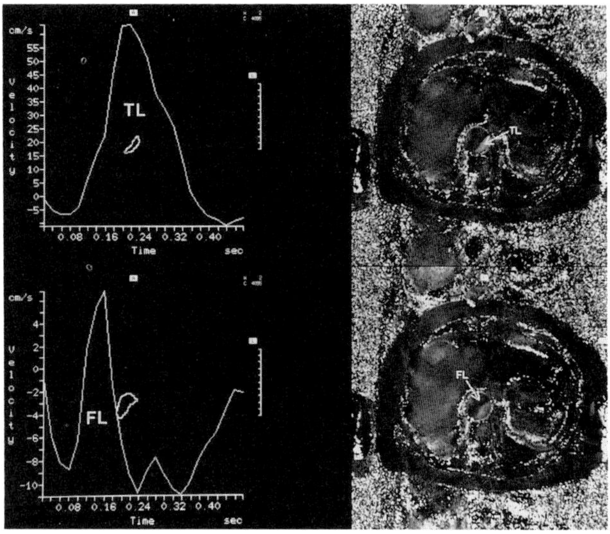

Figure 14. *VELOCITY MAPPING IN AORTIC DISSECTION (VELOCITY MAPPING; TRANSAXIAL). Velocity mapping through the lower descending thoracic aorta produced the following flow velocity curves (left) and the corresponding phase reconstruction images (right). Although there is earlier peaking of velocity within the false lumen (FL) (below), the peak velocity in the false lumen is greatly diminished throughout systole and its diastolic flow is retrograde compared to the flow in the true lumen (TL) (above).*

dissected wall; the overall aortic diameter is usually normal to only slightly enlarged. On the other hand, a relatively normal sized and shaped residual aortic lumen is usually present with a thoracic aortic aneurysm which is partially filled in with the tapering crescentic mural thrombus; the overall aortic diameter is substantially enlarged in either a fusiform or saccular manner. Unfortunately, this morphological method can be limited when the aortic dissection has become aneurysmal, which often applies to chronic cases [6,51]. Other useful guidelines helping in the differentiation of aortic dissection by MRI include the following characteristics: changing position of the thrombus at different levels and longitudinal extension of the thrombus over more than 7 cm [1,2,5,6].

Despite recognized problems and pitfalls [52], the overall effectiveness of MRI for the evaluation of aortic dissection is great [53,54]. The sensitivity of spin-echo MRI for detecting aortic dissection has been shown to be as high as 95% at the 90% specificity level [55]. Improved diagnosis with cine MRI, compared to both CT and spin-echo MRI, has been indicated by initial work [42,43]. The excellent capabilities of MRI to detect cases of type A (Fig. 15) and to distinguish them from type B cases (Fig. 16) have also been de-

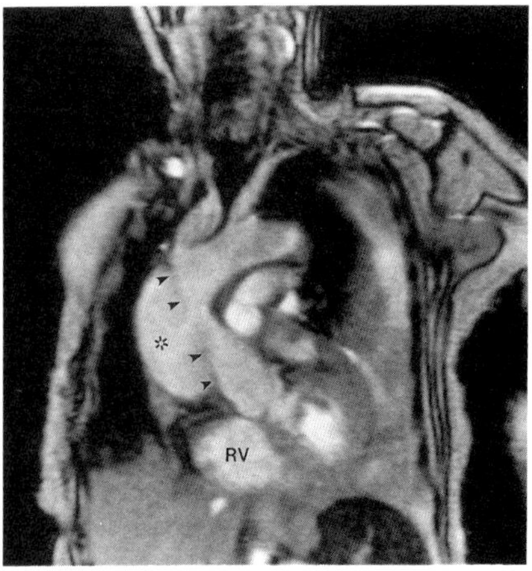

Figure 15. *TYPE A AORTIC DISSECTION (CINE; OBLIQUED). The intimal flap [arrowheads] and false lumen (asterisk) are seen only in the ascending aorta, indicating a limited type A aortic dissection.*

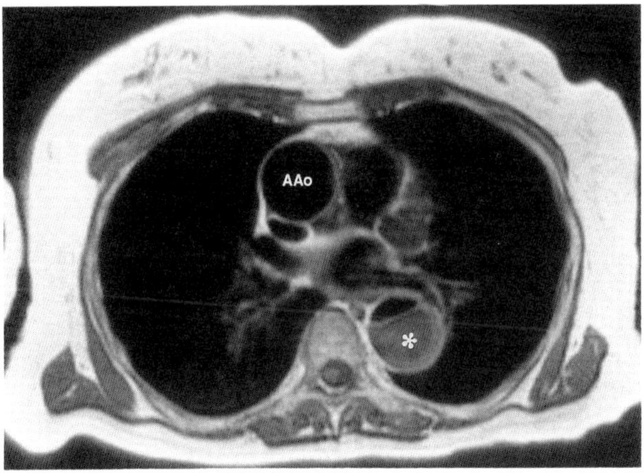

Figure 16. *TYPE B AORTIC DISSECTION (SPIN-ECHO; TRANSAXIAL). There is evidence of aortic dissection involving only the descending thoracic aorta; the ascending aorta is uninvolved. Slow blood flow signal is observed in the large false lumen (asterisk).*

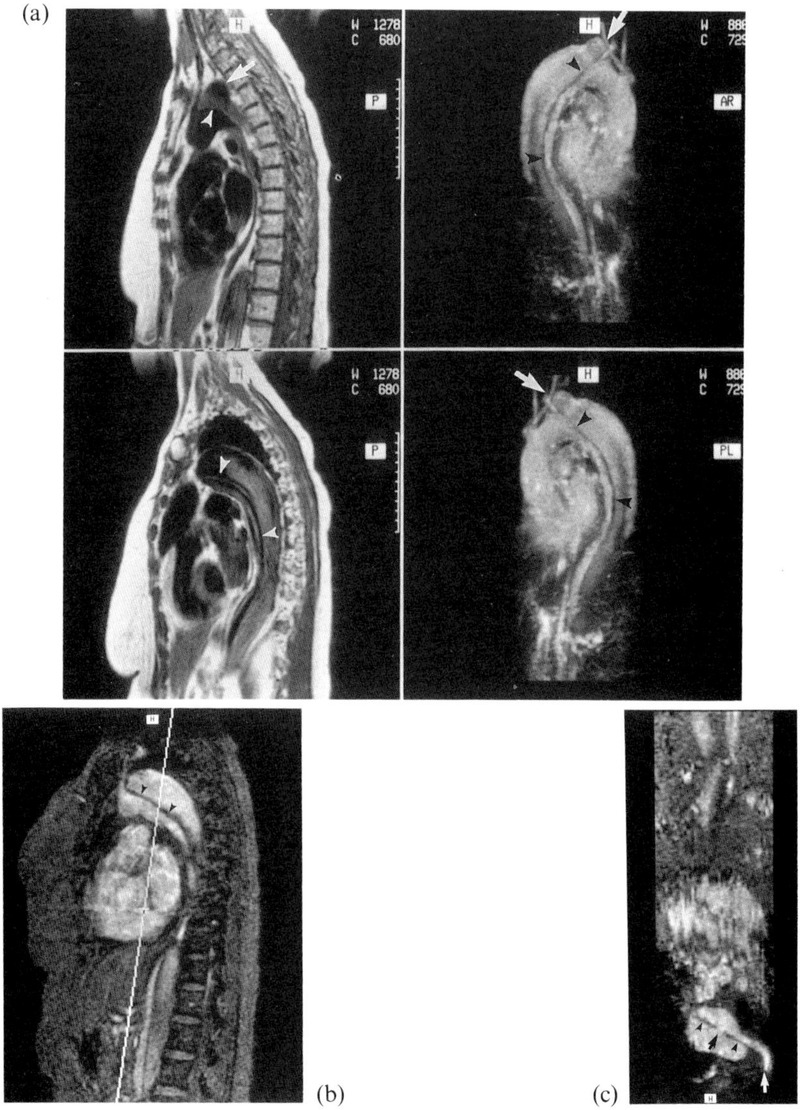

Figure 17. *MRI ANGIOGRAPHIC EVALUATION OF AORTIC DISSECTION (SPIN-ECHO; LONG-AXIS, AND MRI ANGIOGRAPHY WITH MIP AND MPR). Although identified on the spin echo (left image a), evidence of the type B aortic dissection with extension into a dilated anomalous right subclavian artery (white arrows) is easily seen on the MRI angiographic MIP images (right a) in several projections (a). Using a near-coronal angulation (b), an MPR tomographic image (c) was produced to demonstrate the communication between the true and false lumina (black arrow). On all images the intimal flap (arrowheads) is noted.*

scribed [56]. Initial work with MRI angiographic techniques for production of projection images alone or with reconstructed tomographic images has been encouraging (Fig. 17).

MRI can also identify complications related to aortic dissection, including extravasation of blood into the pericardial, pleural, or peri-aortic spaces [1,2,6,38,40]. Since it is possible to distinguish the true lumen from the false lumen, MRI can also effectively determine the lumen of origin of the aortic branches (Fig. 18).

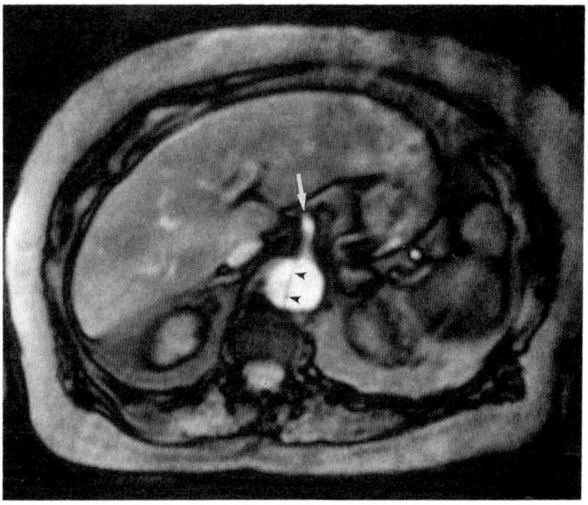

Figure 18. *ORIGIN OF AN AORTIC BRANCH VESSEL IN AORTIC DISSECTION (CINE; TRANSAXIAL). The superior mesenteric artery (arrow) is identified originating from the larger and more signal-enhanced true lumen. The intimal flap (arrowheads) is easily seen.*

MRI has also been used to evaluate cases of aortic dissection after surgical repair or medical therapy; persistent patency of the false lumen has been almost uniformly found [6,48]. The assessment of both the late complications, including aneurysm formation in the false lumen, and postsurgical problems have also been documented [57,58].

Aneurysm of the Thoracic Aorta

The evaluation of thoracic aortic aneurysms requires the demonstration of the following: outer dimension of the aorta; longitudinal extent of the aneurysm; fusiform versus saccular configuration; size of the residual lumen; status of the aortic wall; presence of mural thrombus; relationship of the aneurysm to aortic branches; peri-aortic haematoma; and the effect of the aneurysm on adjacent structures [1,2,6]. These parameters are important clinically for determining prognosis and the need and timing of surgery [59]. MRI is ideally suited for assessing the size, shape, location, aortic branch involvement, secondary effects, and complications of thoracic aortic aneurysms [6,38,54,60]. Spin-echo and cine MRI are capable of defining both the outer wall and the patent lumen of an aneurysm (Fig. 19). Good correlation between descriptions of aneurysm morphology and

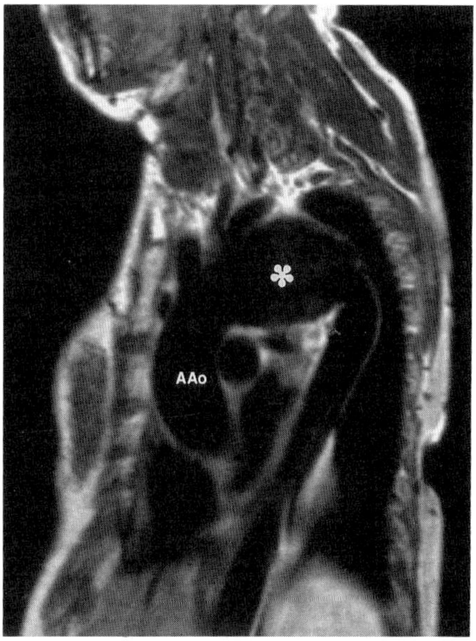

Figure 19. *THORACIC AORTIC ANEURYSM (SPIN-ECHO; LONG-AXIS). A focal aneurysm involving the distal aortic arch (asterisk) is identified. It is fusiform in morphology.*

diameter by MRI and those by other imaging procedures has been established. Also, the ability of MRI to image the proximal thoracic aorta in multiple planes facilitates the differentiation between causes of ascending aortic aneurysm which preserve (e.g. atherosclerotic dilatation) from those resulting in effacement (e.g. aortico-annuloectasia) of the junction of the sinuses and tubular portion (Fig. 20) [61]. MRI angiographic techniques may gain an increasingly important role in the evaluation of thoracic aortic aneurysms.

Identification of different constituents of the aortic aneurysm is also possible with MRI [1,2,6,60]. Thrombus atherosclerotic plaques

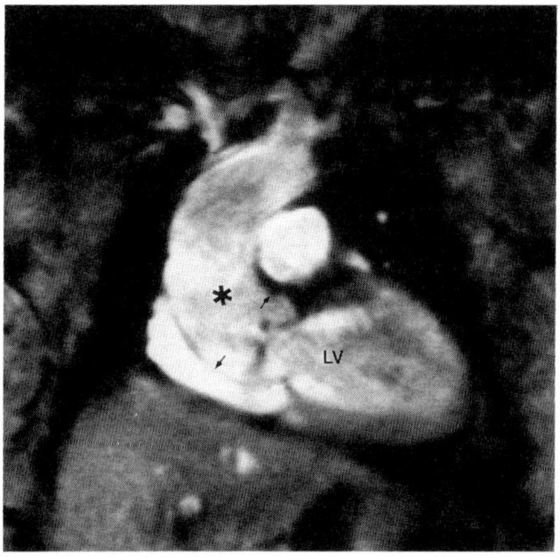

Figure 20. *ACQUIRED AORTICO-ANNULOECTASIA (CINE; CORONAL). There is overall dilatation of the ascending aorta (asterisk), but this is most evident at the level of the aortic root. At this level, there is some early effacement of the sinotubular junction (arrows).*

are both demonstrated as areas of wall thickening. However, on a multiple spin-echo series, thrombus decreases in relative signal intensity while atheromatous material maintains its intensity [38]. Using spin-echo MRI images reflecting the presence or absence of either even echo rephasing or motion dependent phase changes, the differentiation between stagnant blood and fixed mural material in a thoracic aortic aneurysm can be accomplished (Fig. 21). This is also accomplished with cine MRI.

One of the most life-threatening complications of aortic aneurysms is rupture. The ability of MRI to detect penetrating aortic ulcers has been demonstrated (Fig. 22) [62]. MRI also permits the differentiation between haemorrhage versus inflammatory fibrosis surrounding the thoracic aorta which may be problematic for CT [47]. Acute haemorrhage has a spin-echo intensity greater than that of muscle but less than that of fat on a T1-weighted sequence but an intensity similar to that of fat on the T2-weighted sequence. Chronic peri-aortic hematomas, on the other hand, have intensities comparable to fat on both the T1- and T2-weighted sequences. These appearances are quite different from those of peri-aortic inflammatory fibrosis. Based partly on signal intensity changes, MRI has been found to be superior to CT in distinguishing acute intramural haematoma from both atherosclerotic

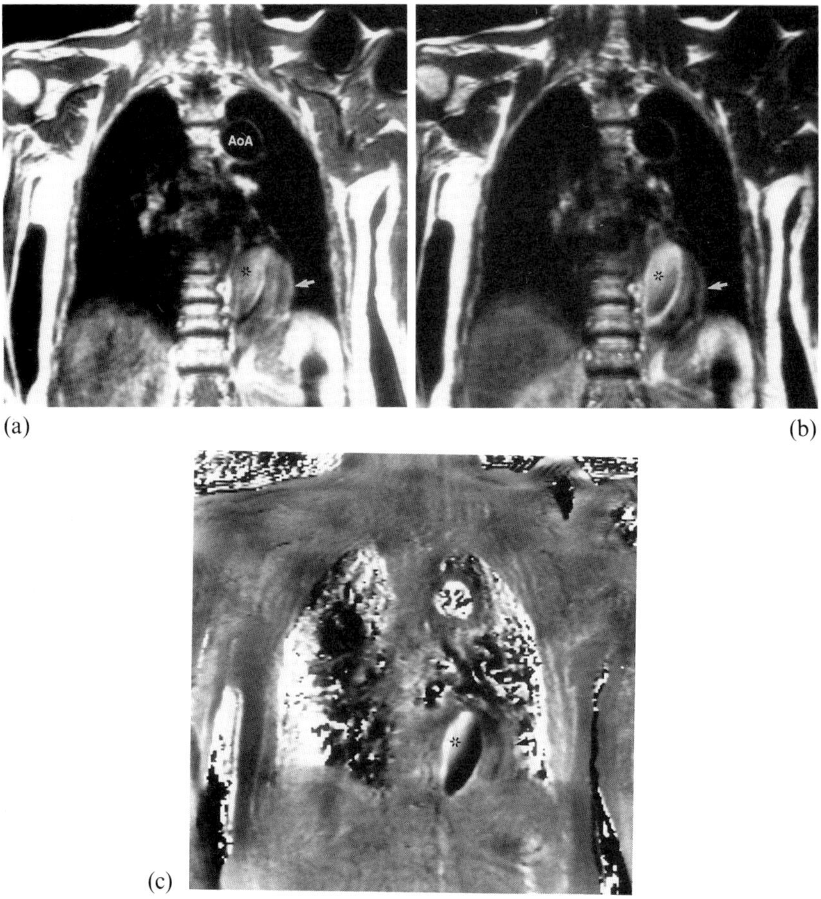

Figure 21. *THORACIC AORTIC ANEURYSM WITH SLOW BLOOD FLOW AND THROMBUS (SPIN ECHO MAGNITUDE AND PHASE-DISPLAY; CORONAL). Because of the presence of both even-echo rephasing from the first-echo (a) to the second-echo (b) image and phase changes on the phase-display image (c) the slow blood flow (asterisks) is properly identified and differentiated from the adherent mural thrombus (arrows). Reprinted from White RD, van Rossum AC. Introduction to the use of magnetic resonance imaging. In: Elliott LP (ed), The Fundamentals of Cardiac Imaging in Children and Adults, J.B. Lippincott, Philadelphia - 1991;206-220.*

plaque and chronic intraluminal thrombus. For related reasons, MRI is also valuable in evaluating many postoperative complications of repair of a thoracic aortic aneurysm (Fig. 23) [58].

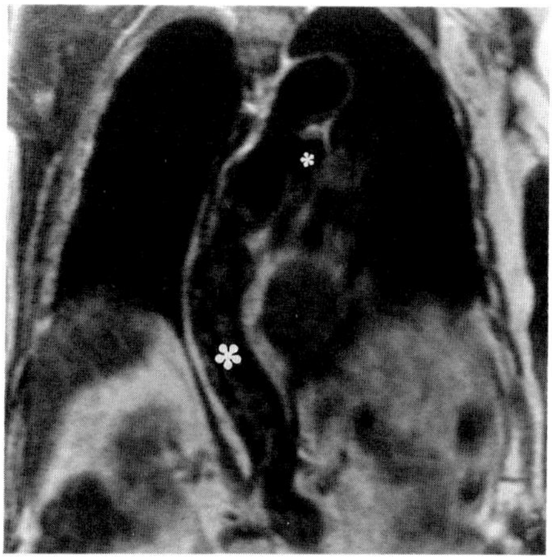

Figure 22. *RUPTURED ATHEROSCLEROTIC PLAQUE (SPIN-ECHO; OBLIQUED). A focal saccular out-pouching from the proximal descending aorta with limited intramural extension represents the product of a penetrating atherosclerotic ulcer (small asterisk). The lower descending and upper abdominal aorta (large asterisk) demonstrates atherosclerotic changes, including thickening of the wall, and evidence of slow intraluminal flow.*

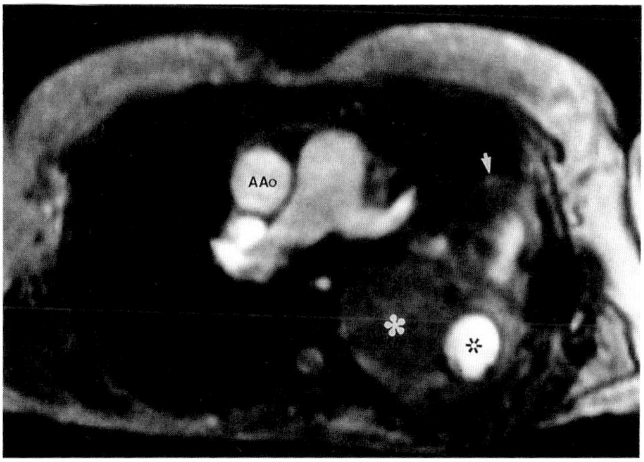

Figure 23. *PERI-AORTIC HAEMATOMA STATUS POST-AORTIC GRAFTING (CINE; TRANS-AXIAL). Signal enhancement of rapidly flowing blood is noted within the grafted descending thoracic aorta (black asterisk). Surrounding the graft is a large peri-aortic collection of organizing haematoma (white asterisk). Anterior to this collection is a more fluidic loculated pleural effusion (arrow).*

Acquired Aortic Root Disease

Acquired disease of the aortic root has several forms [1,2,6]. A sinus of Valsalva aneurysm most commonly involves the right, and least often the left, coronary artery sinus. Non-ruptured sinus of Valsalva aneurysms are usually asymptomatic, but occasionally they may cause either atrioventricular conduction problems or outflow obstruction from the right ventricle due to their mass effect. MRI is effective in detecting this pattern of asymmetric dilatation of the aortic root with focal prominence of a sinus of Valsalva (Fig. 24). In addition, if there is perivalvular abscess formation, MRI can be used to detect and characterize an abscess near the aortic valve (Fig. 25) [6].

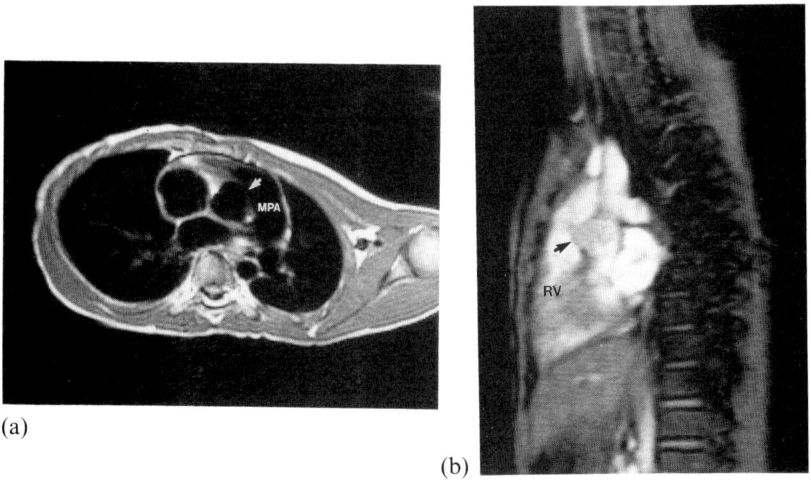

(a) (b)

Figure 24. *ANEURYSM OF RIGHT CORONARY ARTERY SINUS (SPIN-ECHO AND CINE; OBLIQUED). Focal prominence of the right coronary sinus with early aneurysm formation (arrows) is noted. It causes some narrowing of the right ventricle outflow tract. The location and extent of this sinus of Valsalva aneurysm are well demonstrated on both the spin-echo (a) and cine (b) images.*

Acquired aortico-annuloectasia is caused by severe changes of cystic medial necrosis of the wall of the afflicted aorta; the aortic root is most often involved. Consequently, the annulus dilates, carrying the aortic valve leaflets apart and eventually making it impossible for the edges to meet in diastole. The characteristic diffuse dilatation usually associated with effacement of the sinotubular junction and an 'onion-bulb' configuration of the proximal ascending aorta and

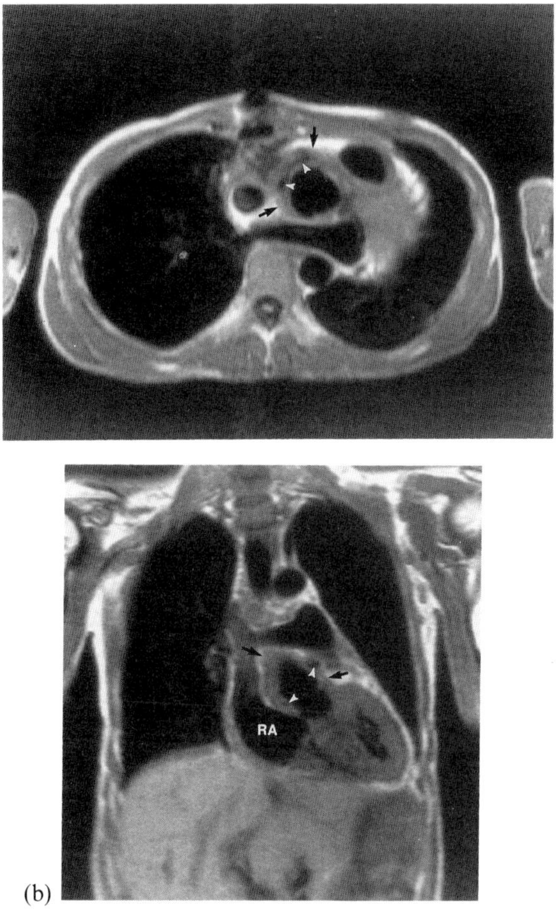

(a)

(b)

Figure 25. *PERI-AORTIC/PERI-AORTIC VALVE ABSCESS (SPIN-ECHO; TRANSAXIAL AND CORONAL). The thickened appearance of the walls of the aortic root and proximal ascending aorta, noted both on the transaxial (a) and coronal (b) images, represents purulent material (arrows). Small rounded areas of signal loss (arrowheads) represent the artefact from the prosthetic aortic valve.*

aortic root is easily seen on MRI. In general, the sinuses of Valsalva are symmetrically dilated in this form of aortic root disease [6,9].

The integrity of the aortic root and aortic valve annulus can also be well assessed using cine MRI [1,2,6,44]. This evaluation is particularly important in cases of type A aortic dissection because 25% of such cases have involvement of the aortic valve annulus, causing aortic insufficiency [45]. Dilatation of the aortic root from acquired aortico-annuloectasia is another common cause of secondary aortic insufficiency.

Cine MRI is capable of detecting direct evidence of such aortic valve disease [9]. Because of signal enhancement of the intracardiac/intravascular blood pools, morphological changes of the aortic valve leaflets may be demonstrated on Cine MRI; due to the dynamic display, abnormal leaflet motion may also be appreciated [13].

The complex nature of retrograde flow through an incompetent aortic valve is manifested by the characteristic signal void jet proximal to the closed valve within the otherwise signal enhanced left ventricle (Fig. 26) [9,13]. The detection of these jets has been shown to be an accurate means of identifying significant aortic insufficiency [63,64]. The assessment of the severity aortic insufficiency using cine MRI has been approached by two methods [65]; one approach

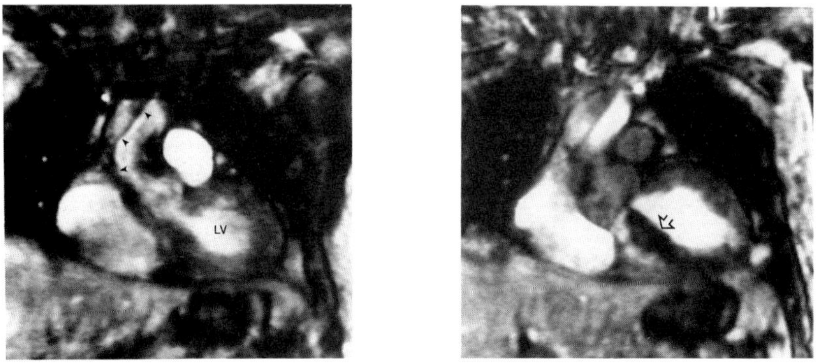

(a) (b)

Figure 26. *SECONDARY AORTIC INSUFFICIENCY FROM AORTIC ROOT AND AORTIC VALVE DISEASE (CINE; CORONAL). A type A aortic dissection with involvement of the aortic root and ascending aorta is well demonstrated on the systolic image (a). The aortic dissection is manifested by an intimal flap (arrowheads). The diastolic image (b) demonstrates aortic insufficiency with a signal-void jet (open arrow).*

emphasizes the size of the regurgitant flow jet and the other the quantitated effects on left ventricle volumes. The size of an aortic insufficiency jet has been evaluated both semiquantitatively and quantitatively according to the area or volume of the region of signal void [66]. Comparison of the stroke volume of the right ventricle with that of the left ventricle provides another quantitative method for defining the severity of aortic insufficiency. In the presence of aortic insufficiency in the absence of right heart valve problems, the aortic insufficiency regurgitant volume can be calculated as the difference in stroke volume (i.e. left ventricle larger than right ventricle), and can be used to determine aortic insufficiency regurgitant fraction [9,67-68].

Traumatic Thoracic Aortic Injury

Complete or partial transection of the thoracic aorta may result from a severe deceleration injury; it has been found in one-sixth of all casualties of automobile accidents [69]. If the individual with thoracic aortic injury survives the initial traumatic event, they often die within the first week from progressive haemorrhage at the site of injury which is usually the aortic isthmus. If the thoracic aorta is only partially transected, a localized pseudo-aneurysm may develop [70]; rupture of these lesions is unpredictable. Thus, immediate and aggressive evaluation and treatment of suspected traumatic thoracic aortic injury is essential.

Potential problems with the use of transaxial imaging in evaluating aortic transection have been previously described [5,6]. Subtle abnormalities in aortic contours due to such injury may be missed on a series of contiguous transaxial images because of non-perpendicular imaging, partial volume averaging, and difficulties in scanning traumatized individuals. MRI has not been found to have a valuable role in the initial evaluation for traumatic injury to the thoracic aorta [1,2,6]. On the other hand, MRI is diagnostically accurate for the evaluation of traumatic pseudo-aneurysms [71].

Aortitis

Aortitis, or inflammation of the aortic wall, relates to several mechanisms including immunological disorders and infections. The spin-echo MRI findings in several types of aortitis have been reported [6,44,60,72]. In cases of Takayasu's disease studied using spin-echo MRI, features consisted of one or a combination of the following: mural thickening involving the thoracic aorta and/or arch vessels; arch vessel occlusion or stenosis; coarctation of the lower thoracic aorta or wall thickening and severe stenosis of the abdominal aorta. Giant cell and bacterial aortitis has also been examined using spin-echo MRI; irregular wall thickening and aneurysmal dilatation of the aorta have been noted (Fig. 27). Although increased signal intensity has been observed in regions of aortic wall thickening, it is unlikely that such inflammatory changes can be reliably distinguished from atherosclerotic plaque or recently formed thrombotic material.

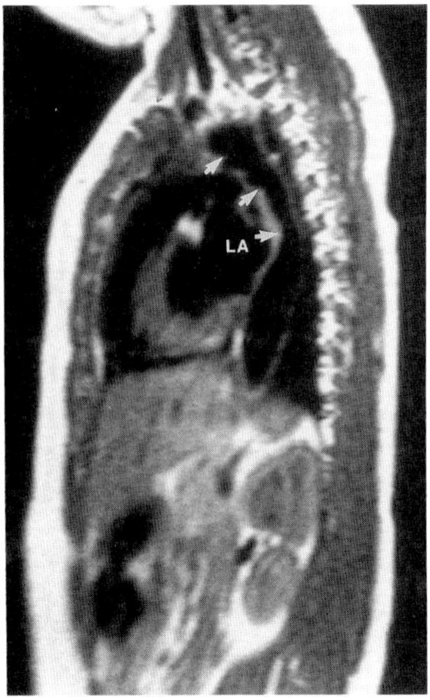

Figure 27. *GIANT CELL ARTERITIS (SPIN-ECHO; LONG-AXIS). Diffuse irregular wall thickening is associated with moderate narrowing of the proximal descending aorta (arrows).*

While MRI could be particularly helpful in cases in which severe stenosis of the arch vessels, descending thoracic aorta, or abdominal aorta complicates catheterization for aortography, limited accuracy of spin-echo MRI for defining stenoses of aortic branch vessels has been noted [72]. MRI angiographic techniques have been showing great promise for the visualization of peripheral vasculature and they may eventually improve the capabilities of MRI for evaluation of aortitis with small and medium sized vessel involvement.

MRI of Congenital Thoracic Aortic Disease

Congenital Thoracic Aortic Stenoses

The value of MRI in the assessment of coarctation, the most common cause of congenital stenosis of the thoracic aorta, was recognized early [73-76]. While coarctation can usually be diagnosed by echocardiography in infants, the wider field-of-view allows it to obtain images of the entire thoracic aorta for the improved diagnosis of coarctation in larger children and adults.

Spin-echo MRI can be used to assess the exact location of the narrowing; a coarctation in the typical juxtaductal location (Fig. 28)

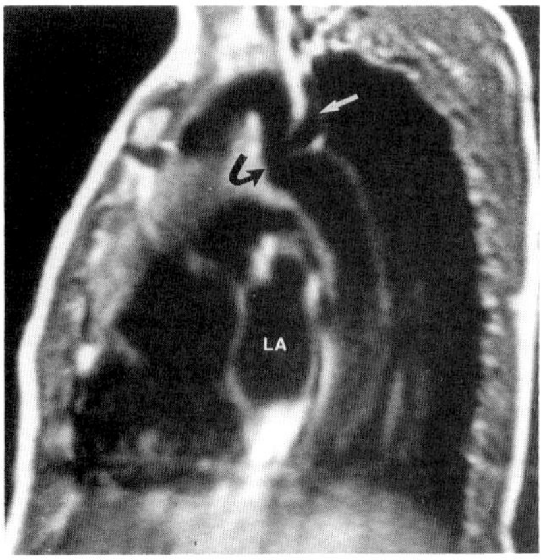

Figure 28. *JUXTADUCTAL COARCTATION (SPIN-ECHO; LONG-AXIS). Moderate narrowing due to a coarctation (curved arrow) is noted in the juxtaductal region. The left subclavian artery (straight arrow) originates from the region of coarctation and shows proximal stenosis.*

can be easily differentiated from a coarctation in other locations [73-76]. Next, the longitudinal extent can be determined, and a discrete short-segment narrowing can be differentiated from a more generalized long-segment narrowing. Finally, the degree of stenosis due to coarctation can be judged. Secondary findings of coarctation include dilatation or stenosis of the left subclavian artery, poststenotic dilation of the descending aorta beyond the level of coarctation large collateral vessels, and left ventricle hypertrophy (Fig. 29).

The accuracy of spin-echo MRI in the evaluation of coarctation has been assessed. In cases with angiographic proof of coarctation, spin-echo MRI has almost universally detected properly the site and type of coarctation. Based on interpretation of images from spin-echo MRI series, sensitivity for detection of thoracic aortic abnormalities including coarctation has been shown to be 94% at a 95% specificity level [77]. A superior accuracy for diagnosis of coarctation using spin-echo MRI (i.e. 91%) compared to echocardiography (i.e. 62%) has been noted [75].

Coarctation has also been evaluated using cine MRI [9,79-81]. Not only does cine MRI provide anatomical information, it offers infor-

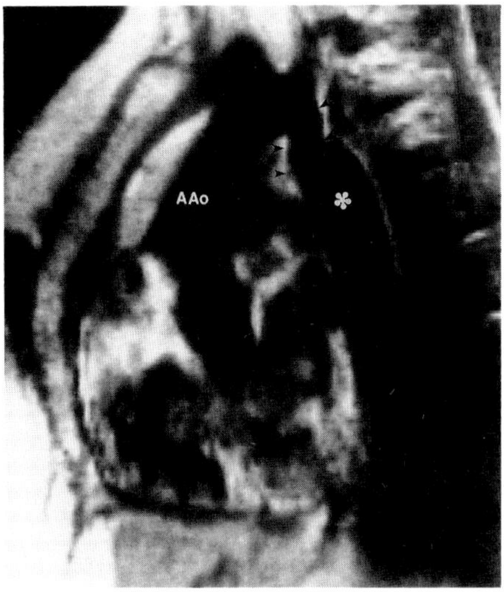

Figure 29. *POSTSTENOTIC DILATATION BEYOND A COARCTATION (SPIN-ECHO; LONG-AXIS). A moderately long segment of narrowing due to coarctation (arrowheads) is followed by a segment of poststenotic dilatation (asterisk) of the descending thoracic aorta.*

mation about the haemodynamics at or beyond the site of coarctation, the anatomy and function of the aortic valve, and the function of the left ventricle. The anatomical severity of coarctation determined with cine MRI has been similar to that assessed with spin-echo MRI, but the haemodynamic observations obtained from cine MRI supply additional physiological information. The smallest diameter of the signal enhanced intra-aortic space noted on cine MRI also showed excellent agreement with the degree of narrowing noted on contrast aortography in proven cases of coarctation [79].

A signal void jet beyond the level of the aortic narrowing has been frequently noted in the setting of coarctation (Fig. 30); this represents complex flow beginning at the site of the narrowing [9,79-81]. Signal void jets have been seen extending distally from the coarctation site in most cases, except those with mild degrees of aortic narrowing or those with severe coarctation but normal flow velocities due to large collaterals. Such jets on cine MRI indicate systolic velocities of greater than 3.5 m/s and end-diastolic velocities greater than 0.8 m/s across the coarctation site [79].

MRI has also been effective for evaluation of coarctation after

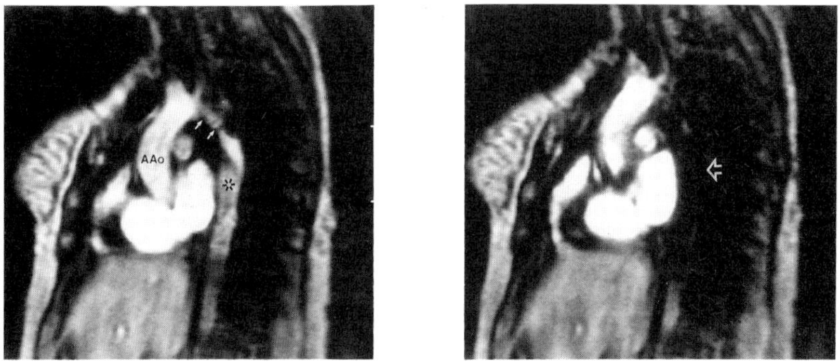

Figure 30. *COARCTATION-INDUCED JET (CINE; LONG-AXIS). On the diastolic image (a), a long segment of coarctation involving the distal arch and upper descending thoracic aorta (arrows) is associated with some poststenotic dilatation [asterisk]. The systolic image (b) shows total signal loss within the descending thoracic aorta (open arrow) due to complex poststenotic flow.*

therapy [78,80-82]. Using spin-echo or cine MRI, the results of surgical repair or balloon angioplasty can be evaluated. Relief of obstruction and/or a decrease in the number and size of collateral vessels have indicated successful therapy.

MRI can also be used to identify restenosis [78]. However, on cine MRI, intra-aortic signal loss beyond the site of repair has not been found to be qualitatively different between cases with and those without a residual gradient [81]. Thus, complex flow resulting in gradient echo signal loss may follow coarctation repair, due either to luminal irregularity or to residual obstruction.

Following coarctation repair, aortic compliance has been measured with MRI from transaxial systolic and diastolic images [81]; it was found to be abnormally low, implicating it as a cause of systolic hypertension after treatment. In addition, complications of coarctation therapy, including aneurysm formation and aortic dissection, have been observed [78,80-82].

MRI may also be used to distinguish between coarctation and complete aortic interruption [6]. The length of absent aortic lumen, with interposed fat or fibrous tissue between the proximal and distal segments, can be assessed. In addition, a patent ductus arteriosus supplying the descending aorta beyond the interruption may be visualized.

Supravalvular aortic stenosis, involving the ascending aorta, can also be readily detected and graded with MRI [6]. The typical 'hour-glass' configuration of the ascending aorta and the poststenotic dilatation can be appreciated (Fig. 31).

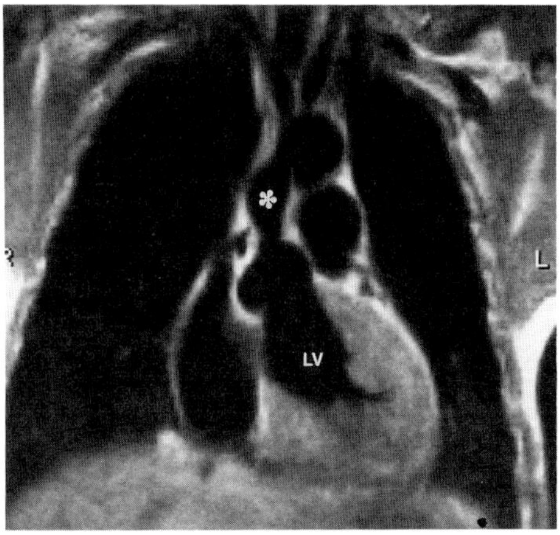

Figure 31. *SUPRAVALVULAR AORTIC STENOSIS (SPIN-ECHO; CORONAL). A long segment narrowing of the mid-ascending aorta (asterisk) gives the ascending aorta an 'hour-glass' configuration. Left ventricle hypertrophy is also noted, reprinted with permission from ref. 2.*

Congenital Aortic Root Disease

MRI has been shown to be particularly valuable in the evaluation of the aortic root and has shown great utility in assessing congenital aortico-annuloectasia, such as from Marfan's syndrome. Using spin-echo MRI, a significantly greater ratio of the aortic root diameter to the pre-arch diameter has been demonstrated in cases with Marfan's syndrome compared to those with ascending aortic enlargement or to normals [83,84]. MRI derived measurements of aortic root diameter have agreed closely with echocardiography measurements [85]. Cine MRI appears to have a significant role in assessing both the anatomical changes and physiological abnormalities (e.g. aortic insufficiency) associated with Marfan's syndrome (Fig. 32).

Cine MRI may also be used to evaluate aortic stenosis due to a bicuspid aortic valve which is often found in association with coarctation of the aorta; the bicuspid nature of the aortic valve can usually be appreciated. If there is aortic stenosis, leaflet thickening and

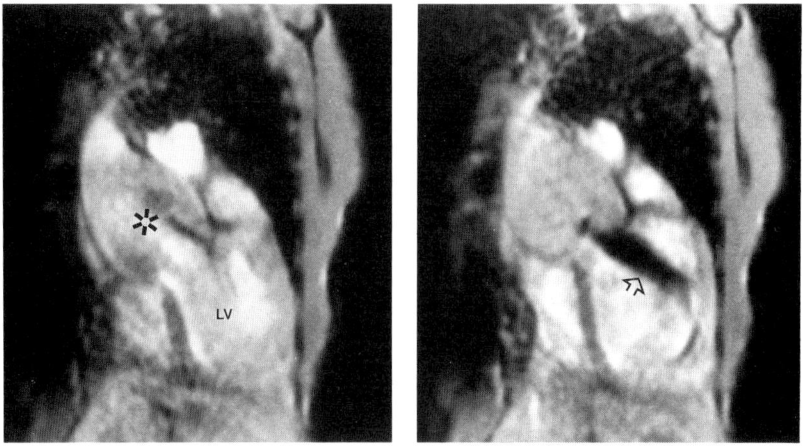

(a) (b)

Figure 32. *AORTIC ROOT DILATATION AND AORTIC INSUFFICIENCY FROM MARFAN'S SYNDROME (CINE; OBLIQUED). The marked of dilatation of the aortic root and proximal ascending aorta with an 'onion-bulb' configuration (asterisk) is well seen on the systolic image (a). The diastolic image (b) shows a signal-void jet of aortic insufficiency (open arrow).*

calcification, both characterized by signal void, may be noted in association with reduced mobility and delayed and limited systolic opening.

Focal pronounced signal void is produced by complex flow through a stenotic aortic valve on cine MRI [6,9]. The resulting signal void jet can be used as a marker for significant aortic stenosis (Fig. 33) [86]. In significant aortic stenosis, the jet extends distally from the level of the aortic valve and expands outward throughout systole until its haemodynamic effects are dissipated and lost within the blood pool of the ascending aorta. Aortic stenosis can be detected and graded using cine MRI [86]. There is good correlation between the severity of pressure drop and the maximal length of the area of the jet within the ascending aorta on cine MRI. However, at pressure gradients above approximately 60 mmHg, no further increase in length is noted.

Aortic Arch Anomalies

Aortic arch anomalies have been effectively evaluated using MRI. The value of MRI has been particularly evident in cases with

(a) 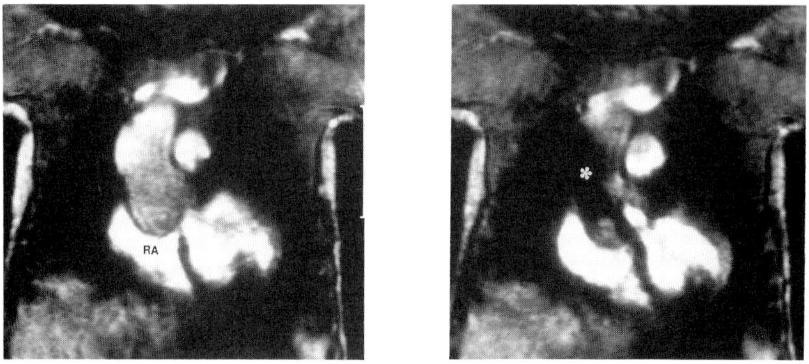 (b)

Figure 33. *BICUSPID AORTIC VALVE WITH AORTIC STENOSIS (CINE; CORONAL). From diastole (a) to systole (b), a signal-void jet (asterisk) appears. It represents significant aortic stenosis related to a bicuspid valve.*

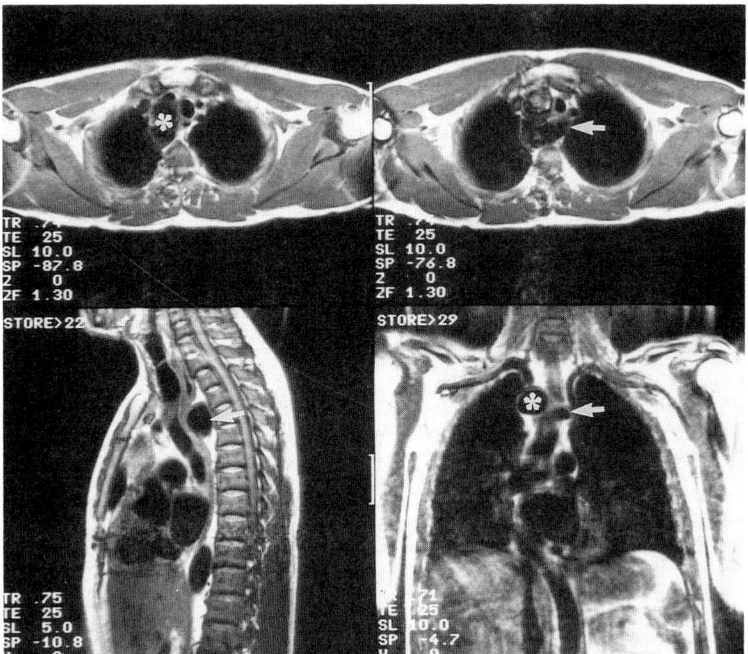

Figure 34. *RIGHT AORTIC ARCH WITH ABERRANT LEFT SUBCLAVIAN ARTERY (SPIN-ECHO; ORTHOGONAL). Originating beyond the right aortic arch (asterisks) is the left subclavian artery from a diverticulum of Kommerell (arrows). It passes retro-oesophageal, causing anterior displacement of the trachea and oesophagus.*

symptoms suggesting tracheo-bronchial compression by the anomaly. Aortic arch anomalies which are assessed well using spin-echo MRI include left aortic arch with an aberrant right subclavian artery, right aortic arch with mirror-imaging branching, right aortic arch with aberrant origin of the left subclavian artery possibly from a ductus diverticulum or diverticulum of Kommerell (Fig. 34), and double aortic arch [75,76,87]. The latter two are of particular note because they are common forms of vascular rings.

While cine MRI does not appear to play a major role in the evaluation of such anomalies, MRI angiographic techniques are very promising (Fig. 35).

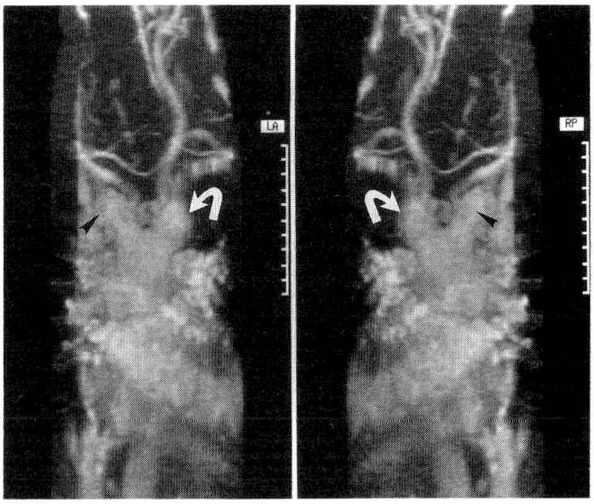

Figure 35. *MRI ANGIOGRAPHY OF AN AORTIC ARCH ANOMALY (MRI ANGIOGRAPHY WITH MIP). Anterior (left) and posterior (right) projections from MIP processing demonstrate the double aortic arch arrangement. The right aortic arch (arrowheads) is higher than the left arch (curved arrows). A complete vascular ring is formed.*

Summary

The combination of anatomical and physiological capabilities of MRI make it particularly suitable for the evaluation of thoracic aortic disease. Its non-invasiveness, its ability to define anatomy by 2-D and/or 3-D schemes, and its ability to evaluate qualitatively and quantitatively motion and intra-aortic flow make MRI the most versatile imaging technique for assessment of disease involving the thoracic aorta. Accordingly, MRI has become the procedure of choice in many institutions.

References

1. White RD, Dooms GC, Higgins CB. Advances in imaging thoracic aortic disease. *Invest Radiol* 1986;**21**:761-778.
2. White RD, Higgins CB. In: Pohost GM, Higgins CB, Nanda NC (eds). *Evaluation of thoracic aortic disease with CT and MRI: reappraisal of the imaging procedure of choice. New concepts in cardiac imaging,* pp 143-168. Chicago: Year Book Publishing, 1989.
3. Hayashi K, Meaney TF Zelch JV. Aortographic analysis of aortic dissection. *AJR* 1974;**122**:769-782.
4. Engberding R, Bender F, Grosse-Heitmeyer W. Identification of dissection or aneurysm of the descending thoracic aorta by conventional and trans-esophageal two-dimensional echocardiography. *Am J Cardiol* 1987;**59**:717-719.
5. White RD, Lipton MJ, Higgins CB. Non-invasive evaluation of suspected thoracic aortic diseasc by contrast-enhanced computed tomography. *Am J Cardiol* 1986;**57**:282-290.
6. Whitc RD, Higgins CB. Magnctic rcsonancc imaging of thoracic vascular discasc. *J Thorac Imag* 1989;**4**:34-50.
7. Higgins CB. MR of the heart: anatomy, physiology, and metabolism. *AJR* 1988;**151**:239-248.
8. Koutcher JA, Burt T. Principles of nuclear magnetic resonance. *J Nucl Med* 1984;**25**:101-111.
9. White RD, Paschal CB, Tkach JA. Functional cardiovascular evaluation by magnetic resonance imaging. *Topics Magn Reson Imag* 1990;**2**:31-48.
10. Lanzer P, Barta C, Botvinick EH. ECG-synchronized cardiac MR imaging: method and evaluation. *Radiology* 1985;**155**:681-686.
11. Crooks LE, Hylton NM, Ortendahl DA. The value of relaxation times and density measurements in clinical MRI. *Invest Radiol* 1987;**22**:158-169 .
12. Haase A, Frahm J, Matthaei D. FLASH imaging: rapid NMR imaging using low flip angle pulses. *J Magn Reson* 1986;**67**:258-266.
13. Sechtem U, Pflugfelder PW, White RD. Cine MR imaging: potential for the evaluation of cardiovascular function. *AJR* 1987;**148**:239-246.
14. Glover GH, Pelc NJ. In: Kressel HY, (ed). *A rapid-gated cine MRI technique.* Magnetic Resonance Annual, pp 299-333. New York: Raven Press, 1988.

15. Lenz GW, Haacke EM, White RD. Retrospective cardiac gating: a review of technical aspects and future directions. *Magnet Reson Imag* 1989;**7**:445-455.
16. Bradley WG, Waluch V. Blood flow: magnetic resonance imaging. *Radiology* 1985;**154**:443-450.
17. von Schulthess GK, Higgins CB. Blood flow imaging with MR: spin-phase phenomenon. *Radiology* 1985;**157**:687-695.
18. von Schulthess GK. *Morphology and function in MRI: Cardiovascular and renal systems*, Berlin:Springer-Verlag, 1989.
19. White EM, Edelman RR, Wedeen VJ. Intravascular signal in MR imaging: use of phase display for differentiation of blood-flow signal from intraluminal disease. *Radiology* 1986;**161**:245-249 .
20. Bradley WG, Waluch V. NMR even echo rephasing in slow laminar flow. *J Comput Assist Tomogr* 1984;**8**:594-598.
21. Moran PR. A flow velocity zeugmatographic interface for NMR imaging in humans. *Magn Reson Imag* 1982;**1**:197-203.
22. Bryant DJ, Payne JA, Firmin N. Measurement of flow with NMR imaging using a gradient pulse and phase difference technique. *J Comput Assist Tomogr* 1984;**8**:588-593.
23. Nayler GL, Firmin DN, Longmore DB. Blood flow imaging by cine magnetic resonance. *J Comput Assist Tomogr* 1986;**10**:715-722.
24. Underwood SR, Firman DN, Klipstein RH. Magnetic resonance velocity mapping: clinical application of a new technique. *Br Heart J* 1987;**57**:404-412.
25. Feiglin DH, George CR, MacIntyre WJ. Gated cardiac magnetic resonance structural imaging: optimization by electronic axial rotation. *Radiology* 1985;**154**:129-132.
26. Edelman RR, Mattle HP, Atkinson DJ, Hoogewould HM. MR angiography. *AJR* 1990;**154**:937-946.
27. Edelman RR, Wentz KU, Mattle H. Protection arteriography and venography: initial clinical results with MR. *Radiology* 1989;**172**:351-357.
28. von Schulthess GK, Fisher MR, Crooks LE. Gated MR imaging of the heart: intracardiac signal in patients and healthy subjects. *Radiology* 1985;**156**:125-132.
29. von Schulthess GK, Augustiny N. Calculation of T2 values versus phase imaging for the distinction between flow and thrombus in MR imaging. *Radiology* 1987;**164**:549-554.
30. Higgins CB, Holt W, Pflugfelder P. Functional evaluation of the heart with magnetic resonance imaging. *Magn Reson Med* 1988;**6**:121-139.
31. Evans AJ, Hedlund LW, Herfkens RJ. Evaluation of steady and pulsatile flow with dynamic MRI using limited flip angles and gradient refocused echoes. *Magn Reson Imag* 1987;475-482.
32. Cranney GB, Gunter BC, Pohost GM. *Mechanism of gradient echo and MR signal loss in a stenotic phantom-influence of flow rate and echo time.* Abstract book from 8th Annual Meeting of SMRM, 1989;203.
33. Evans AJ, Blinder RA, Herfkens RJ. Effects of turbulence on signal intensity in gradient echo images. *Invest Radiol* 1988;**23**:512-518.
34. Podolak MJ, Hedlund LW, Evans AJ. Evaluation of flow through simulated vascular stenoses with gradient echo magnetic resonance imaging. *Invest Radiol* 1989;**24**:184-189.
35. van Rossum AC, Sprenger M, Visser FC. An in-vivo validation of quantitative blood flow imaging in arteries and veins using magnetic resonance phase-shift techniques. *Eur Heart J* 1991;**12:**117-126.
36. Daily PO, Trueblood HW, Stinson EB. Management of acute aortic dissections. *Ann Thorac Surg* 1970;**10**:237-247.

37. Svensson LG, Crawford S, Hess KR, Coselli JS, Safi HJ. Dissection of the aorta and dissecting aortic aneurysms. *Circulation* 1990;**82**:IV23-IV46.
38. Glazer HS, Gutierrez FR, Levitt RG. The thoracic aorta studied by MR imaging. *Radiology* 1985;**157**:149-155.
39. Geisinger MA, Risius B, O'Donnell, JA. Thoracic aortic dissections: magnetic resonance imaging. *Radiology* 1985;**155**:407-412.
40. Amparo EG, Higgins CB, Hricak H. Aortic dissection: magnetic resonance imaging. *Radiology* 1985;**155**:399-406.
41. Spritzer C, Gamsu G, Sostman HD. Magnetic resonance imaging of the thorax: techniques, current applications, and future directions. *J Thorac Imag* 1989;**4**:1-18.
42. Sechtem U, Theissen P, Deider S. Acute and chronic aortic dissection: demonstration of intimal tears and blood flow with MR imaging. *Radiology* 1989;**173**:321.
43. Sonnabend SB, Colletti PM, Pentecost MJ. Demonstration of aortic lesions via cine magnetic resonance imaging. *Magn Reson Imag* 1990;**8**:613-618.
44. Tempany CMC, Zerhouni EA. Clinical magnetic resonance imaging of the vascular system. *Top Magn Reson Imag* 1990;**2**:13-30.
45. Dinsmore RE, Willeron JT, Buckley NJ. Dissecting aneurysms of the aorta : aortographic features affecting prognosis. *Radiology* 1972;**105**:567-572.
46. Dinsmore RE, Wedeen VJ, Miller SW. MRI of dissection of the aorta: recognition of the intimal tear and differential flow velocities. *AJR* 1986;**146**:1286-1288.
47. Fisher MR. Utility of magnetic resonance imaging in critical care patients. *Am J Cardiac Imag* 1990;**4**:287-297.
48. White RD, Ullyot DJ, Higgins CB. MR imaging of the aorta after surgery for aortic dissection. *AJR* 1988;**150**:87-92.
49. Underwood SR, Bogren HG, Rees RSO. Cine magnetic resonance velocity mapping in aortic dissection. *Mag Reson Imag* 1988;**6(Suppl. 1);**51.
50. van Rossum AC, Sprenger M, Valk J. (1989). Clinical application of quantitative flow imaging with magnetic resonance phase-shift techniques in patients with aortic diseases: current value and limitations. Abstract book from 8th Annual Meeting of SMRM, 317.
51. Pernes JM, Grenier P, Desbleds MT. MR evaluation of chronic aortic dissection. *J Comput Assist Tomogr* 1987;**11**:975-981.
52. Solomon SL, Brown JJ, Glazer HS. Thoracic aortic dissection: pitfalls and artefacts in MR imaging. *Radiology* 1990;**177**:224-228.
53. Goldman AP, Kotler MN, Scanlon MH. The complementary role of magnetic resonance imaging, Doppler echocardiography, and computed tomography in the diagnosis of dissecting thoracic aneurysms. *Am Heart J* 1986;**111**:970-981.
54. Dinsmore RE, Liberthson RR, Wismer GL. Magnetic resonance imaging of thoracic aortic aneurysms: comparison with other imaging methods. *AJR* 1986;**146**:309-314.
55. Kersting-Sommerhoff BA, Higgins CB, White RD. Aortic dissection: sensitivity and specificity of MR imaging. *Radiology* 1988;**166**:651-655.
56. Hill JA, Lambert CR, Akins EW. Ascending aortic dissection: detection by MRI. *Am Heart J* 1985;**110**:894-896.
57. DiCesare E, DiRenzi P, Pavone P. Post-surgical follow-up with MR imaging of aortic dissections. *Radiology* 1989;**173**:105.
58. Auffermann W, Olofsson P, Stoney R. MR imaging of complications of aortic surgery. *J Comput Assist Tomogr* 1987;**11**:982-989.
59. Joyce JW, Fairbairn JF, Kincaid OW. Aneurysms of the thoracic aorta: a clinical study with special reference to prognosis. *Circulation* 1964;**29**:176-181.
60. Amparo EG, Higgins CB, Hoddick W. Magnetic resonance imaging of aortic disease: preliminary results. *AJR* 1984; **143**:1203-1209.

61. Rehr RB, Filipchuk NG, Malloy CR. Magnetic resonance imaging in aortic valve, ascending aortic and isthmic aortic disease. *Am J Cardiol* 1985;**55**:1243-1244.
62. Yucel EK, Steinberg FL, Egglin TK. Penetrating aortic ulcers: diagnosis with MR imaging. *Radiology* 1990;**177**: 779-781.
63. Utz JA, Herfkens RJ, Heinsimer JA. Valvular regurgitation: dynamic MR imaging. *Radiology*;**168**:91-94.
64. Schiebler M, Axel L, Reichek N. Correlation of cine MR imaging with two-dimensional pulse Doppler echocardiography and valvular insufficiency. *J Comput Assist Tomogr* 1987;**11**:627-632.
65. Auffermann S, Wagner S, Holt W. Evaluation of valvular regurgitation by cine magnetic resonance. *Am J Cardiac Imag* 1989;**3**:27-33.
66. Pflugfelder PW, Landzberg JS, Cassidy MM. Comparison of cine MR imaging with Doppler echocardiography for the evaluation of aortic regurgitation. *AJR* 1989;**152**:729-735.
67. Wagner S, Auffermann W, Buser B. Diagnostic accuracy in estimation of severity of valvular regurgitation from the signal void on cine magnetic resonance images. *Am Heart J* 1989;**118**:760-766.
68. Sechtem U, Pflugfelder PW, Cassidy MM. Mitral or aortic regurgitation: quantitation of regurgitant volumes with cine MR imaging. *Radiology* 1988;**167**:425-430.
69. Fisher RG, Hadlock F, Ben-Menachem Y. Laceration of the thoracic aorta and brachiocephalic arteries by blunt trauma. *Radiol Clin* 1981;**19**:91-110.
70. Bennett DE, Cherry JK. The natural history of traumatic aneurysms of the aorta. *Surgery* 1967;**61**:516-523.
71. Moore EH, Webb WR, Verrier ED. MRI of chronic post-traumatic false aneurysms of the thoracic aorta. *AJR* 1984;**143**:1195-1196.
72. Miller DL, Reinig JW, Volkman DJ. Vascular imaging with MRI: inadequacy in Takayasu's arteritis compared with angiography. *AJR* 1986;**146**:949-954.
73. Amparo EG, Higgins CB, Shafton EP. Demonstration of coarctation of the aorta by magnetic resonance imaging. *AJR* 1984;**143**:1192-1194.
74. von Schulthess GK, Higashino SM, Higgins SS. Coarctation of the aorta: MR imaging. *Radiology* 1986;**158**:469-474.
75. Fletcher BD, Jacobstein MD. MRI of congenital abnormalities of great arteries. *AJR* 1986;**146**:941-948.
76. Gomes AS, Lois JF, George B. Congenital abnormalities of the aortic arch: MR imaging. *Radiology* 1987;**165**:691-695.
77. Kersting-Sommerhoff BA, Diethelm L, Teitel DF. Magnetic resonance imaging of congenital heart disease: sensitivity and specificity using receiver operating characteristic curve analysis. *Am Heart J* 1989;**118**:155-161.
78. Boxer RA, LaCorte MD, Singh S. Nuclear magnetic resonance imaging in evaluation of follow-up with children treated coarctation of the aorta. *J Am Coll Cardiol* 1986;**7**:1095-1098.
79. Simpson IA, Chung KJ, Glass RF. Cine-magnetic resonance imaging for evaluation of anatomy and flow relations in infants and children with coarctation of the aorta. *Circulation* 1988;**78**:142-148.
80. Lion J, Lee JKT, Canter C. Imaging evaluation of post surgical repair of aortic coarctation: value of cine MR imaging. *Radiology* 1989;**173**:320.
81. Rees S, Somerville J, Ward C. Coarctation of the aorta: MR imaging and late post-operative assessment. *Radiology* 1989;**173**:499-502.
82. Bank ER, Aisen AM, Rocchini AP. Coarctation of the aorta in children undergoing angioplasty: pretreatment and post-treatment MR imaging. *Radiology* 1987;**162**:235-240.

83. Kersting-Sommerhoff BA, Sechtem UP, Schiller MB. MR imaging of the thoracic aorta in Marfan patients. *J Comput Assist Tomogr* 1987;**11**:633-639.
84. Soulen RL, Fishman EK, Pyeritz RE. Marfan syndrome: evaluation with MR imaging versus CT. *Radiology* 1987;**165**:697-702.
85. Schaeffer S, Peshock RM, Malloy CR. Nuclear magnetic resonance imaging in Marfan's syndrome. *JACC* 1987;**9**:70-74.
86. Mitchell L, Jenkins JPR, Watson Y. Diagnosis and assessment of mitral and aortic valve disease by cine-flow magnetic resonance imaging. *Magn Reson Med* 1989;**12**:181-197.
87. Didier D, Higgins CB, Fisher MR. Congenital heart disease: gated MR imaging in 72 patients. *Radiology* 1986;**158**:227-235.

Computed tomography and magnetic resonance imaging in acquired heart disease

Rainer Rienmüller
Department of Radiology, Klinikum Großhadern, University of Munich, Munich, Germany

---

Introduction

The methodological requirements in the clinical evaluation of patients with cardiac disease are based on the multifaceted interrelations of cardiac functional and morphological parameters. Functional determinants such as pre-load, after-load, contractility and heart rate depend on morphological parameters such as the status of pericardium, myocardium and endocardium; the status of cardiac valves and chambers; and the status of the coronary arteries as well as the shape and contents of the entire chest. The functional and morphological parameters are essentially influenced by factors such as coronary blood flow and myocardial perfusion and metabolism. Thoracic processes, systemic diseases, endocrine and neurohumoral mechanisms may also play an important role.

Based on fundamental methodological and technical considerations, it does not appear realistic to assume that only one diagnostic procedure will suffice for investigation of the multifaceted interrelations which are characteristic of cardiac function and disease [1]. This chapter deals with cross-sectional imaging of the heart in the clinical evaluation of patients with acquired heart disease.

Computed Tomography of the Heart

For the evaluation of the heart, computed tomography (CT) studies should be performed first as non-enhanced scans and then after i.v. contrast enhancement (50 - 150 ml contrast agent) continuously from the diaphragm to the aortic arch (Fig. 1). Thus intracardiac cavities

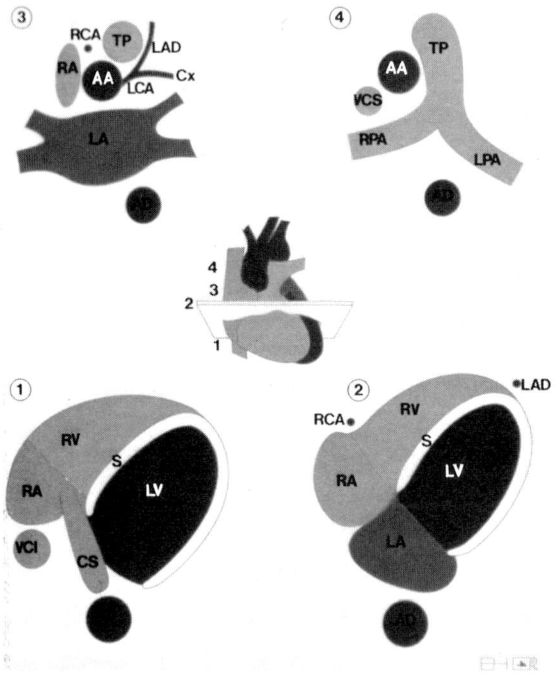

Figure 1. *THE FOUR (MOST) DIAGNOSTIC TRANSVERSE CT SCANS OF THE HEART. Slice 1: just above the diaphragm. Slice 2: through the middle of the heart where the left ventricle shows its maximum circumference. Slice 3: just above the base of the heart including proximal coronary arteries. Slice 4: through the region of the great arteries. VCI - inferior vena cava; VCS - superior vena cava; TP - pulmonary trunk; AA - ascending aorta; AD - descending aorta; LPA - left pulmonary artery; RPA - right pulmonary artery; LCA - main left coronary artery; LAD - left anterior descending coronary artery; CX - left circumflex artery; RCA - right coronary artery; CS - coronary sinus; LA - left atrium; LV - left ventricle; RA.- right atrium; RV - right ventricle; S - ventricular septum.*

(atria and ventricles) including their walls and lumina, great vessels and proximal coronary arteries may be visualized simultaneously and without superimposition. They may be differentiated not from one another but also from the surrounding cardiac, peri- and para-cardial structures. Precontrast scanning is recommended because otherwise it may be difficult to identify calcifications from contrast enhanced structures.

Newer CT equipment shortens the exposure times from 4 to 5 s to 1 s/scan. Electrocardiography (ECG) gating in cardiac CT has not been practical. Modern CT units such as ultrafast CT have decreased exposure to time 50 ms allowing acquisition of images at 17 scans/s. Ultrafast CT studies should start with the volume mode and then, depending upon the clinical problems, in the cine- and/or flow-modes [2].

Magnetic Resonance Imaging of the Heart

ECG triggering is necessary in all magnetic resonance imaging (MRI) studies of the heart to obtain diagnostic image quality. Data acquisition for each image occurs at the same point of the cardiac cycle. In MRI the rotating multislice technique in the spin echo mode should be applied. As in CT the imaging volume should include the complete heart from the diaphragm to the aortic arch. When necessary coronal and/or sagittal scans should also be done.

For qualitative and quantitative image analysis the four chambers of the heart should be visualized with the same trigger delay [3]. We repeat the T1-weighted sequences for each slice, step by step using a 40-, 140-, 240-, 340-, 440- and 540 ms trigger delay after the R-wave. The slices of the heart may be then analyzed at identical phases of the heart cycle. To obtain direct haemodynamic information, gradient echo-sequences, (cine-MR) may be used, especially to determine the direction and the speed of blood flow or to distinguish between intracavitary masses and slow blood flow phenomena. To improve delineation of tumor masses to increase tissue contrast, intravenous gadolinium-diethylene-triaminoacetate (Gd-DTPA) may be applied [4].

Advantages and Limitations of CT and MR

Both cross sectional techniques are non-invasive, imaging the heart free of superimposed cardiac and non-cardiac structures, enabling qualitative and quantitative evaluation of the morphological and functional parameters of the heart.

In contrast to conventional and ultrafast CT, MRI of the heart is somewhat limited by the requirement for ECG triggering to create images of good quality as well as by the long duration of the technique (1 - 1.5 hours) and by difficulties in evaluating areas of low signal intensity which may be due to air, calcification, fibrotic tissue or flowing blood. Furthermore patients with pacemakers should be excluded from MRI as should patients with paramagnetic implants. In comparison to echocardiography and ventriculography both methods allow superior visualization of pericardium, myocardium and the determination of left ventricular muscle mass/end-diastolic volume ratio (LVMM/EDV).

The main disadvantage in imaging the heart using CT is the need for administration of contrast agents to delineate intracavitary and intraluminary volumes and the radiation exposure. The problem of movement artefacts caused by exposure times from 1 - 5 s in conventional CT may be overcome by using ultrafast CT.

Determinants of Cardiac Function

The following functional and morphological parameters are useful in the evaluation of cardiac function:

Functional parameters

1. Pre-load: degree of extension of myocardial fibres measurable as EDV, left-ventricular end-diastolic pressure (LVEDP), diastolic wall stress (TDIAST) and compliance.

2. After-load: sum of the resistances to ejection during systole measurable as systolic wall stress (TSYST).

3. Contractility: extent and velocity of the contraction of myocardial fibres) measurable as ejection fraction (EF) and velocity of pressure increase.

The volume of the left ventricle in conventional CT of the heart corresponds to the EDV as determined by levocardiography [5,6].

The LVMM is more easily and more precisely determined by conventional CT than by levocardiography [6].

The results of various research groups show that with ultrafast CT and MRI it is possible to calculate the following volumes of the left ventricle: EDV, end-systolic volume (ESV), stroke volume (SV), EF, LVMM and their derivatives with a degree of accuracy comparable to ventriculography [2,6,7]. Both methods allow the assessment of valvular regurgitation and intracardiac shunts as well as global and regional variations in the functional status, including the changes of the myocardial wall thickness during cardiac cycle [8-10]. All of the volumes mentioned can be assessed either by applying the formula of a rotating ellipsoid or by the method of Simpson.

Special attention should be given to the possibility of determination of the LVMM/EDV ratio using CT or MRI. This is because of the well known close relationship between decreasing LVMM/EDV ratio and increasing systolic wall stress in patients with various cardiac diseases [11]. The increasing systolic wall stress is accompanied by an increase demand for oxygen and if this demand cannot be satisfied, myocardial ischaemia or infarction may be the result (Fig. 2).

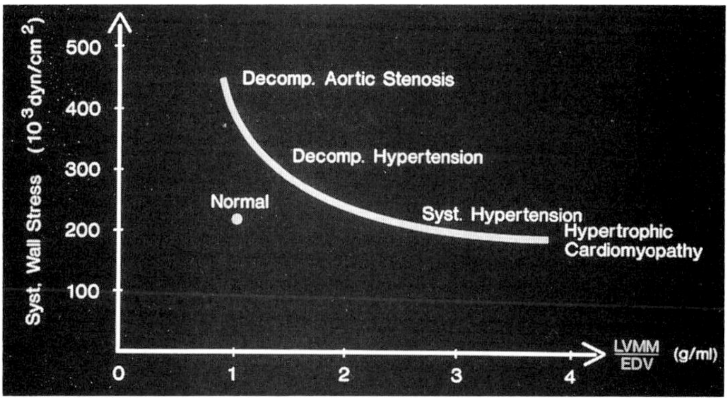

Figure 2. *RELATIONSHIP BETWEEN SYSTOLIC WALL STRESS AND LEFT VENTRICULAR MUSCLE MASS/END-DIASTOLIC VOLUME (LVMM/EDV).*

Comparison (quantitative and qualitative) of the circumferences of the great vessels as inferior vena cava (IVC) vs. descending aorta (DA), superior vena cava (SVC) vs. DA, ascending aorta (AA) vs.

pulmonary trunk (PT) and of the left vs. right atria or ventricles, respectively, gives important information on the state of the cardiac haemodynamics. These comparisons are especially recommended if conventional CT is used [6].

Morphological Parameters

In the evaluation of the morphological parameters (anatomy) of the heart, CT, especially ultrafast CT, and MRI currently offer similar information [1,12]. The LV myocardial wall and the interventricular septum (IVS) can be visualized with both methods and the extent of myocardial hypertrophy and/or atrophy can be qualitatively and quantitatively assessed. Because of the lower spatial and temporal resolution using conventional CT the right ventricular (RV) myocardial wall is only visible if hypertrophied, i.e. in cases of chronic volume and/or pressure overload. By means of ultrafast CT and MRI, RV myocardium is routinely visualized.

The interatrial septum (IAS) is almost never completely visualized because of its position and limited thickness either method. Calcified valves are easily visualized by CT, however, they are difficult to identify with MRI. Conversely, the visualization of uncalcified valves is better with MRI [13], followed by ultrafast CT.

The normal peri-epicardium can be delineated with both methods in all patients as a pencil-thin line in front of the right heart and additionally with MRI along the left heart, the diaphragm and in the area of the superior junction. The normal endocardium is not identifiable with any of these methods.

Intra- and para-cardiac tumours can be visualized if they are over ca. 1.0 cm in diameter [14-16].

Coronary Heart Disease

The term 'coronary heart disease' describes a collective name for myocardial changes as sequelae of insufficient blood, oxygen and metabolite supply to the myocardium. Of this disease entity, 80 - 95% of cases are caused by atherosclerotic narrowing or occlusion of the extramural coronary arterial vessels. With a frequency of 5 - 20% 'small vessel disease' may be considered as a second most common reason, followed by very rare inflammatory processes or anomalies of the coronary arteries.

Coronary Vessels

CT methods are superior to any other modality in the identification of calcified vessels, and ultrafast CT even allows quantification of coronary calcification [17] (Fig. 3). The evaluation of coronary arteries and bypass grafts using non-enhanced and contrast-enhanced conventional CT allows for only the following: if the vessel is

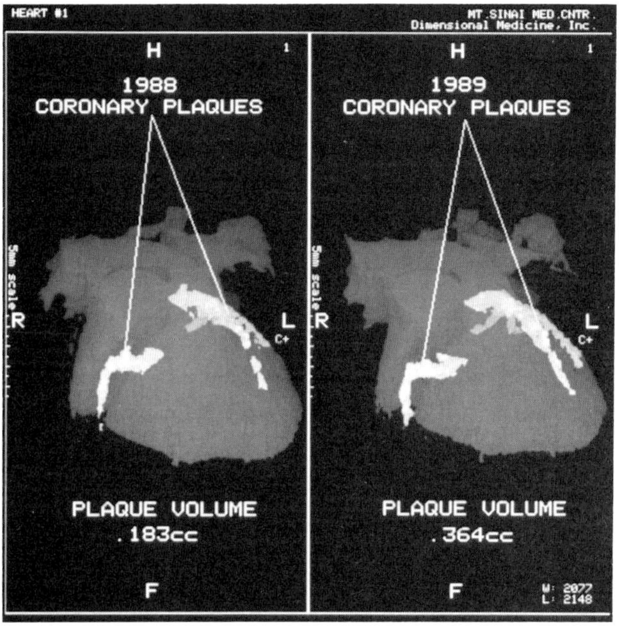

Figure 3. *ULTRAFAST CT IMAGES WITH PROGRESSIVE CORONARY CALCIFICATION FROM 1988 TO 1989 (courtesy of DP. Boyd).*

contrast-enhanced it is open; if it is not contrast-enhanced than it is closed. No other information of clinical significance may be obtained. With ultrafast CT, however, not only the visualization of the coronary arteries and bypass grafts is facilitated, but it is also possible to measure the actual time-density curves of the intraluminary contrast agent flow, yielding a quantitative index of coronary flow [2,18].

Although the visualization of the coronary arteries using MRI may occasionally be excellent, their detection rate at present is less than with CT [13]. Improvements may be expected by routine application of gradient echo sequences. Presently, selective coronary angiography remains the method of choice in the evaluation of coronary artery disease.

Myocardium

Sequelae of transmural infarction can be detected as thinning and/or bulging of the myocardial wall, using either CT or MRI with similar results to levocardiography [13,19,21]. With MRI, coronal and sagittal projections improve the visualization of transmural infarction near the base of the heart or at the posterior myocardial wall. Both methods enable a quantitative assessment of the size of the infarcted and of the normal myocardium, important information before aneurysmectomy.

Myocardial ischaemia is not detectable by conventional CT. However, at present, ultrafast CT may be superior to MRI in the detection of myocardial ischaemia because of the capability to analyse time-density curves after contrast agent application in different parts of the myocardium [18]. Ultrafast CT and MRI also allow the quantitative measurement of myocardial wall thickening and motion, which may be altered as a result of regional or global myocardial ischaemia [22].

Promising results have been published using ultrafast CT to evaluate myocardial perfusion quantitatively [18]. Similar results have been reported for MRI using paramagnetic agents as Gd-DTPA [23].

Complications and accompanying sequelae of myocardial infarctions such as intracavitary thrombi (Fig. 4), rupture of the myocardial wall, pericardial effusions, peri-epicardial and fibrotic wall calcifications are easy to detect with both methods.

Cardiomyopathy

The cardiomyopathies are defined as heart muscle disease of unknown cause by exclusion of coronary heart disease, valvular or congenital heart disease, systemic and pulmonary hypertension. They are divided into three categories:

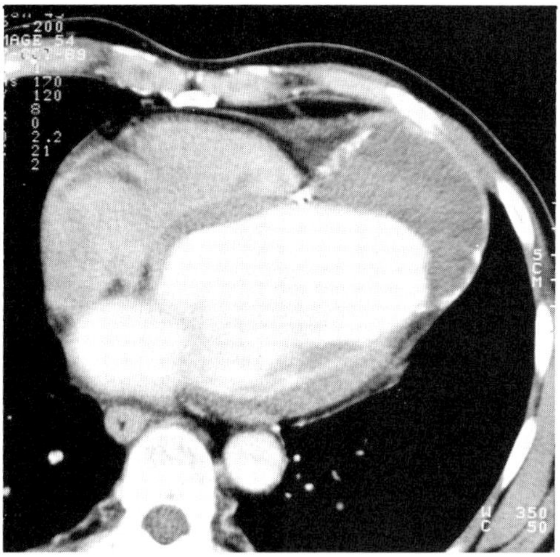

Figure 4. *Conventional CT image trough the mid-portion of the left ventricle after i.v. contrast enhancement with calcified thrombus-filled aneurysm at the apex of the left ventricle.*

1. Dilative cardiomyopathy: characterized patho-anatomically by dilatation of one or both ventricles with myocardial hypertrophy, and haemodynamically by elevated LVEDP and reduced EF (Fig. 5)

2. Hypertrophic cardiomyopathy: characterized by asymmetric or concentric hypertrophy of the IVS or other myocardial walls or of both. Haemodynamically they may show no obstruction or intraventricular obstruction of varying severity with diminished myocardial compliance (Fig. 6)

3. Restrictive cardiomyopathy: restrictive filling of one or both ventricles, e.g. endomyocardial fibrosis.

Specific heart muscle diseases are all heart muscle diseases in which the cause is supposed to be known. These are distinguished from the cardiomyopathies.

In the clinical diagnostic work up of patients with known or suspected cardiomyopathy both CT and MRI contribute to excluding or confirming those morphological and functional findings which are or are not characteristic of the cardiomyopathies, as defined above. Both methods are of special interest in those cardiac diseases with similar

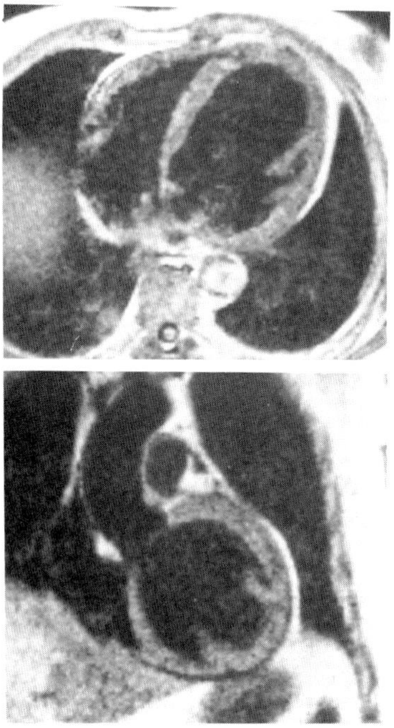

Figure 5. *MRI transverse (upper) and coronal (lower) slices through the mid-portion of the dilated, hypertrophic left ventricle of a patient with dilative cardiomyopathy.*

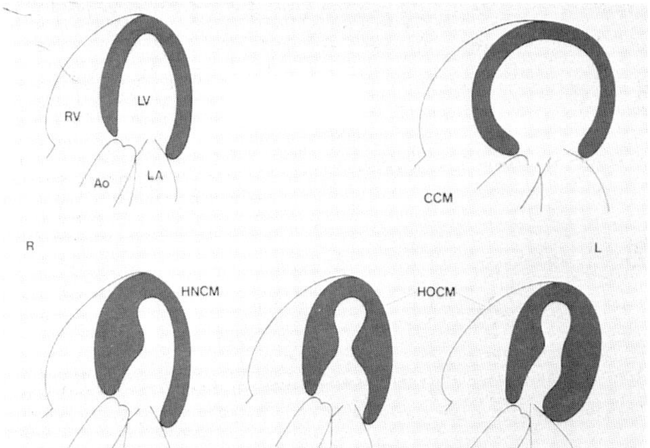

Figure 6. *PATTERN OF VARIOUS FORMS OF LEFT VENTRICULAR CARDIOMYOPATHIES. RV - right ventricle; LV - left ventricle; LA - left atrium; AA - ascending aorta; CCM - dilative cardiomyopathy; HNCM - hypertrophic non-obstructive cardiomyopathy with asymmetric hypertrophy of the inter-ventricular septum; HOCM - hypertrophic obstructive cardiomyopathy (left, with mid-ventricular obstruction; right, with subvalvular outflow obstruction).*

haemodynamics such as restrictive cardiomyopathy and constrictive pericarditis. In this situation the lack of specific pericardial and cardiac changes in CT or MRI is suggestive for restrictive cardiomyopathy [4,20].

Among the patients with specific heart muscle diseases only in those with iron or certain types of glycogen storage disease (such as Pompe's disease) the myocardial involvement may be detected non-invasively by CT techniques (Fig. 7). The qualitative and quantitative evaluation of myocardial CT densities shows an elevation of CT values making this method not only suitable for detection but also for follow up studies of these patients during therapy [24].

Up to the present, the quantitative evaluation of myocardial signal intensities or of myocardial T1 or T2 values have not been useful in identifying or excluding any type of cardiomyopathies or specific heart muscle diseases.

Pericardial Disease

Any enlargement of the peri-epicardial line above the previously mentioned criteria, are suggestive of an acute (if smooth contour) or chronic (if irregular contour) pericardial disease. If there is enlargement of the pericardial space greater than 1 cm, then it is possible by measuring the CT densities or by analysis of MRI signal intensities to distinguish between solid, liquid, semi-liquid and haemorrhagic processes [4].

Pericardial Effusion

Because any type of pericardial effusion may cause pericardial tamponade it is also necessary to analyse CT and/or MRI images under this aspect. In a comparative catheter and conventional CT study of patients with pericardial fluid, the following morphological patterns of pericardial tamponade were found (Fig. 8):

- pericardial effusion around the heart
- non-visualization of the subepicardial space
- reduction of the size of the heart chambers
- enlargement of the diameters of the IVC and SVC vs. the descending aorta over 2:1 and 1:1 respectively [20].

(a)

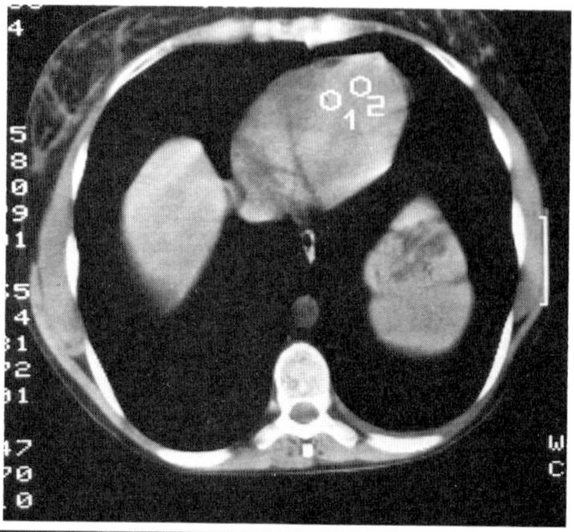

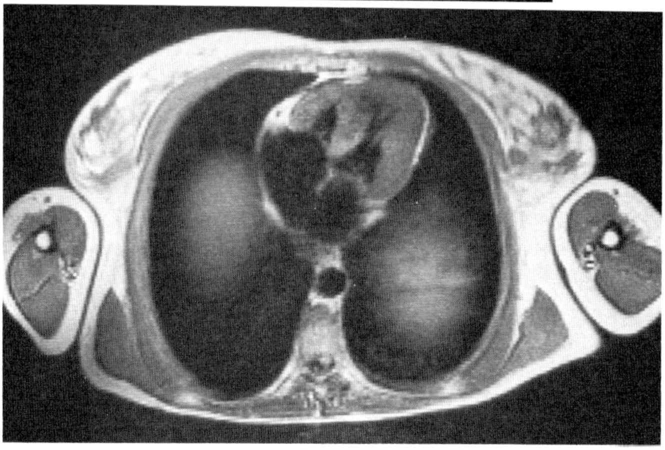

(b)

Figure 7. *(a) Transverse CT scan without i.v. contrast enhancement through the mid-portion of the left ventricle shows increased CT. Density of the ventricular septum (1 = 63.8 HU) and normal density of the intraventricular blood (2 = 55.4 HU). (b) Transverse MRI scan through the mid-portion of the left ventricle of the same patient as in (a) with biventricular myocardial hypertrophy as known in patients with Pompe's disease.*

Constrictive Pericardial Disease

The term 'constrictive pericardial disease' is applied to inflammatory or non-inflammatory disorders that involve one or both layers of the pericardium and lead to constriction and compression of the underlying cardiac chambers. It is characterized by scarring and/or calcification of the peri- and/or epi-cardium, which thereby loses its compliance and restricts the diastolic filling of the heart.

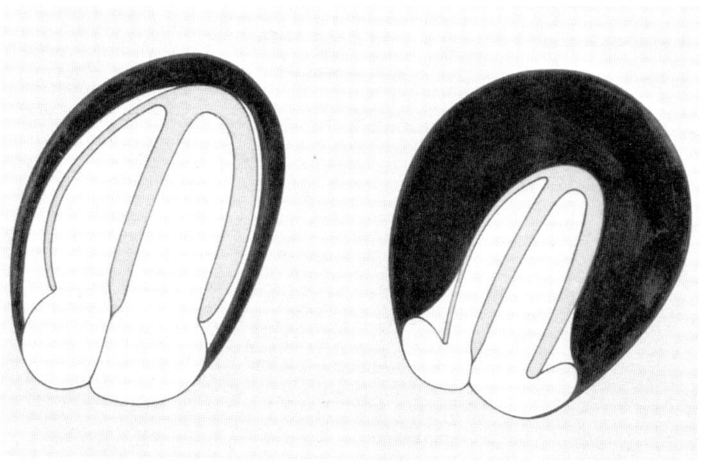

Figure 8. *PATTERN OF A PERICARDIAL EFFUSION WITHOUT TAMPONADE (left) AND WITH TAMPONADE (right).*

In patients with constrictive pericardial disease, total or partial pericardiectomy is the only treatment that may normalize or at least improve cardiac haemodynamics. The current mortality of the surgical procedures ranges from 4 to 32% [25-27].

Using catheter and angiocardiographic data only it is difficult and maybe even impossible:

- to distinguish constrictive from restrictive cardiac diseases (both diseases required different treatments)
- to determine the type and the extent of constriction which determines the surgical approach
- to exclude patients from surgery with myocardial atrophy and/or fibrosis.

In a comparative study of catheter and angiocardiographic studies vs. CT and MRI in patients with pericardial diseases the following diagnostic criteria of constrictive pericardial disease were found [25,26]:

- enlargement and/or calcification of the peri-epicardial line
- narrowing (tube-like configuration) of one or both ventricles
- enlargement of one or both atria
- narrowing of one or both atrioventricular grooves
- enlargement of the diameters of the IVC and SVC in comparison with the descending aorta.

When all of these morphological criteria are present the diagnosis of constrictive pericardial disease proved to be certain. In contrast to constrictive pericardial diseases, in restrictive cardiomyopathies (with similar cardiac haemodynamic) there is neither any thickening of the peri-epicardium nor any tube-like configuration of either ventricles (Fig. 9).

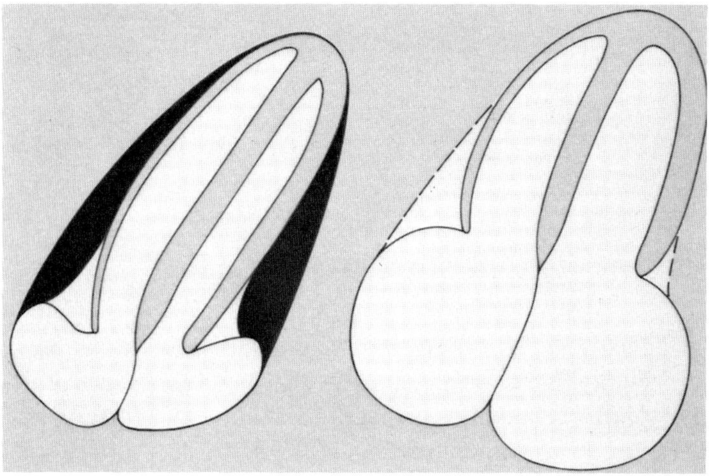

Figure 9. *Pattern of global pericardial constriction (left) with peri-epicardial thickening along both ventricles, which have a tube-like configuration and pattern of restrictive cardiomyopathy (right) with normal peri-epicardial line and enlarged atria.*

Using only analysis of the morphological appearance of the visualized cardiac and pericardial structures it is possible to distinguish between:

- global or general constrictive pericardial disease
- localized constrictive pericardial disease
- annular constrictive pericardial disease
- right-sided constrictive pericardial disease
- left-sided constrictive pericardial disease
- surrounding the aortic and/or pulmonary roots constrictive pericardial disease
- effusive constrictive pericardial disease
- occult forms or variants of constrictive pericardial diseases

By qualitative and quantitative analysis of the pericardial and myocardial structures it is possible to identify CT and/or MRI criteria of myocardial atrophy or fibrosis (Fig. 10) as demonstrated in the table [25,26].

Table. *CT and/or MRI criteria of myocardial atrophy or fibrosis*

Left ventricular	Right ventricular
Interventricular septum < 1 cm	Peri-epicardium not separable from ventricular wall
Ventricular wall < 1 cm	Irregular wall thickening
Systolic/diastolic wall thickness changes < 40%	
LVMM/EDV ratio < 1.1	

The diagnostic and prognostic validity of CT and MRI is a based on:

1. Exclusion of patients with restrictive cardiac diseases from 'diagnostic surgery'.

2. Determination of the surgical approach and extent of necessary pericardiectomy by pre-operative definition of the different forms or variants of the constrictive pericardial disease.

3. Exclusion of patients with constrictive pericardial diseases from surgery with evidence of myocardial atrophy or fibrosis as defined above.

Cardiac Tumours

Until 1950 only five intracardiac tumours had been described. Since the first angiocardiographic demonstration of an intracardiac tumour by Goldberg in 1952 and later by the introduction of sonography among the cardiological diagnostic modalities, this situation has changed drastically. Because of its easy handling, excellent results in comparison with angiocardiography, and wide-spread availability,

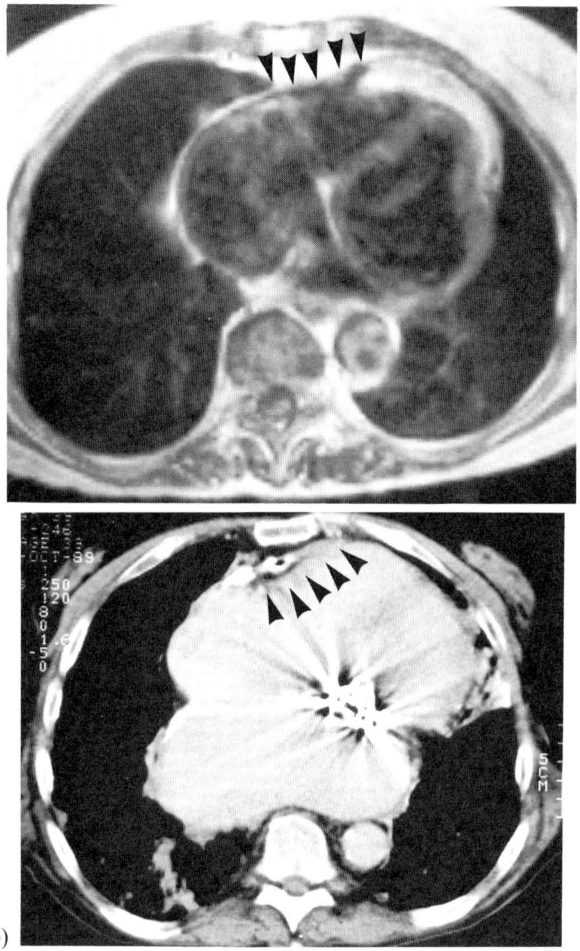

(a) (b)

Figure 10. *(a) MRI transverse scan through the mid-portion of the ventricles with calcified pericardial constriction (arrows), small compressed right ventricle, enlarged right atrium and thinning of the inter-ventricular septum and of the myocardial wall, suggesting myocardial atrophy; furthermore there is an aneurysm of the posterior lateral wall of the left ventricle close to the base of the heart. (b) CT transverse scan after i.v. contrast enhancement slightly above the mid-portion of the ventricles with irregular calcified peri-epicardial line in-front of the right heart with non-separable irregular configurated right ventricular wall (arrows) suggesting myocardial fibrosis.*

echocardiography is today considered the method of choice in the evaluation of intracardiac tumours [16,28], but there are still some well known methodical limitations. In contrast to echocardiography, CT and MRI are able to visualize not only the entire heart but also all of the mediastinal, pulmonary, pleural, and chest-wall structures in a single image. Consequently, CT and MRI should be used when ever echocardiography has failed.

In suspected or known cardiac neoplasm the following questions are of clinical interest [28]:

- to demonstrate or to exclude tumour
- to define the exact localization, the size, and the extent of a tumour mass
- to evaluate a haemodynamic effect of the tumours
- to distinguish benign and malignant, primary and secondary processes
- to determine the optimal treatment.

CT and MRI are useful in the planing of surgical treatment, evaluation of therapeutical complications, and in follow up of patients with various cardiac neoplasms treated by surgery, drugs and/or radiation. They are also useful in determining inoperability of the tumour.

As previously mentioned solid, fatty or cystic tumours, are easily identified with both methods. Calcified tumours in contrast to fibrous tumours are more easily recognized by CT than by MRI. A recent study [16] revealed that MRI is inferior to echocardiography in the detection of intramural rhabdomyomas; however, it is superior in delineation of the intra- and extra-cardiac extension of non-rhabdomyomal tumors (Fig. 11). With both method it is at present time not possible to distinguish between benign and malignant, primary or secondary tumours. However a careful image analysis, patient history, and additional clinical data help to restrict the array of differential diagnoses.

Valvular (Acquired) Heart Disease

Morphological changes of the heart, its chambers and its great vessels as a consequence of chronic pressure and/or volume overload caused by valvular heart disease can be visualized using CT and/or MRI [29,30]. Using ultrafast CT and/or gradient echo-sequences in MRI it is also possible to demonstrate regurgitant and shunt lesions and to quantify the volumes of these lesions [29,31,32].

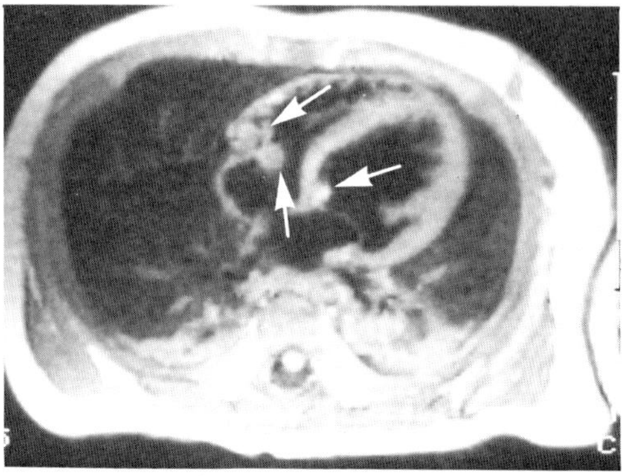
(a)

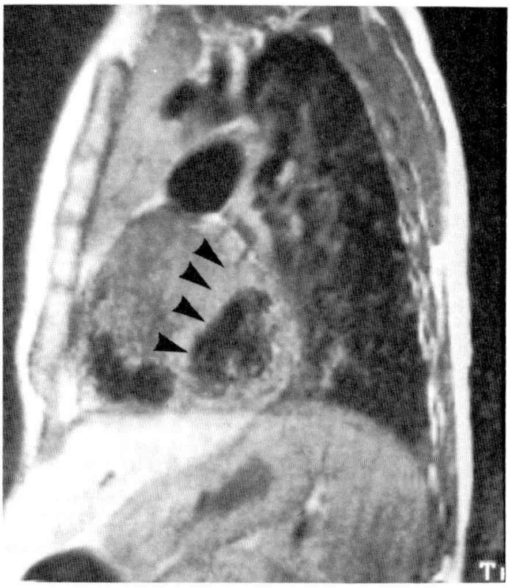
(b)

Figure 11. *(a) MRI transverse scan through the mid-portion of the ventricles during diastole in a patient with three rhabdomyomas (arrows). (b) MRI sagittal scan through the mid-portion of the left ventricle with a fibroma in the out-flow tract of the right ventricle clearly delineated in the interventricular septum (arrowheads).*

The direct evaluation of valvular changes or anomalies is still best performed by echocardiography. CT may contribute in the preoperative differentiation between the extent of valvular ring calcifications and leaflet calcifications.

The demonstration of morphological changes (position, size, configuration, cavitary dilatation, myocardial hypertrophy) and the application of the principles of sequential analysis enable the assessment of the type and extent of the acquired or congenital heart disease using CT and/or MRI with a high degree of accuracy.

Transplanted Heart

The survival rates of patients after cardiac transplantation are now 85 and 65% at 1 and 5 years respectively. Worldwide practice in the postsurgical monitoring of these patients consists of a number of non-invasive and invasive methods including cardiac catheterization and biopsy. This is because acute and chronic rejection, accelerated atherosclerosis, systemic hypertension, drug toxicity and denervation of the heart may cause alteration of the cardiac function in transplanted hearts [33, 34]. The development of coronary artery disease and changes of the myocardium and its function as a result of chronic rejection are severe complications after transplantation which limit the survival time (Fig. 12).

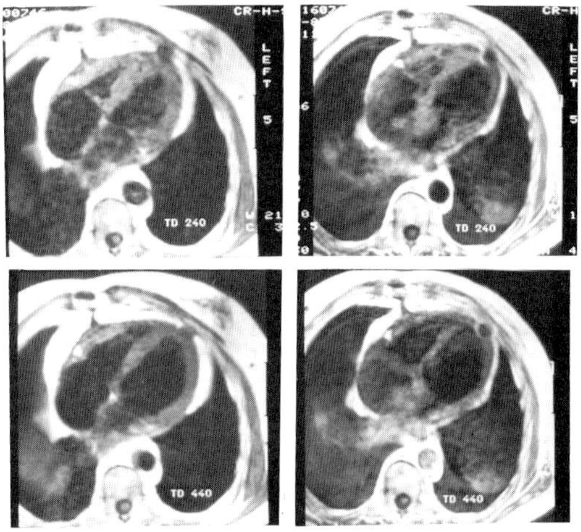

(a) (b)

Figure 12. *(a) MRI transverse scan through the mid-portion of the left ventricle in diastole (TD = trigger delay 440 ms) and in systole (TD = trigger delay 240 ms) 1 year after heart transplantation with a LVMM = 190 g and an EDV = 90 ml and a LVMM/DV ratio = 2.1. (b) 1.5 years later the LVMM decreased to 100 g and the EDV remained with 90 ml unchanged. The LVMM/EDV ratio = 1.1. The patient died on the next day and the autopsy revealed diffuse fibrosis of the myocardium.*

In a 4-year follow-up-study of patients with cardiac transplants using MRI the following findings were made [8]:

- the diastolic volume of the left ventricle remains in the normal range and does not change
- the ejection fraction remains in the normal range and does not change (Fig. 13)
- the left ventricular muscle mass remains elevated in transplanted hearts compared with normals (not significant)
- the LVMM/EDV ratio is elevated at 1.7 in comparison to normals with 1.3. (Fig. 14)

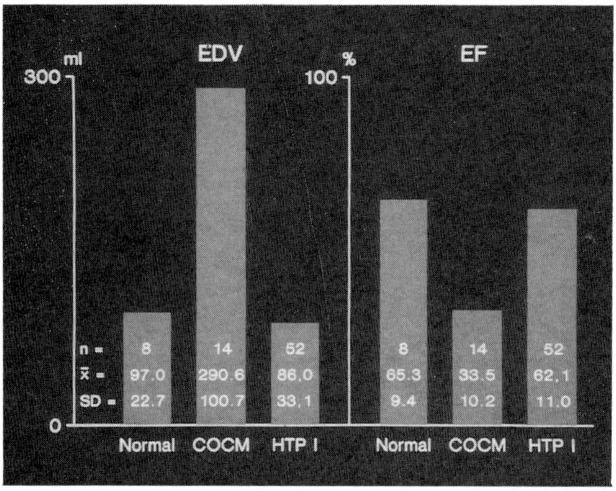

Figure 13. *Results (mean ± SD) of EDV and EF 1 year after heart transplantation (HTPI) and in healthy volunteers (normal) and in patients with dilative cardiomyopathy (COCM).*

Close relationship was found between the frequency of rejection episodes and the decrease of the left ventricle muscle mass if the diastolic volume remained unchanged (Fig. 15). From these results the following conclusions may be drawn:

- if the LVMM/EDV ratio remains constant at ≥ 1.3 the angiographic and biopsy controls may be extended to the next year
- if the LVMM/EDV ratio is decreasing, a coronary angiography and biopsy should be performed, regardless of the clinical status of the patient or the data from the next invasive studies
- if the LVMM/EDV ratio ≤ 1.1, than a retransplantation may be considered as indicated.

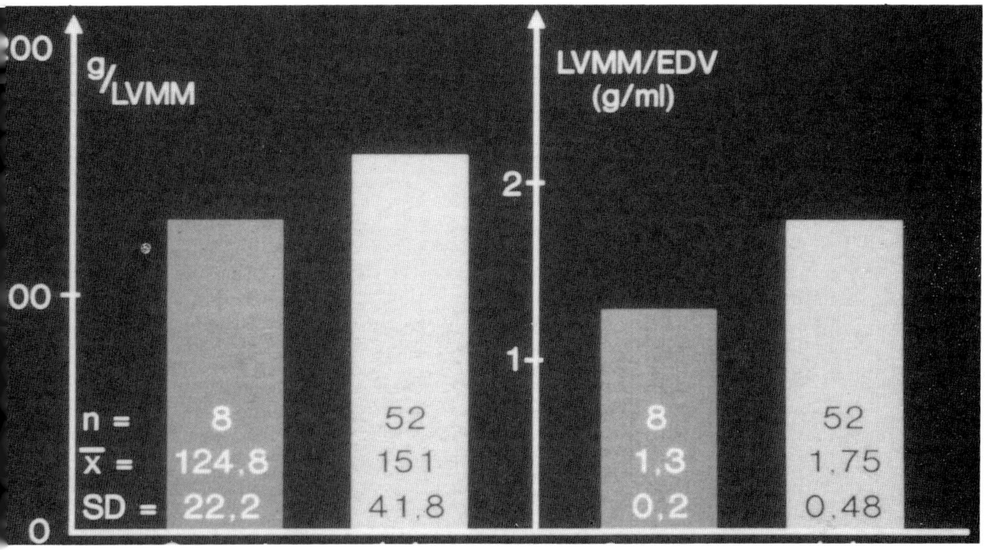

Figure 14. *LVMM and its relationship to EDV (LVMM/EDV, mean ± SD) 1 year after heart transplantation (HTPI) and in healthy volunteers (normal).*

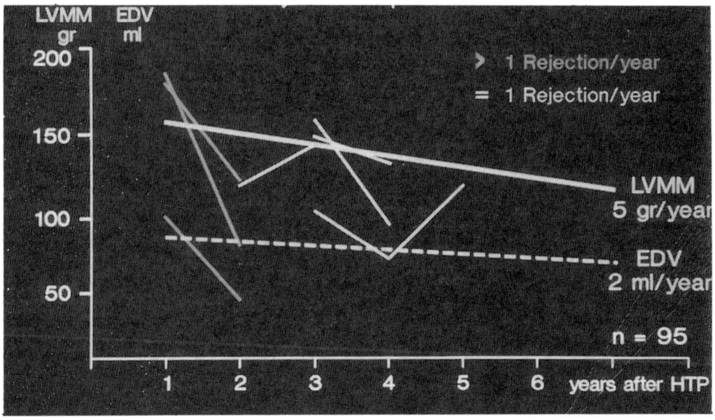

Figure 15. *Changes of the LVMM in transplanted hearts with histologically-verified rejection episodes.*

As, in acute rejection, experimental and clinical MRI findings and results are very controversial, MRI is presently only of limited value in this situation. Since it is possible with ultrafast CT to quantify the amount of coronary atherosclerosis [17] this method might be used for the postoperative evaluation of these patients. Accelerated atherosclerosis is a severe problem in transplanted hearts.

References

1. Rienmüller R. Computertomographie versus Kernspintomographie in der klinischen Diagnostik kardialer Erkrankungen. *Internist* 1990;**31**:321-332.
2. Lipton MJ, Brundage BH, Higgins CB, Boyd DP. Clinical applications of dynamic computed tomography. *Prog Cardiovasc Dis* 1986;**38**:349-366.
3. Aellig WM. Nuclear magnetic resonance in clinical pharmacology and measurement of therapeutic response. *Br J Clin Pharmacol* 1990;**29**:157-167.
4. Rienmüller R. Herz. In *Klinische Kernspintomographie.* Lissner J, Seiderer M (eds). Stuttgart:Ferdinand Enke Verlag, 1990;425-444..
5. Rienmüller R, Lissner J, Kment A, Bohn J, Strauer BE, Hellwig D, Erdmann E, Cyran J, Steinbeck G, Höss D, Hofling B. Das enddiastolische Volumen des linken Vetrikels in der Computertomographie im Vergleich zur Herzkatheterventrikulographie. *Computertomographie* 1981;**1**:62-67.
6. Rienmüller R, Baumer A, Kirsch CM, Strauer BE. Quantification of left ventricular function by computed tomography. In *Advances in non-invasive cardiology.* Meyer J, Schweizer P, Eberl R, (eds). Boston:Martinus Nijhoff Publishers, 1983;109-121.
7. Miller SW, Brady TJ, Dinsmore RE, Edelman RR, Johnston DL, Okada RD, Rosen BR, Stark DD, Stratemeier EJ, Thompson R, Van Wedeen J, Wismer GL. Cardiac magnetic resonance imaging: the massachusetts general hospital experience. *Radiol Clin North Am* 1985;**23**:.
8. Rienmüller R, Gartner Ch, Lloret JL, Schütz A, Tiling R, Kemkes BM, von Scheidt J. MR-Ergebnisse einer 4 jähriger Studie in der postoperativen Nachsorge herz-transplantierter Patienten. In *MR '89, 3. Internationales Kernspintomographie Symposium.* Lissner J, Doppmann JL, Margulis AR. (eds). Köln:Deutscher Arzte Verlag 1990;166-175.
9. Lanzer P, Garrett J, Lipton MJ, Gould R, Sievers R, O'Connell W, Botvinick E, Higgins CB. Quantitation of regional myocardial function by cine computed tomography: pharmacologlc changes in wall thickness. *J Am Coll Cardiol* 1986;**8**:682-692.
10. Farmer D, Lipton MJ, Higgins CB, Ringertz H, Dean PB, Sievers R, Boyd DP. In vivo assessment of left ventricular wall and chamber dynamics during transient myocardial ischemia using cine computed tomography. *Am J Cardiol* 1985;**55**:560-565.
11. Strauer BE. Hypertensive heart disease. Heidelberg;Springer Verlag Berlin, 1980..
12. Rienmüller R, Schmidt HC, Gärtner Ch, Erdmann E, Kemkes BM. CT vs. MRI in the clinical evaluation of cardiac diseases. *Hospimedica* 1987;**5**:37-45.
13. Rienmüller R, Schultheiss HP, Baierl P, Strauer BE. Myokardiale und perikardiale Wandveränderungen in der Kernspintomographie und der Computertomographie. Eine klinische Studie. In *MR '85.* Lissner J, Doppman JL, (eds). Konstanz:Schnetztor Verlag GmbH, 1985;158-165..
14. Nair CK, Sketch MH, Mahoney PD, Lynch JD, Mooss AN, Kenney NP. Detection of left ventricular thrombi by computerized tomography. *Br Heart J* 1981;**45**:535-41.
15. Niehues B, Heuser L, Jansen W, Hilger HH. Non-invasive detection of intracardiac tumors by ultrasound and computed tomography. *Cardiovasc Intervent Radiol* 1983;**6**:30-36.

16. Rienmüller R, Lloret JL, Tiling R, Groh J, Manert W, Muller KD, Seifert K. MR imaging of pediatric cardiac tumors previously diagnosed by echocardiography. *J Comput Assist Tomogr* 1989;**13**:621-626.
17. Agatson AS, Janowitz WR, Hildner FJ, Zusmer NR, Viamonte M, Detrano R. Quantification of coronary artery calcium using ultrafast computed tomography. *JACC* 1990;**15**:827-832.
18. Marcus ML, White CW. Coronary flow reserve in patients with normal coronary an angiograms. *JACC* 1985;**6**:1254-6.
19. Rienmüller R, Ontyd J, Krappel W, Strauer BE. Infarktbedingte Veränderungen des linksventrikulären Myokards in der kardialen Computertomographie. *Fortschr Röntgenstr* 1983;**138**:403-411.
20. Rienmüller R, Seiderer M, Doliva R, Kemkes BM, Lissner J. Pericardial and congestive heart failure diagnostic with CT- and MR-imaging. *Ann Radiol* 1986;**29**:95-100.
21. Rabkin L, Ovtchinnikov V, Judin A. Computed tomographic evaluation of morphological and functional condition of left ventricle in heart aneurysm. *Europ J Radiol* 1986;**6**:15-20.
22. Higgins CB, Lanzer P, Stark D, Botvinick E, Schiller B, Crooks L, Kaufman L, Lipton MJ. Imaging by nuclear magnetic resonance in patients with chronic ischemlc heart disease. *Circulation* 1984;**69**:523-531.
23. De Roos A, Doornbos J, Vander Wall EE, van Voorthuisen AE. MR imaging of acute myocardial infarction: value of Gd-DTPA. *Am J Radiol* 1988;**150**:531-534.
24. Rienmüller R. Computertomographische Untersuchungen bei Patienten mit Hämochromatose. *Bayerischer Internist* 1984;**4**:74-80.
25. Rienmüller R, Doppman JL, Lisner J, Kemkes BM, Strauer BE. Constrictive pericardial diseases: prognostic significance of a nonvisualized left ventricular wall. *Radiology* 1985;**156**:753-755.
26. Rienmüller R, Schmidt HC. CT und MR in der präoperativen Diagnostik konstriktiver Perikarderkrankungen. In *Neues im Kontrastbild Herz und große Gefäße*. Felix R, Wolf KJ, Zeitler E, (eds). Berlin:Fa.Schering, 1987;123-130.
27. Doppman JL, Rienmüller R, Lissner J, Cyran J, Bolte HD, Strauer BE, Hellwig H. Computed tomography in constrictive pericardial disease. *J Comput Assist Tomogr* 1981;**5**:1-11.
28. Rienmüller R, Tiling R. MR and CT for detection of cardiac tumors. *Thorac cardiovasc Surgeon* 1990;**38**:168-172.
29. Higgins CB, Byrd III BF, Farmer DW, Osaki L, Silverman NH, Cheitlin MD. Magnetic resonance imaging in patients with congenital heart disease. *Circulation* 1984;**70**:851-860.
30. Rienmüller R. Gefäßanomalien des Mediastinums in der Computertomographie. In *5. Radiologische Woche*, Lissner J, (eds). pp. 247-263. Konstanz:Schnetztor Verlag GmbH, 1983.
31. MacMillan RM, Rees MR, Eldredge WJ, Maranhao V, Clark DL. Quantitation of shunting at the atrial level using rapid acquisition computed tomography with comparison with cardiac catheterization. *JACC* 1986;**7**:946-948.
32. Brundage BH, Rich S, Spigos D. Computed tomography of the heart and great vessels: Present and future. *Ann Int Med* 1984;**101**:801-809.
33. Kemkes BM, Reichenspurner H, Osterholzer G, Angermann C, Schad N, Erdmann E, Rienmüller R, Gokel JM. Hemodynamic Results after orthotopic heart-transplantation (HTx). *Transplantation Proceedings* 1986;**18(Suppl. 3)**:31-34.
34. Schütz A, Kemkes BM, Kugler Ch, Angermann C, Schad N, Rienmüller R, Fritsch S, Anthuber M, Neumaier P, Gokel JM. The influence of rejection episodes on the development of coronary artery disease after heart transplantation. *Eur J cardio-thorac Surg* 1990;**4**:300-30.

Magnetic resonance imaging of congenital heart disease

Charles B. Higgins
University of California, San Francisco, USA

Introduction

The capability of magnetic resonance imaging (MRI) for the diagnosis of CHD has now become apparent [1-5]. MRI can define cardiovascular patho-anatomy with the precision of angiocardiography. Because MRI requires neither ionizing radiation nor contrast medium, it is a completely non-invasive technique for evaluation of CHD. This non-invasive nature of MRI is very important in examining children with CHD, since the success in surgical management of even the most complex anomalies requires serial repeated evaluation of such patients during follow-up studies after palliative or definitive surgical procedures. MRI may supplant or at least substantially decrease the total number of angiocardiographic procedures performed in patients with CHD.

Echocardiography is currently being used as the initial non-invasive imaging study for nearly all patient suspected of having CHD. MRI is not likely to supplant echocardiography as the first diagnostic procedure because of the portability, universal availability, and low cost of echocardiography. However, MRI and echocardiography are considered to be complementary rather than competitive. Because MRI can depict precise patho-anatomy without the limitation of acoustic windows or ultrasound penetration of the body, the morphology of some regions, such as the supra-cardiac region and posterior aspect of the heart, can be more clearly shown with MRI than echocardiography. Furthermore, MRI can provide tomographic images in any imaging plane and with a wide field of view.

The capability of MRI for cardiovascular diagnosis is not limited to the anatomical diagnosis alone. With recent development of gradient-echo techniques (cine MRI), evaluation of cardiac function with MRI has now become practical [6-10]. Cine MRI attains a temporal resolution almost equal to cine angiography, which is sufficient to isolate images corresponding to end-diastole and end-systole and thus provides accurate measurements of stroke volume, ejection fraction, regional ventricular wall motion and wall thickening dynamics [6-10]. Furthermore, new MRI flow techniques (velocity encoded cine MRI) can produce functional images depicting a map of blood flow velocity of all cardiovascular structures on the multiple cine MR images acquired throughout a cardiac cycle [11-15]. By multiplying averaged cross sectional velocity and cross sectional area, blood flow volume through the vessel can be quantified. Cine MRI and velocity encoded cine MRI can be used to assess ventricular dimensions and function and blood flow in the central circulation.

Technique

Electrocardiographic (ECG)-gated multislice spin-echo sequences are used for evaluation of patho-anatomy of CHD. Cine MRI is also employed when functional information is required. A recent report of 51 MRI studies of patients with CHD indicated that diagnostic image quality was obtained in 94% of patients [16]. Major reasons for reduced image quality are patient motion and respiratory artefacts.

Children older than 5 or 6 years usually can be studied without sedation. For younger children, sedation is usually required. For this purpose, we have used chloral hydrate (75 - 100 mg/kg) administered orally approximately 45 min prior to entry into the magnet. An alternative sedation is pentobarbital (5 - 7 mg/kg) administered parenterally. In order to minimize disturbance of a sleeping child, the ECG leads are attached prior to sedation. ECG signal is monitored and respiration is observed throughout the imaging procedure.

The standard imaging plane is the transverse; 5 mm transverse images are acquired from above the aortic arch to and including the upper abdomen. These images are used to define segmental cardiac anatomy: visceroatrial situs, atrioventricular connections, ventricular loop, and arterioventricular connections (Fig. 1). Coronal and sagittal images or oblique sagittal images are used for specific purposes.

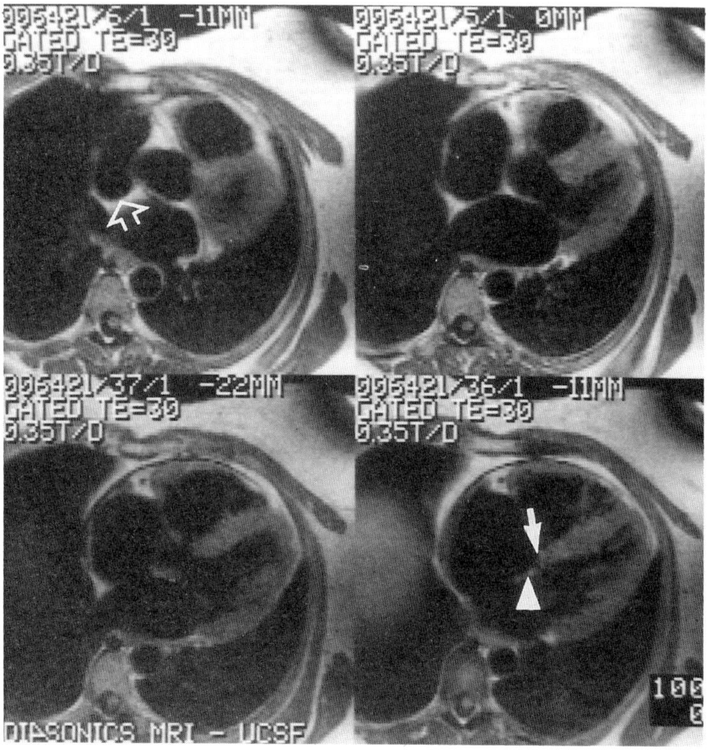

Figure 1. *TRANSVERSE SPIN-ECHO IMAGES EXTENDING FROM THE BASE OF THE HEART (upper left panel) TO THE MIDDLE OF THE VENTRICLES (lower right panel). The portion of the atrial septum separating the superior vena cava from the left atrium is the sinus venosus portion of the atrial septum (open arrow). The portion of the atrial septum at the level of the atrioventricular valves (lower left panel) is considered the primum portion (arrowhead) of the septum. The remainder of the atrial septum is essentially the secundum portion. There is a defect in the secundum portion of the atrial septum. The outlet portion of the ventricular septum separates the aorta from the right ventricle. The inlet portion of the ventricular septum is that portion located at the level of the tricuspid and mitral valves (arrow). The atrioventricular septum separates the left ventricle from the right atrium (small arrows).*

MRI of Specific Anomalies

Abnormalities of Arterioventricular Connections

This is a diverse group of abnormalities in which the great arteries are not connected to their appropriate ventricle (transposition) or both great arteries are predominantly connected to one ventricle (double outlet left and double outlet right ventricle) or only a single large trunk connects to the ventricle (truncus arteriosus). Spatial relationship of the great arteries to each other at the base of the heart and the connections to the ventricles are clearly depicted on transverse images through the base of the heart. The arterial relationships are also depicted on sagittal and coronal images.

Arterioventricular connections can be concordant or discordant. Concordant connections are aorta with left ventricle and pulmonary artery with right ventricle. Discordant connections are pulmonary artery with left ventricle and aorta with right ventricle (complete transposition). Corrected transposition has discordant arterioventricular relationship and discordant atrioventricular relationships.

Transposition of Great Arteries

Several reports have indicated the effectiveness of MRI for defining the patho-anatomy of transposition and other positional anomalies of the great vessels [1,16,17]. Transverse images at the base of the heart demonstrate the aorta anterior to the pulmonary artery; it is to the right of the pulmonary artery in D-transposition and to the left of the pulmonary artery in L-transposition (Fig. 2). When examining transverse images in great-vessel anomalies, one must distinguish the aorta and pulmonary artery; the pulmonary artery is identified by examining transverse images extending to the level of the pulmonary arterial bifurcation. The aorta can be recognized by identifying the arch and following the ascending aorta caudally to the base of the heart. Transverse or coronal scans at the base of the heart will reveal the origin of the aorta from the right ventricle, and the pulmonary artery from the left ventricle in transposition. In complete transposition, sequential transverse images show the right-sided aorta arising from a normally positioned right ventricle (rightward in relation to the left ventricle, D bulboventricular loop). In corrected transposition, the aorta is leftward and arises from the right ventricle, inverted to a

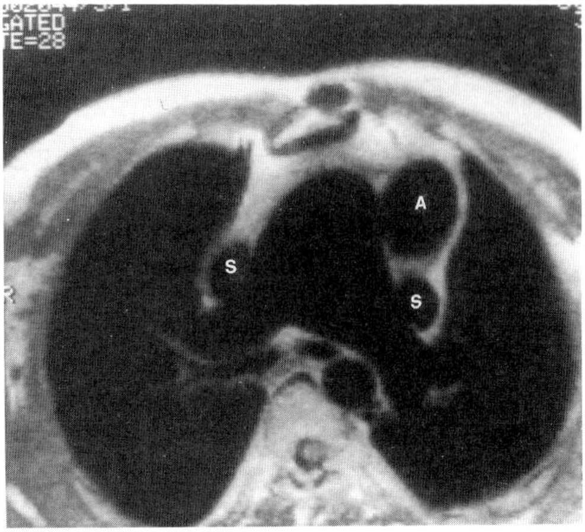

Figure 2. *TRANSVERSE IMAGES IN A PATIENT WITH L-TRANSPOSITION OF THE GREAT ARTERIES. Note that the aorta (A) is located anterior and to the left of the pulmonary artery. The pulmonary artery is recognized by the bifurcation of it. There are bilateral superior vena cavae (S).*

position leftward from the morphologic left ventricle (L bulboventricular loop).

The anomalies associated with transposition are also depicted on MR images. Transverse images can define the presence and severity of atrial and ventricular septal defects and valvular and subvalvular pulmonic stenosis. In transposition with severe pulmonary stenosis or pulmonary atresia, MRI is indicated in order to determine and measure the size of the central pulmonary arteries. MRI can also precisely define the size of the interatrial communication after either balloon or blade septostomy or after partial surgical excision of the atrial septum. MR images reveal reversal in shape and muscle thickness of the right ventricle in relation to the left ventricle, which is characteristic for transposition of great arteries. When the mural thickness of the left ventricle is equal to that of the right ventricle, this should suggest severe pulmonary arterial hypertension or pulmonary outflow obstruction in patients with complete transposition.

Double Outlet Right Ventricle (DORV)

The side-by-side relationship of the great vessels at the semilunar valve level characterizes this anomaly on transverse MR images.

Sequential transverse images reveal the origins of both vessels from the anteriorly located right ventricular outflow tract. The site of a ventricular septal defect in relation to the semilunar valves can be defined by transverse MR images. Coronal images confirm the side-by-side relationship of the semilunar valves, the origins of both great vessels from the right ventricle, and isolation of the left ventricle from the site of the semilunar valves. The anatomical features of DORV on MR images have been reported [17].

The position of the great arteries is not always side-by-side at the base of the heart. In some cases the aorta is anterior to the pulmonary artery and located either to the left anterior or right anterior aspect of the pulmonary artery.

A critical finding on transverse images is that neither semilunar valve is in direct fibrous continuity with the mitral valve. A complete rim of muscle intervening between both semilunar valves and the anterior leaflet of the mitral valve is a diagnostic feature. Side by side circles of myocardium in the outflow region of the right ventricle may be observed on transverse MR images acquired at the base of the heart.

The relationship of the ventricular septal defect (VSD) to either or both of the great arteries can usually be defined by transverse images. The defect may lie immediately beneath the aortic valve (subaortic VSD); pulmonic valve (subpulmonic VSD); both semilunar valves (doubly committed VSD); or displaced from both semilunar valves (non-committed VSD).

Subvalvular or valvular stenosis of the pulmonary artery occurs in some patients with DORV, especially in those with a subaortic VSD. The angiographic and clinical features of this type of DORV may be difficult to distinguish from tetralogy of Fallot. Transverse MR tomograms readily establish the diagnosis of this type of DORV by showing a complete circle of muscle separating the aortic from the mitral valve. The advantage of MRI is that it provides direct visualization of the myocardium rather than inferring its presence by the distance separating the aortic and mitral valves, as shown on left ventriculography.

Truncus Arteriosus

Transverse and sagittal images at the base of the heart can demonstrate a large truncus arising above the ventricular septal defect and aligned over both the right and left ventricles. In type I truncus, the origin of a main pulmonary artery from the truncus can be defined. Transverse scans can reveal the relative sizes of the two ventricles. A large single vessel arising from the base of the heart can also be observed on sagittal images in pulmonary atresia. Differentiation between truncus and pulmonary atresia is done by showing a small infundibular chamber on transverse images in the latter anomaly. Sagittal images are useful for depicting the truncus and demonstrating the origin of the pulmonary arteries from the truncus. MR images, usually thin (3 mm) tomograms, are used to assess the size of the right and left pulmonary arteries. MRI in transverse and sagittal planes is also used to evaluate the calibre of anastomoses after placement of a Rastelli conduit for the repair of truncus. Demonstration of focal stenosis of the distal anastomosis or of the central pulmonary artery requires thin transverse tomograms.

Tetralogy of Fallot

Sagittal and transverse tomograms are used to assess tetralogy. Sagittal images demonstrate the narrowing of the right ventricular outflow region. The transverse tomograms depict the ventricular septal defect and the infundibular, annular, and/or pulmonary arterial stenosis.

Transverse MR images can reveal disparity in the sizes of the aorta and pulmonary artery in tetralogy; there tends to be a reciprocal relationship in the sizes of the great vessels in this anomaly. Sequential transverse images can be used to determine stenosis of the main pulmonary artery and pulmonary annulus and obstruction of the infundibulum. This can also be depicted on sagittal images. On MR images, tetralogy of Fallot is characterized by an enlarged anteriorly displaced aorta, small pulmonic annulus, multilevel narrowing of the infundibulum, and perimembranous ventricular septal defect.

Important information provided by MR images concerns the sizes of the main and central pulmonary vessels in patients with severe stenosis or pulmonary atresia. Depiction of the size of the right and left pulmonary arteries requires very thin tomograms (3 mm slice thickness). Usually an initial series of 5 mm thick tomograms is obtained through the entire heart and then 3 mm thick ones at the pulmonary arterial level. Because it is not necessary to opacify the pulmonary arteries for visualization by MRI, determination of the presence of central pulmonary arteries and a central confluence of the right and left pulmonary arteries is a unique capability of MRI [18].

Assessment of blood supply to the lungs is achieved on both transverse and coronal images. On transverse images at the level of the carina and immediately below, it is usually possible to distinguish between pulmonary and bronchial arteries. Pulmonary arteries are situated ventral to the bronchi, whereas bronchial arteries are located posterior to the bronchi. Occasionally, a bronchial artery arising from subclavian arteries may be located ventral to the bronchi. The origin of bronchial arteries from the descending aorta can be observed on transverse and coronal images.

Pulmonary Atresia

Pulmonary atresia is depicted on transverse MR images as a solid layer of muscle in the region of the right ventricular outflow tract at the base of the heart; this represents the blind-ended infundibulum (Fig. 3). Continuity of the lumen of the right ventricle cannot be traced into the main pulmonary artery on sequential transverse MR images. The length of atresia may be shown to be extensive or focal at the valve level (Fig. 3). Focal membranous valvular atresia may not always be discernible as such on transverse tomograms due to partial volume inclusion of the patent lumen above or below the focal atresia on 5 or 10 mm sections. Consequently, valvular atresia and stenoses may not be distinguishable on spin-echo images. However, the presence or absence of flow across the valve can be determined on cine MR image in the transverse or sagittal planes. The length of the atresia of the main pulmonary artery as well as the infundibulum is demonstrated on sequential transverse tomograms.

In pulmonary atresia the aorta is usually markedly enlarged. There is generally a reciprocal relationship between the diameters of the aorta and pulmonary artery in patients with right ventricular outflow tract obstruction.

The aortic valve straddles a large ventricular septal defect in pulmonary atresia with ventricular septal defect (severe form of tetralogy of Fallot). A ventricular septal defect is not observed in the form of pulmonary atresia with intact ventricular septum. In the latter variety, MR is effective for determining the size of the right ventricle, which varies from severely hypoplastic to enlarged.

The most useful information provided by MRI in patients with pulmonary atresia is the determination of the status of the main and central pulmonary arteries distal to the atresia (Fig. 4). The right pulmonary artery is sought in the image containing the right main

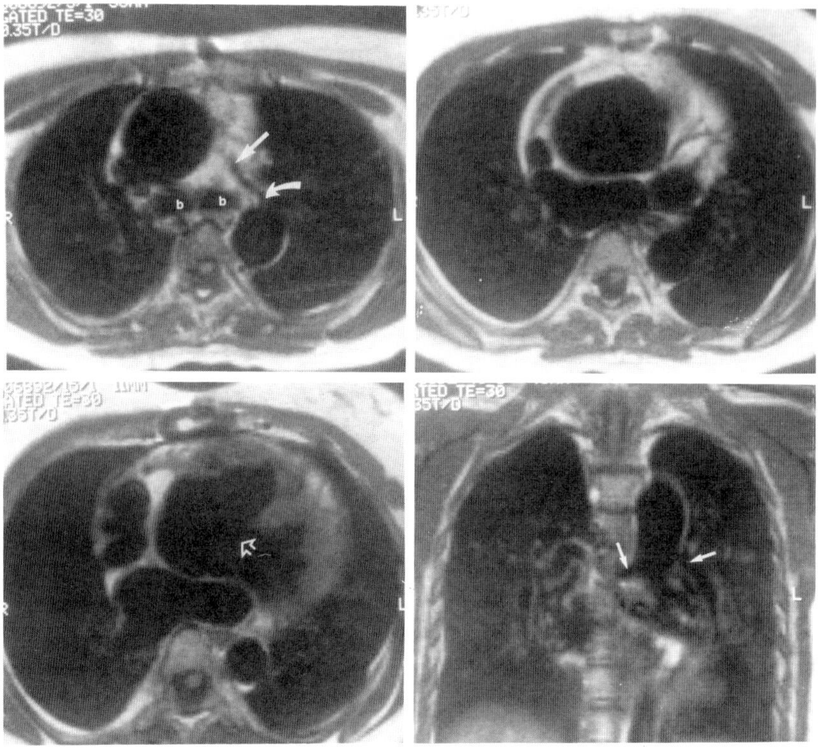

(a) (b) (c) (d)

Figure 3. *SERIES OF TRANSAXIAL IMAGES EXTENDING FROM CRANIAL (a) TO CAUDAL (c) IN A PATIENT WITH PULMONARY ATRESIA AND VENTRICULAR SEPTAL DEFECT. The main (closed arrow) and left pulmonary arterial segments (curved arrow) are very small in size. Note that the central pulmonary arteries are located ventral to the bronchi (b). There is a large ventricular septal defect (open arrow). Coronal image (d) demonstrates several enlarged bronchial arteries arising from the descending aorta in a patient with pulmonary atresia. The bronchial arteries (arrows) originate from both sides of the descending aorta.*

bronchus: it courses in front of the right bronchus. The left pulmonary artery courses over the left bronchus and is observed on the same tomogram as the proximal left bronchus or the one just cranial to the left bronchus. It is useful to determine if a main pulmonary artery or a central confluence between the pulmonary arteries exists. A recent report indicated that MRI is at least as accurate as angiography in defining the presence of main and central pulmonary arterial segments in patients with pulmonary atresia [18]. The pulmonary

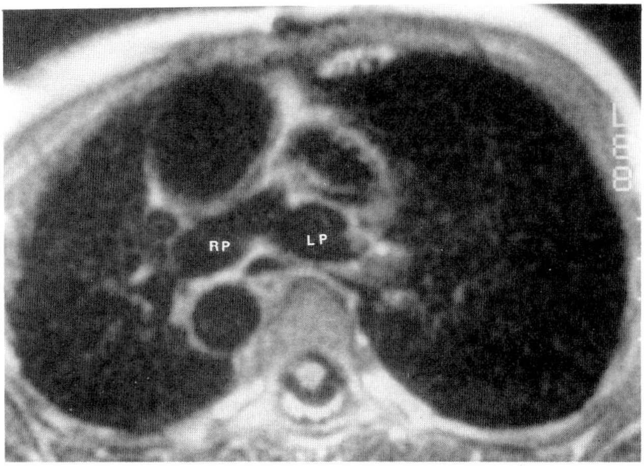

Figure 4. *TRANSVERSE IMAGE AT THE LEVEL OF THE PULMONARY ARTERIES IN A PATIENT WITH RIGHT-SIDED ISOMERISM, ASPLENIA AND PULMONARY ATRESIA. There is a central confluence between the right (RP) and left pulmonary (LP) arteries. The right and left pulmonary arteries have a normal size. No significant stenoses are recognized along the course of the right pulmonary artery.*

arteries frequently are hypoplastic to varying degrees or contain stenoses at the origin of the right, left, or segmental pulmonary arterial segments in patients with pulmonary atresia and ventricular septal defect. The pulmonary arteries are usually normal or nearly normal in diameter and usually do not contain stenoses in patients with pulmonary atresia with intact ventricular septum.

The presence of both right and left pulmonary arteries, their diameter. and whether there is a central confluence can be accurately defined by MRI. Adequate diameters of the central pulmonary arteries and the presence of a central confluence identifies a patient as a good candidate for a Rastelli procedure while the opposite finding indicates a poor candidate.

MR images also effectively display the bronchial arterial supply to the lungs. MR can be used to monitor the size of the surgically constructed systemic-to-pulmonary shunts, either by direct anastomosis or through an interposed graft. Distortion or stenosis of the pulmonary arteries caused by construction of these shunts is also depicted on images. The evaluation of the main and central pulmonary arterial segments is accomplished by transverse and coronal MR images, generally using the spin-echo sequence. Oblique coronal images ('sit up view') can be used to depict the length of the main pulmonary artery and bifurcation [19]. The region of the main and central pulmonary arterial segments is usually studied with 3 mm thick tomograms, frequently using four excitations (averages) in order to minimize partial volume averaging and enhance the accuracy of quantification of arterial diameter.

MR imaging is an effective method for monitoring the size and growth of the pulmonary arteries after surgical procedures intended to augment blood flow into them. Stenoses in pulmonary artery segments distal to surgical shunts, conduits, and anastomoses have been shown by MRI.

Ventricular Septal Defect

MRI can identify the presence and site of VSD. Transverse images are the most useful for this purpose, because they separate the inflow and outflow portions of the ventricular septum. In our initial group of patients with CHD evaluated by MRI, VSD was identified in 20 of 22 patients [20].

Using adjacent transverse images, the various components of the ventricular septum can be identified. The most frequently encountered defect is the perimembranous VSD. These can be clearly identified on transverse scans just below the aortic cusps. A transverse section located 1 cm caudal to the base of the aorta will demonstrate perimembranous VSD. The extensiveness of large perimembranous VSDs extending into the inlet and/or the outlet septa can be defined by adjacent transverse MR images. The position of perimembranous VSDs below the crista supraventricularis of the right ventricle can be discerned on both transverse and sagittal images. Aneurysm of the ventricular septum associated with a membranous VSD can also been demonstrated on transverse scans.

VSDs involving the inlet septum (atrioventricular-canal-type VSD) have been demonstrated in patients with complete endocardial cushion defects. The other components of the endocardial cushion defect, namely, ostium primum atrial septal defect and common atrioventricular valve, can also be visualized on transverse images positioned at a level to include all four chambers. Endocardial cushion defect is now usually called the atrioventricular septal defect.

Defects involving the outlet septum can be identified on transverse, sagittal, and coronal images. These defects include subpulmonic

VSDs and malalignment VSDs associated with truncus arteriosus, tetralogy of Fallot, and double-outlet right ventricle. Most malalignment VSDs studied by MRI have been large and associated with dilatation of the overlying great vessel. They have been demonstrated effectively on both transverse and sagittal images.

Another terminology for describing the location of VSDs relates to their location in relation to the crista supraventricularis. Distinction between infracristal and supracristal locations can be established on transverse or short-axis images through the right ventricular outflow tract. These images define cristal muscle between the pulmonary valve and the defect, indicating an infracristal VSD. Absence of muscle between the pulmonary valve and the defect is observed for the supracristal VSD. In the latter anomaly, the defect appears to directly connect the right ventricular outflow tract to the aorta. Cine MR images assist in locating the site of the VSD by showing a signal void at the defect which extends into the right ventricle in left-to-right shunts.

The bulboventricular foramen connecting the predominant ventricular chamber with the hypoplastic outflow chamber in the left ventricular type of single ventricle have also been identified and their dimensions assessed by MRI. The ideal imaging plane for demonstrating the foramen depends on the orientation of the foramen, which can vary considerably. Sometimes the septum in such cases of single ventricle is oriented in the sagittal plane, so that the foramen is depicted best on a coronal image.

Complex Ventricular Abnormalities

The components of complex ventricular abnormalities may be difficult to unravel using any imaging technique. In these complex lesions, transverse MR images can clearly define the visceroatrial situs, the type of bulboventricular loop, the relationship of the great arteries; and the position of the cardiac apex. A recent paper showed that the information provided by MRI was more complete than that obtained by angiography [21]. Evaluation of these complex anomalies should be done by sequential analysis in order to formulate a complete description of the abnormal cardiovascular morphology. Abnormalities of arterioventricular connection, atrioventricular connection and situs are frequently concomitant with complex ventricular anomalies. Abnormalities of arterioventricular connection include transposition and double outlet ventricles. Abnormalities of atrioventricular connection include: double inlet ventricle, atresia of one of the atrioventricular valves, over-ride or straddling of one of the arterioventricular valves, criss-cross atrioventricular connections, and common atrioventricular valve (Fig. 5).

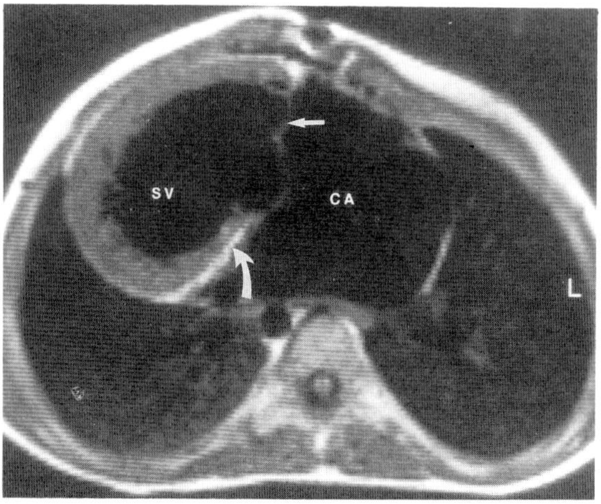

Figure 5. *TRANSAXIAL IMAGE OF THE MIDDLE OF THE VENTRICLE IN A PATIENT WITH MITRAL ATRESIA. Note the large common atrium (CA) and the single ventricular (SV) chamber. This single ventricle receives the tricuspid valve, which is located anteriorly (arrow). In the posterior portion of the ventricle there is a solid bar of muscle (curved arrow) separating the ventricle from the atrium, which indicates the presence of mitral atresia.*

On angiography it may not always be possible to differentiate among the various types of complex ventricular anomalies such as single ventricle (double inlet ventricle), hypoplasia of one ventricle with atresia of its atrioventricular valve, common atrioventricular valve with asymmetric relationship of the valve to the ventricular system (Fig. 6), and common ventricle (essentially absence of a ventricular septum, with each ventricle receiving an atrioventricular valve). In the analysis of these complex anomalies. MR can define the presence and connections of the atrioventricular valves, the size of the ventricular septal defect or bulboventricular foramen, the size of the two ventricles, the size of the ventricular septum, and the arterioventricular connections.

Differentiation of tricuspid atresia or mitral atresia with a very large VSD from single ventricle necessitates demonstration of the

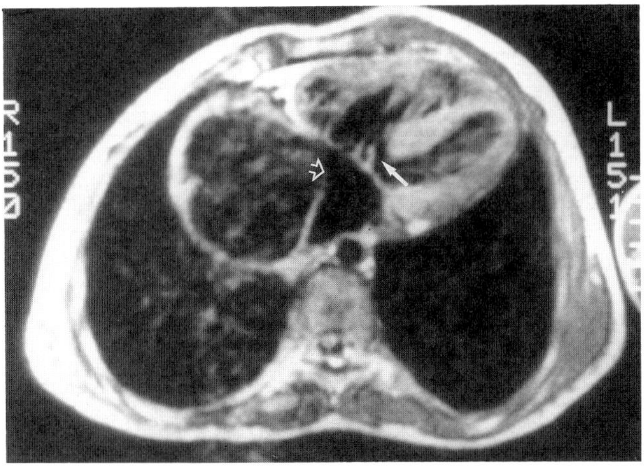

Figure 6. *TRANSAXIAL IMAGE AT THE MIDDLE OF THE VENTRICLES IN A PATIENT WITH COMPLETE ATRIOVENTRICULAR CANAL DEFECT. This entity is also referred to as the atrioventricular septal defect. Note the large primum atrial septal defect (open arrow) and large inlet ventricular septal defect (arrow). The atrioventricular valve spans the two ventricles.*

atretic valve region (Fig. 5). Atresia of an atrioventricular valve has been shown on transverse MR images as a layer of muscle separating the atrium from the ventricle at the expected level of the valve. The MR images also display the hypoplasia or absence of the inflow portion of the afflicted ventricle.

Atrial Abnormalities

Transverse or short axis MR images clearly display the sinus venosus, secundum, and primum portions of the atrial septum. The thinned region at the site of the fossa ovalis may produce little or no MR signal and can be misinterpreted as a secundum atrial septal defect (ASD). The septum gradually thins toward the site of signal absence in this circumstance, rather than the thickened edge of the septum adjacent to the true secundum defect. Cine MR images can be used to demonstrate that the septum is intact in the fossa ovalis region and to exclude a signal void at an atrial septal site, which could occur in the presence of a left-to-right shunt through a defect.

Spin-echo MRI has been found to be accurate for detection and determination of the site of ASDs. We have found greater than 90%

sensitivity at the 90% specificity level for MRI in identifying defects at any level of the atrial septum [22]. Our criteria for stating the definite presence of an ASD is to visualize a defect at two adjacent levels on multislice transverse images or to visualize the defect at multiple phases of the cardiac cycle at the same anatomic level. Dinsmore et al. [23] utilized images in the short-axis plane to estimate the size of the defect; MRI measurements correlated well with measurements made at operation. However, another report indicated only moderate sensitivity and specificity of gated MRI for detecting ASDs [24].

Pulmonary Venous Abnormalities

Partial anomalous pulmonary venous connection occurs in nearly all patients with sinus venosus defects and also occurs with an increased frequency in other types of ASD as well. Because MRI can clearly define the connection of the pulmonary veins to the left atrium, it is important to locate the connection of these veins in patients with ASD. These connections are nearly always clearly defined on transverse images. Coronal images can also be used to demonstrate this anatomy.

Transverse images show the right upper pulmonary vein entering the superior vena cava above its junction with the right atrium with partial anomalous connection. Transverse MR images display the coronary sinus; a dilated sinus may be a sign of anomalous connection to this structure. MR images in transverse, sagittal and coronal planes have shown the connection of a common right-sided pulmonary vein to the inferior vena cava in patients with the scimitar syndrome.

Systemic Venous Abnormalities

Several anomalies of the systemic venous system have been depicted by MRI (Fig. 7). Transverse images can reveal persistent left superior vena cava lying lateral to the main pulmonary artery. Transverse images can also show the enlarged vertical and horizontal limbs of the coronary sinus. The persistent left superior vena cava is variable in size; its diameter is reciprocal to the size of the right superior vena cava. In the rare instance of atretic right superior vena cava, the left cava and coronary sinus are markedly enlarged. Venous anomalies, including left superior vena cava, may raise concern regarding a

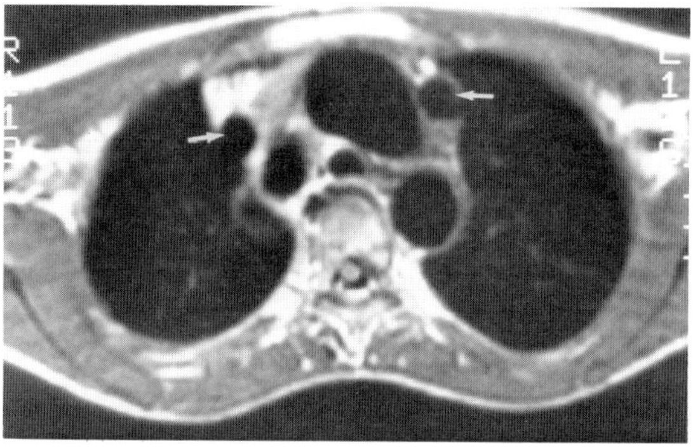

(a)

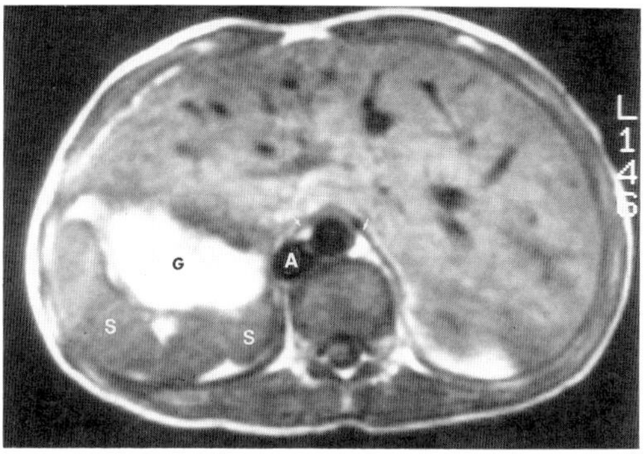

(b)

Figure 7. *TRANSAXIAL IMAGES AT THE LEVEL OF THE AORTIC ARCH (a) AND LIVER (b) IN A PATIENT WITH BILATERAL SUPERIOR VENA CAVAE AND INTERRUPTION OF THE INFERIOR VENA CAVA. Note the bilateral superior vena cavae (arrows). There is absence of the intra-hepatic portion of the inferior vena cava. Note that dorsal to the diaphragm (arrowheads) there is a markedly enlarged azygous vein (A). Note also the multiple spleens (S) in this patient with abdominal situs inversus. The liver is located on the left side and the stomach (G) on the right side.*

superior mediastinal mass on plain chest radiograph. MRI provides a simple non-invasive method for identifying this vascular anomaly and excluding a mediastinal mass. Transverse MR images have demonstrated the substantially enlarged coronary sinus into which the persistent left superior vena cava drains in most patients. Drainage of the left superior vena cava directly into the left side of the atrium has been observed in patients with the asplenia syndrome (unroofed coronary sinus defect) .

Interruption of the inferior vena cava (IIVC) with azygous continuation is clearly recognized on MR images (Fig. 7). MR has been used to clearly diagnose this anomaly when the enlarged azygous vein has suggested a posterior mediastinal mass on plain chest radiograph. Identification of this anomaly prior to catheterization can also be useful in facilitating this procedure. The IIVC occurs as an isolated anomaly or is associated with complex congenital heart disease. IIVC is a characteristic anomaly in the polysplenia syndrome; it occurs in a majority of patients with the polysplenia syndrome.

Thoracic Aortic Anomalies

MRI has been found to be effective for the definitive diagnosis of a number of thoracic aortic abnormalities. For thoracic aortic abnormalities, MRI should be considered the preferable imaging technique and can usually be substituted for the traditional reliance upon angiography. For most abnormalities, it provides diagnostic information at least equivalent to that obtained with angiography.

Arch Anomalies

MRI has demonstrated aortic arch anomalies, including double aortic arch and right aortic arch with retro-oesophageal left subclavian artery [25,26]. MRI displays both the vascular anomaly and the compression of the airway (Fig. 8). Compression of the airway is displayed optimally on the sagittal images. In right aortic arch, transverse MR images show the arch lying to the right of the trachea and the proximal descending aorta on the right aspect of the vertebral bodies. Usually, the right arch crosses to the left of the spine in the upper thoracic region; however, this crossing site is variable and is readily defined by MRI. Transverse images readily show the diameter of the right and left arches in double aortic arch. Transverse images also reveal the diameter of the retro-oesophageal subclavian artery. Usually, right retro-oesophageal subclavian artery (with left arch) has a normal diameter, whereas left retro-oesophageal subclavian artery (with right arch) has a focal dilatation at the site of origin from the descending aorta and consequently narrows the trachea and oesophagus.

Aortic Coarctation

The most frequently encountered congenital anomaly of the thoracic aorta is coarctation. MRI has been found to be effective for evaluating coarctation initially and after treatment. For evaluation of coarc-

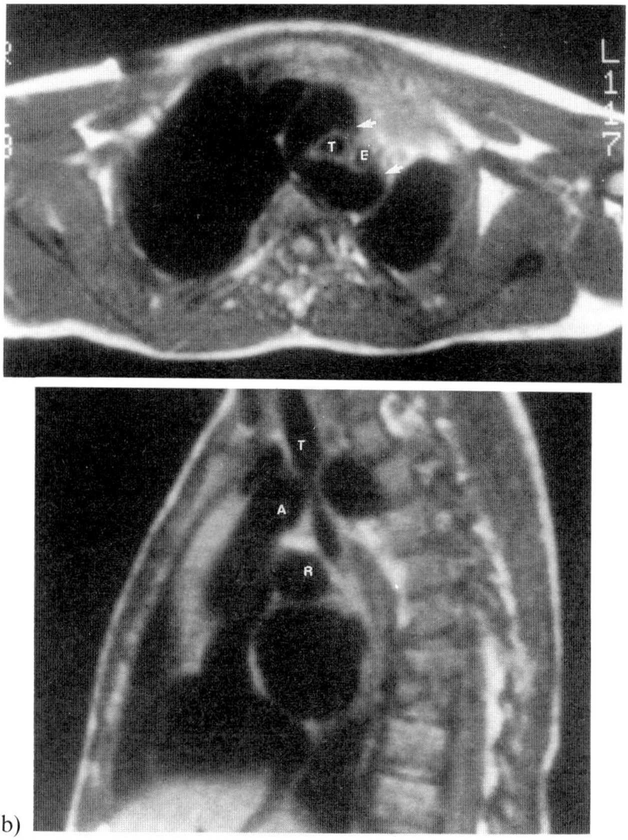

(a) (b)

Figure 8. *TRANSAXIAL (a) AND SAGITTAL (b) IMAGES IN A PATIENT WITH A DOUBLE AORTIC ARCH. The sagittal image demonstrates compression of the trachea (T) by the double aortic arch. The transaxial image demonstrates the large right aortic arch and the anterior and posterior component of the smaller left aortic arch (arrows). A = aorta; E = oesophagus; R = right pulmonary artery.*

tation and other thoracic aortic anomalies, gated images are obtained in planes perpendicular to each other. The imaging planes utilized when this diagnosis is suspected are the transverse and the sagittal, or a plane reproducing the 'LAO view'. The latter view is obtained by elevating the right shoulder 30° and imaging in the sagittal plane or angulating the slice-selective gradient so that it cuts through the middle of the arch. Identification of the stenotic segment sometimes is easier using the sagittal or LAO-equivalent plane than in the transaxial planes, because these planes are perpendicular to the coarctation, and thereby the narrowing is less obscured by partial-volume effects. These partial-volume effects encountered in the transverse plane may lead to underestimation or overestimation of the severity of coarctation. A 3 mm thick sagittal image centered in the middle of the coarctation should be used to measure the luminal diameter of the coarctation site (Fig. 9).

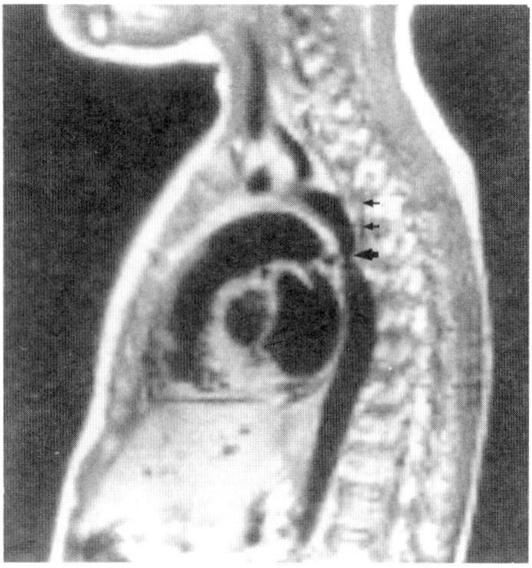

Figure 9. *SAGITTAL MR IMAGES IN A PATIENT WITH COARCTATION OF THE AORTA. The marked narrowing of the proximal portion of the descending thoracic aorta (arrow) is demonstrated. There is also a prominent collateral artery (small arrows).*

A report of results of MRI in 15 patients with coarctation of the thoracic aorta showed that this modality identified all but one coarctation and also showed the site, extent, and involvement of the arch vessels by the coarctation [27]. In addition, MRI was able to visualize poststenotic dilatation and dilated collaterals. Cine MR images can demonstrate the abnormal flow pattern caused by the aortic coarctation; a signal void originates from the site of the coarctation (Fig. 10). A recent study has shown the capability of a velocity-sensitive cine MR technique for estimating the gradient across the coarctation [28].

Postoperative Evaluation

A recent paper has indicated the value of MRI in comparison to angiography for the evaluation of complex surgical procedures for cyanotic CHD [29]. MRI has attributes for the monitoring of patients after operations for congenital heart disease. These are: the attractiveness of performing repeated studies with a technique free of the

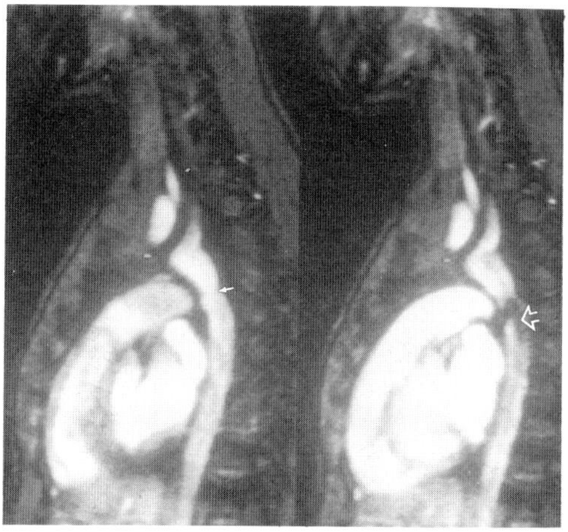

Figure 10. *CINE MR IMAGES IN A PATIENT WITH COARCTATION OF THE AORTA. The image on the left was obtained during diastole. The image on the right was obtained during systole. A transverse lucency across the descending thoracic aorta is recognized in diastole (small arrow). At the site of the coarctation a flow void (open arrow) is recognized due to high velocity turbulent flow across the coarctation site.*

concerns of radiation exposure or contrast media, the capability for displaying extracardiac anatomy as well as intracardiac anatomy, the capability of unequivocally demonstrating patency of shunts and the blood flow rate in systemic pulmonary shunts and conduits. The availability of echocardiography and MRI should substantially decrease the use of angiography for the postoperative evaluation of congenital heart disease. The potential advantage of MRI compared to echocardiography in this evaluation is the reliable and nearly unequivocal demonstration of conduits and anastomoses at the level of the great vessel and the quantitative assessment of the dimensions of the central and hilar pulmonary arterial segments.

MRI has been shown to be effective for demonstrating patency of systemic to pulmonary shunts (Fig. 11). In general these shunts are depicted optimally on transverse images. In some cases a long segment of a graft may be depicted very well on the coronal images. The major complications are occlusion, stenosis, pseudoaneurysm of an anastomosis, lymphocele, seroma or chyloma surrounding a graft, and distortion of the pulmonary artery at the anastomotic site or proximal to it.

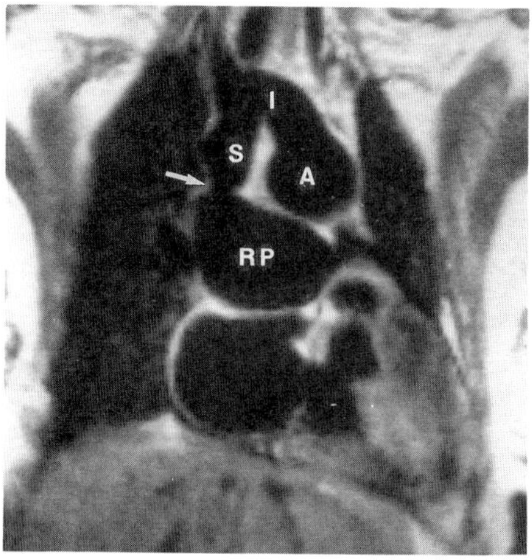

Figure 11. *CORONAL IMAGE IN A PATIENT WITH A RIGHT SUBCLAVIAN TO RIGHT PULMONARY ARTERY ANASTOMOSIS (ARROW). Note the aneurysmal dilatation of the right pulmonary artery (RP). A = aortic arch; I = innominate artery; S = right subclavian artery.*

Operations involving supracardiac anastomoses are very well demonstrated by MRI [29]. The surgical procedures in which MRI has been found to be very useful are the Rastelli, Fontan, Damus, Jatene, and Norwood procedures (Fig. 12). Each of these operations involves grafts and/or anastomoses performed above the level of the cardiac chambers; consequently MRI is particularly useful. MRI has also been used to assess intracardiac reconstructions such as the Mustard and Senning procedures, repairs of the right ventricular outflow tract in tetralogy of Fallot, and intraventricular baffles used in the repair of double outlet ventricles.

Assessment of Function - Cine MR and Blood Flow Measurement

Quantification of central cardiovascular function is a necessary step in the complete evaluation of CHD. Recent advances have rendered MRI as a comprehensive technique for depicting morphology and for measuring ventricular dimensions, mass and function. Moreover, velocity-sensitive imaging sequences provide measurement of flow velocity and flow volume in the vena cavae, pulmonary veins, pulmonary artery, and aorta. Abnormal flow velocities and profiles can be identified using cine MRI; recognition of disturbed flow patterns facilitates the diagnosis of valvular stenosis and regurgitation and the site of cardiovascular shunts.

Cine MRI permits the segmentation of the cardiac cycle into multiple time-resolved images. In order to isolate images corresponding to end diastole and end systole, gradient echo pulses are

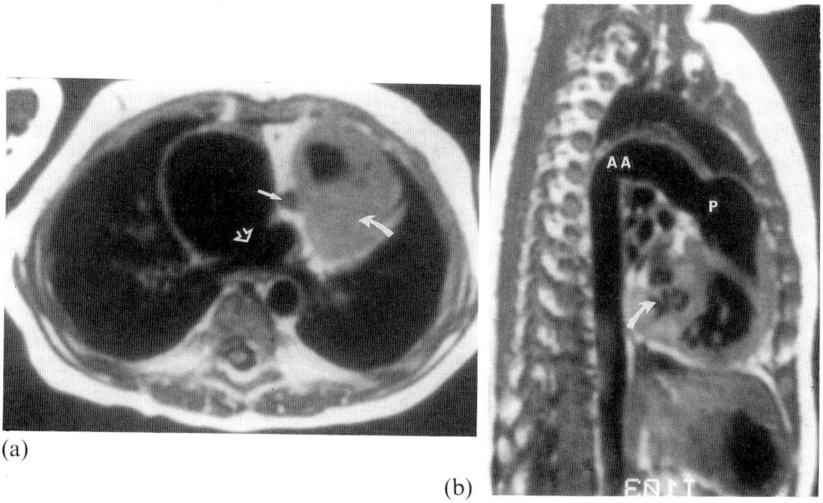

(a) (b)

Figure 12. *TRANSAXIAL (a) AND SAGITTAL (b) IMAGES IN A PATIENT AFTER THE FIRST STAGE OF THE NORWOOD PROCEDURE FOR PALLIATION OF HYPOPLASTIC LEFT HEART SYNDROME. The sagittal image demonstrates the connection of the main pulmonary artery to the aortic arch and continuing into the descending aorta. The transaxial view demonstrates the large interatrial communication (open arrow) connecting the large right atrium to the small left atrium. The left ventricular cavity is nearly completely obliterated by muscle (curved arrow). The base of the ascending aorta is very hypoplastic (small arrow). AA = aortic arch; P = pulmonary artery.*

performed at a rate to produce 15 to 30 images per cardiac cycle. When such sequences are repeated so that they encompass both ventricles, it is possible to measure the area of the blood volume of the right and left ventricles. Measurements done on the stack of tomograms acquired at end-diastole and end-systole provide end-diastolic (EDV) and end-systolic (ESV) volumes, stroke volume (SV = EDV - ESV) and ejection fraction (SV/EDV) for both the right (RV) and left (LV) ventricles. Studies have indicated that the stroke volumes are equivalent for the right and left ventricles in normal subjects. Stroke volume is greater for one of the ventricles in circumstances of volume overload lesions of a ventricle, such as valvular regurgitation and shunts. The stroke volume of the left ventricle exceeds that of the right ventricle in aortic and mitral regurgitation; the total regurgitant volume of the left ventricle is the difference in stroke volume of the two ventricles. In tricuspid or pulmonic regurgitation, the stroke volume of the right ventricle exceeds that of the left ventricle in the same manner.

Using volume quantification of the stack of cine MR images it is possible to estimate the volume of some shunt lesions. For patent ductus arteriosus, the LVSV exceeds the RVSV by an amount equal to the net left-to-right shunt. The RVSV exceeds the LVSV by an amount equal to a left-to-right shunt at the atrial level. The opposite relationship holds for net right-to-left shunts at the various levels.

Parameters of global systolic function of the two ventricles are readily derived from the stack of cine MR images. The most useful parameter of global function of the ventricle is ejection fraction. Ejection fractions for each ventricle using cine MRI have been established [10]. A study has also shown the reproducibility of volume and functional measurements of the ventricles between sequential studies in patients with normal, hypertrophied, and dilated ventricles [30,31].

The velocity-encoded cine MRI technique can be used to measure blood flow in the central circulation. The phase (velocity) image can discriminate between forward and retrograde blood flow [14] (Fig. 13). Regurgitant flow in the pulmonary artery and aorta can be recognized and appropriate accommodation made for it in the volume flow calculation in the great arteries. Left and right ventricular stroke volumes can be measured by integrating the flow values from the multiple images acquired during the cardiac cycle from regions of interest encompassing the proximal aorta and main pulmonary artery. This technique measures the effective forward flow from each ventricle if the aortic or pulmonary valves are competent. In the absence of aortic or pulmonary regurgitation, this technique also can be used to measure the volume of shunts. For instance, calculated LVSV exceeds RVSV by a volume equal to the net left-to-right shunt of a patent ductus arteriosus. On the other hand, calculated RVSV exceeds LVSV by a volume equal to the net left-to-right shunt of atrial septal defect, partial anomalous pulmonary venous connection, and ventricular septal defect. It should be noted that the volumetric calculations of the ventricles obtained by planimetry of the stack of cine MR images measures the volume of blood pumped by each ventricle (total stroke volume), while the velocity encoded cine MR technique measures the volume of blood ejected from the ventricles into the great arteries (effective stroke volumes).

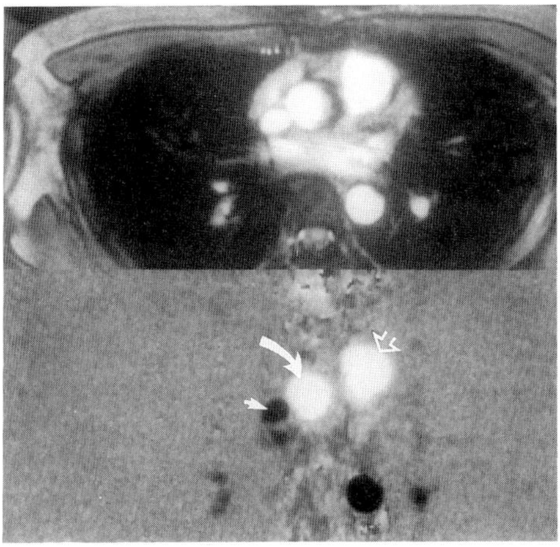

Figure 13. *MAGNITUDE (upper panel) AND PHASE (lower panel) IMAGES THROUGH THE REGION OF THE GREAT VESSELS. The phase image indicates that only regions within the image with blood flow are visible. Each pixel within the blood vessel provides a measurement of velocity at that site. Note that the direction of blood flow is indicated by the reverse polarity in the superior vena cava (arrow) and descending aorta in comparison to the ascending aorta (curved arrow) and pulmonary artery (open arrow).*

Role of MRI in Diagnosis of CHD

At this point, several limitations of MRI still exist for the evaluation of CHD. Valvular lesions and abnormalities of the subvalvular tensor apparatus are difficult to demonstrate clearly on spin-echo MRI. For example, cleft of the atrioventricular valves cannot be directly visualized on MR images. This limitation is caused by partial volume averaging of cardiac structures within the slice thickness. Although cine MRI partially solves this problem, spatial resolution still may not be enough to depict such structures effectively.

Another limitation of MRI is related to its relatively long time of examination. To accomplish a full examination of patients with CHD requires about 60 minutes. This requires full sedation for infants and small children. Recently, ultrafast imaging sequences have been developed, such as echo-planar and turbo-flash sequences. By using these techniques, eight or 16 images per cardiac cycle can be obtained within 20 seconds. Although these techniques are currently limited by relatively low spatial resolution, future technical development may enable them to be applied to small children.

MRI has advantages over other imaging techniques in terms of non-invasiveness, high image contrast and resolution, and accessibility to any site in the body. The role of MRI for diagnosis of CHD is still evolving. In the near future, full utilization of MRI may decrease or partially supplant angiography for the diagnosis of CHD.

Acknowledgement

Portions of this chapter are modified from Higgins CB. Congenital Heart Disease. In: Higgins CB, Hricak H, Holmes C (eds). Magnetic Resonance Imaging of the Body. Second Ed. Raven Press, New York, 1991.

References

1. Higgins CB, Byrd BF III, Farmer DW, Osaki L, Silverman NH, Cheitlin MD. Magnetic resonance imaging in patients with congenital heart disease. *Circulation* 1984;**70:**851-860.
2. Fletcher BD, Jacobstein MD, Nelson AD, Riemenschneider TA, Alfidi RJ. Gated magnetic resonance imaging of congenital cardiac malformations. *Radiology* 1984;**150**:137-140.
3. Didier D, Higgins CB, Fisher MR, Osaki L, Silverman NH, Cheitlin MD. Congenital heart disease: gated MR imaging in 72 patients. *Radiology* 1986;**158**:227-235.
4. Julsrud PR, Ehman RL, Hagler DJ, Ilstrup DM. Extracardiac vasculature in candidates for Fontan surgery: MR imaging. *Radiology* 1989;**173**:503-506.
5. Canter CE, Gutierrez FR, Mirowitz SA, Martin TC, Hartmann AF. Evaluation of pulmonary arterial morphology in cyanotic congenital heart disease by magnetic resonance imaging. *Am Heart J* 1989;**118**:347-354.
6. Hasse A, Frahm J, Matthaei D, Hänicke W, Merboldt KD. FLASH imaging: rapid NMR imaging using low flip angle pulses. *J Magn Res* 1986;**67**:258-266.
7. Sechtem U, Pflugfelder PW, White RD, Gould RG, Holt W, Lipton MJ, Higgins CB. Cine MRI: potential for the evaluation of cardiovascular function. *AJR* 1987;**148**:239-246.
8. Pflugfelder PW, Sechtem UP, White RD, Higgins CB. Quantification of regional function by rapid cine MR imaging. *AJR* 1988;**150**:523-529.
9. Utz JA, Herfkens RJ, Heinsimer JA, et al. Cine MR determination of left ventricular ejection fraction. *AJR* 1987;**148**:839-843.
10. Sechtem U, Pflugfelder P, Gould R, Cassidy MM, Higgins CB. Measurement of right and left ventricular volumes in healthy individuals with cine MR imaging. *Radiology* 1987;**163**:697-702.
11. Moran PR, Moran RA, Karstaedt NK. Verification and evaluation of internal flow and motion. *Radiology* 1985;**154**:433-441.

12. van Dijk P. Direct cardiac NMR imaging of heart wall and blood flow velocity. *J Comput Assist Tomogr* 1984;**8**:429-436.
13. Nayler GL, Firmin DN, Longmore DB. Blood flow imaging by cine magnetic resonance. *J Comput Assist Tomogr* 1986;**10**:715-722.
14. Kondo C, Caputo GR, Semelka R, Foster E, Shimakawa S, Higgins CB. Right and left ventricular stroke volume measurements with velocity encoded cine NMR imaging: in vitro and in vivo validation. AJR 1991 (submitted).
15. Underwood SR, Firmin DN, Klipstein RH, Rees RS, Longmore DB. Magnetic resonance velocity mapping: clinical application of a new technique. *Br Heart J* 1987;**57**:404-412.
16. Kersting-Sommerhoff BA, Diethelm L, Teitel DF, Sommerhoff CP, Higgins SS, Higashino SS, Higgins CB. Magnetic resonance imaging of congenital heart disease: sensitivity and specificity using receiver operating characteristic curve analysis. *Am Heart J* 1989;**118**:155-161.
17. Mayo JR, Roberson D, Sommerhoff B, Higgins CB. MRI of double outlet right ventricle. *J Comput Assist Tomogr* 1990;**14**:336-339.
18. Kersting-Sommerhoff BA, Sechtem U, Higgins CB. Evaluation of pulmonary blood supply by nuclear magnetic resonance imaging in patients with pulmonary atresia. *JACC* 1988;**11**:166-171.
19. Chung KJ, Simpson IA, Glass RF, Sahn DJ, Hesselink JR. Cine magnetic resonance imaging after surgical repair in patients with transposition of the great arteries. *Circulation* 1988;**77**:104-109.
20. Didier D, Higgins CB. Identification and localization of ventricular septal defects by gated magnetic resonance imaging. *Am J Cardiol* 1986;**57**:1363-1368.
21. Kersting-Sommerhoff BA, Diethelm L, Stander P, Dery R, Higashino SM, Higgins SS, Higgins CB. Evaluation of complex congenital ventricular anomalies with magnetic resonance imaging. *Am Heart Journal* 1990.
22. Diethelm L, Dery R, Lipton MJ, Higgins CB. Atrial level shunts: sensitivity and specificity of MR in diagnosis. *Radiology* 1987;**162**:181-186.
23. Dinsmore RE, Wismer GL, Guyer D, Thompson R, Liu P, Stratemeir E, Miller S, Okada R, Brady T. Magnetic resonance imaging of the interatrial septal and atrial septal defects. *AJR* 1985;**145**:697-703.
24. Lowell DG, Turner DA, Smith SM, et al. The detection of atrial and ventricular septal defects by gated MRI. *Circulation* 1986;**73**:89.
25. Bisset GS III, Strife JL, Kirks DR, Bailey WW. Vascular rings: MR imaging. *AJR* 1987;**149**:251-256.
26. Kersting-Sommerhoff BA, Sechtem UP, Fisher MR, Higgins CB. MR imaging of congenital anomalies of the aortic arch. *AJR* 1987;**149**:9-13.
27. von Schulthess GK, Higashino SM, Higgins SS, Didier D, Fisher MR, Higgins CB. Coarctation of the aorta: MR imaging. *Radiology* 1986;**158**:469-474.
28. Rees S, Somerville J, Warad C. Martinez J, Mohiakkin RH, Underwood R, Longmore DB. Coarctation of the aorta: MR imaging in late postoperative assessment. *Radiology* 1989;**173**:499-502.
29. Kersting-Sommerhoff BA, Seelos KC, Hardy C, Kondo C, Higgins SS, Higgins CB. Evaluation of surgical procedures for cyanotic congenital heart disease using MR imaging. *AJR* 1990;**155**:259-266.
30. Semelka RC, Tomei E, Wagner S, Mayo J, Kondo C, Suzuki J-I, Caputo G, Higgins CB. Normal left ventricular dimensions and function: interstudy reproducibility of measurements with cine MR imaging. *Radiology* 1990;**174**:763-768.

31. Semelka RC, Tomei E, Wagner S, Mayo J, Caputo G, O'Sullivan M, Parmley WW, Chatterjee K, Wolfe C, Higgins CB. Interstudy reproducibility of dimensional and functional measurements between cine magnetic resonance studies in the morphologically abnormal left ventricle. *Am Heart Journal* 1990;**119**:1367-1373.

Blood flow measurements with magnetic resonance imaging

Chisato Kondo, Gary R. Caputo and Charles B. Higgins
Department of Radiology, University of California Medical Center, San Francisco, CA, USA

Introduction

The importance of MR signal changes associated with flow was recognized in the early stage of magnetic resonance imaging (MRI) [1]. MR flow studies were accomplished with conventional spin-echo sequences and intended to employ flow-related signal intensity changes as an indicator of flow velocity [2-5]. Using this technique, the signal intensity may be influenced by various complex factors, including the flow velocity, direction, and flow profile in a vessel [5]. Consequently, spin-echo sequences have played a limited role in measuring blood flow.

With recent development of MR techniques, such as radiofrequency (RF) presaturation, gradient-echo sequences, and flow compensation, MR flow signal can be manipulated so as to measure flow velocity accurately, and flow measurements have become practical in clinical medicine. These techniques have contributed to the development of MR angiography as well [6]; therefore, MR may be utilized to provide morphological and functional information of blood flow. This article will review several principles and techniques utilized for MR flow measurements and current clinical applications.

MR Flow Effects

Signal intensity observed in MRI is influenced by motion of spins. To produce MR tomographic images, selective excitation of spins in a defined slice is accomplished by using a combination of an RF excitation pulse and a magnetic field gradient during excitation. The spins in the excited slice gain transverse magnetization which produces MRI signal. On the other hand, longitudinal magnetization of the spins is partially lost or saturated at the instance of next RF excitation. Flow or motion of spins affects these longitudinal and/or transverse magnetizations of MR signal. All MR flow phenomena arise only from one of two basic properties: (1) the changes in position of spin magnetization (time-of-flight effect), and (2) the changes in the phase of the transverse magnetization induced by motion along the magnetic field gradient (flow phase effects). These flow-related effects are very important to understand various MR techniques for flow quantification.

Time-of-Flight Effects

The principle of time-of-flight effects was reviewed by Axel [7] and recently by Wehrli [8]. Flowing spins produce velocity-dependent changes in signal intensity; with increasing velocity, the signal first increases and then decreases. This class of flow effects is simply caused by the changes in space of excited or saturated spins. The increase in signal is related to the washout of spins partially saturated by previous RF excitation and to the replenishment of fresh unsaturated spins from upstream (Fig. 1). Fresh spins first entering the imaging slice produces intense signal because they have not been affected by previous RF pulses and thus not been saturated. This effect (flow-related enhancement) is most pronounced in the entrance slice in multi-slice acquisition [9]. A competing effect is caused by the washout of excited spins from the imaged slice during imaging process, since the excitation and detection of an MR signal is not instantaneous. When images are obtained with spin echo sequences, only spins exposed to both the 90° and 180° pulses can produce signal (Fig. 2). With increasing flow velocity, washout effects tend to dominate, so that flowing blood appears dark. Consequently, the signal from flowing material first increases by flow-related enhance-

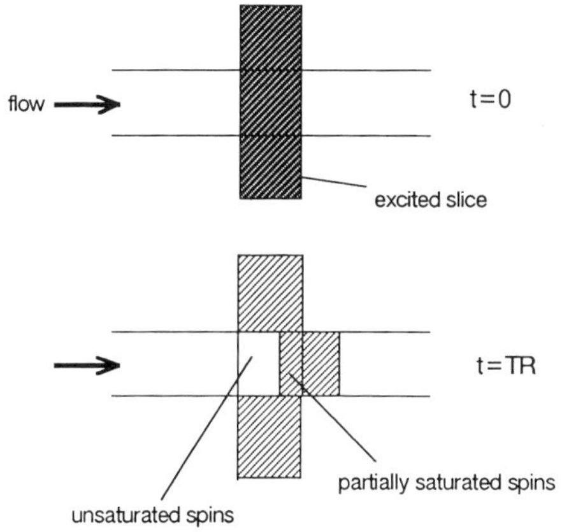

Figure 1. *DIAGRAMS OF FLOW-RELATED ENHANCEMENT. At the next RF excitation at TR, partially saturated spins within the imaging slice or stationary tissues produce only limited amount of signal, while fresh unsaturated spins produce intense signal.*

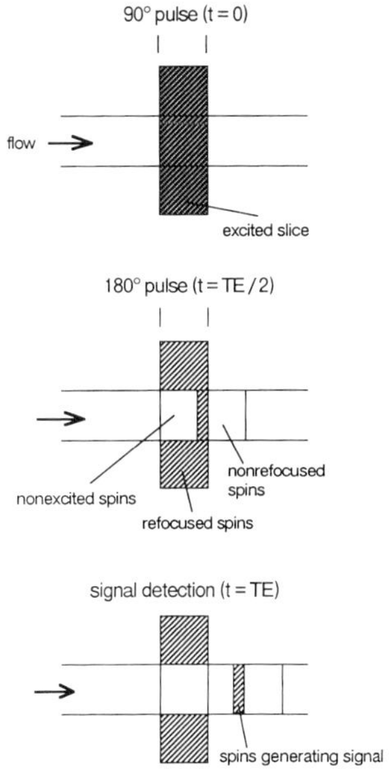

Figure 2. *DIAGRAMS OF WASHOUT OF EXCITED SPINS BETWEEN 90° AND 180° RF PULSES. Only spins exposed to both 90° and 180° pulses generate signal.*

ment mechanism, followed by its reaching a peak, and, thereafter, decreases by the washout of excited spins.

Flow Phase Effects

The second class of MR flow effects is phase effects, which arise from changes in phase of transverse magnetization induced as the spin moves along a magnetic field gradient. The phase of a spin moving in a field gradient along x evolves proportionally to the magnetic field strength; therefore, the amount of accumulated phase shifts during the time τ is;

$$\phi(\tau) = \gamma \int_0^{\tau} G(t)\, x(t)\, dt$$

where $\phi(\tau)$ is the phase shifts, G(t) is the time dependent gradient along x, γ is the gyromagnetic ratio, and x(t) is the position along the x coordinate. This equation can be applied to any type of movement of spins. Different locational changes of spins due to different velocity or higher order term of position results in different phase shifts. For moving spins with constant velocity (V), $x(t) = x_0 + Vt$, where x_0 is the initial position of spins. Therefore, phase shifts of flowing spins are influenced by its initial location and velocity. If sequential two square gradient pulses with same amplitude and duration but opposite polarity (bipolar gradient pulses; Fig. 3) are applied, spin phase shifts are simply given by $\phi = \gamma V A_G T$, where A_G is the area of one lobe of the flow encoding gradient and T is the time between centres of two lobes [10]. This relation indicates that the phase shift is linearly proportional to the spin velocity, and, therefore, can be utilized for flow quantification [11-14]. This simple relation holds true for constant velocity. If higher order of motion such as acceleration, jerk etc., is present in spin movement, these factors also influence the spin phase shift.

Spatial misregistration is the circumstance when spin position on images is different from where the spin actually is. Spatial misregistration may cause overlapping flow signal on adjacent stationary tissues and lead to errors in phase velocity quantification. This spatial

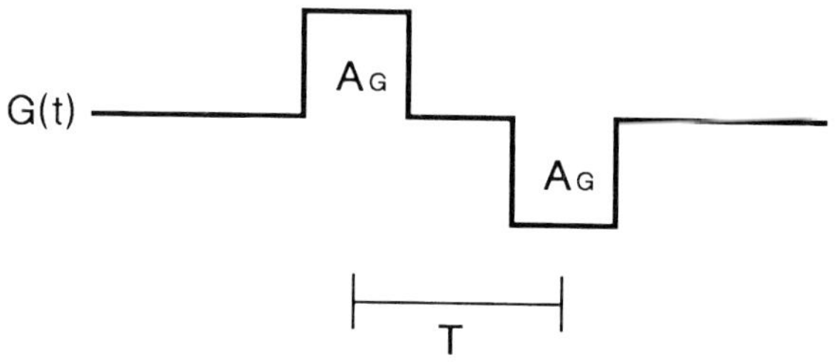

Figure 3. *BIPOLAR GRADIENT PULSES EMPLOYED FOR PHASE VELOCITY ENCODING. Two pulse lobes with opposite polarity are separated at a time interval T.*

misregistration can also be considered from two aspects: time-of-flight effects and flow phase effects. Spin warp imaging with two dimensional Fourier transformation determine the location of spins in space by sequential imaging steps with selective slice excitation, phase and frequency encoding. Because these steps are not instantaneous, any spin locational changes between these steps cause spatial misregistration [15]. An example of this effect is in-plane misregistration. If in-plane flow is obliquely directed to both phase encoding and frequency encoding direction, the temporal difference between phase encoding and readout results in the shift of spin signal in the direction of flow along the frequency encoding direction (Fig. 4). The similar misregistration also occurs in obliquely passing flow through the plane between selective slice excitation and readout. Spin phase effects are also responsible for spatial misregistration [16-17]. By motion-related phase shifts under gradient magnetic field, the position of flowing spins along phase encoding direction is artificially different from its true location. If the variation in velocity is present among voxels in a vessel (e.g. parabolic flow), the signal from blood is smeared out along the phase encoding direction.

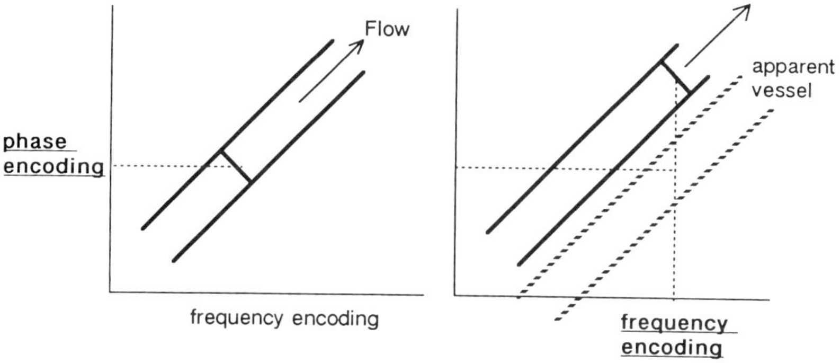

Figure 4. *DIAGRAMS OF SPATIAL MISREGISTRATION. Flowing spins are initially phase encoded, and thereafter frequency encoded. The time difference between these two encoding steps result in misregistration of a vessel along frequency encoding direction.*

Techniques for MR Flow Imaging

Presaturation techniques, which incorporate one or more additional

RF pulses prior to imaging sequences, are employed to label a restricted region of blood producing a dark signal region in a blood stream [18-19]. The principle is that an extra RF pulse (typically 90°) can be applied to saturate longitudinal magnetization of spins in a restricted region (presaturation tag). The labelled or tagged flowing region can be tracked precisely during the RF tagging and image formation. The presaturation technique is classified as time-of-flight flow methods in MR flow measurements.

Flowing blood appears to be very bright by the use of gradient-echo sequences. The nature of the flow enhancement on the gradient echo sequences is very important in terms of flow quantification, because the capability of MR flow measurements is based upon the presence of signal from flowing material; the signal enables the measurement of the movement of a flow bolus or spin phase shifts due to flow. The mechanism for the enhancement is thought to be that: (1) Fully relaxed spins continuously enter the imaging slice between subsequent RF excitations (flow-related enhancement). In contrast signal from stationary spins is relatively suppressed by very short TR of the gradient-echo sequences. (2) The signal is detected irrespective of the location of the moving spins because a non-slice selective gradient reversal is used for refocussing of the signal. Therefore, washout effects of excited spins are negligible in gradient-echo sequences. (3) TE employed on gradient-echo sequences is relatively short compared to T2 of blood, resulting in maintaining the signal from blood [20]. The enhancement of flowing blood on gradient-echo sequences, however, is interfered with by phase shifts due to flow across the magnetic field gradients.

Flow phase effects decrease signal intensity by two mechanisms: intravoxel phase dispersion and phase shift of a voxel [21]. Across the lumen of the vessel, there is usually a gradient of velocities; higher velocities exist in the center and lower velocities at the periphery of the lumen (Fig. 5). Such dispersion of the velocities produces corresponding dispersion of the phases and thus phase coherence within a voxel is lost, with a resultant decrease in amplitude of the signal. The second mechanism, a phase shift of a voxel, is that phase coherence is maintained within a voxel but is not constant among voxels. This effect leads to the spatial misregistration of signal from a voxel and spread out of flow signal as an artifact along the phase encoding direction.

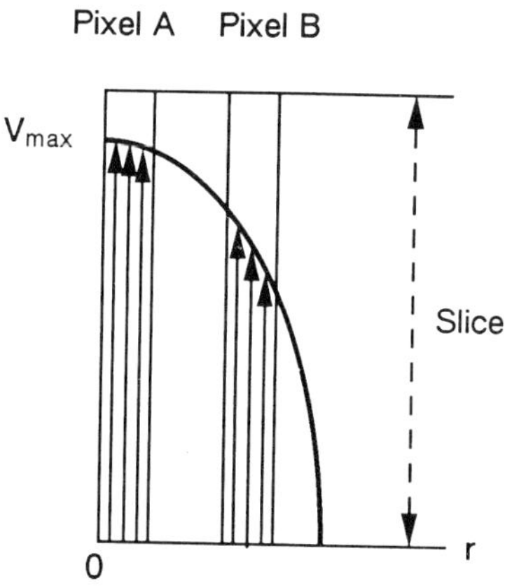

Figure 5. *DIAGRAM SHOWING VELOCITY INHOMOGENEITY WITHIN A VOXEL IN PARABOLIC FLOW. Progressing toward the periphery of a vascular cross-section, the degree of the velocity dispersion increases, resulting in corresponding phase dispersion within a voxel.*

To minimize the flow-related signal loss caused by phase effects, flow compensation techniques are applied [22-23]. The pulse sequence is modified by adding one or more gradient pulses, which are designed to reduce or eliminate phase shifts from both stationary and flowing spins. The flow compensation sequences can be designed so that the phase is zero at the echo for all velocities or so that incomplete refocusing occurs and yet enough signal remains so that sufficient phase information persists to measure velocity. There are two approaches for flow compensation. The first technique employs complex time-varying gradient wave forms to eliminate phase shifts due to the first few successive derivatives of position of spins [24]. A flow compensated gradient wave can be added for compensation of every derivative. The tradeoff of this technique is the prolongation of the length of the sequence and resultant decreasing time resolution. The second approach is more simple. A bipolar gradient pulse is combined with the bipolar pulse with its mirror image, resulting in three lobe pulse gradients [25] (Fig. 6). The flow induced phase shift of the first half of the lobed pulse is cancelled by the second half of the three lobed pulse. By using this technique, the phase effects due to odd order of derivatives of spin position can be eliminated [25]. The simplicity of the sequence can minimize the effect of even order derivatives by shortening of the length of the sequence.

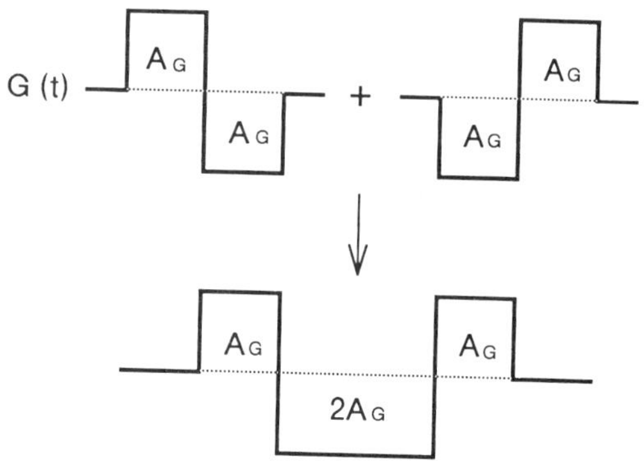

Figure 6. *THREE LOBE PULSE GRADIENTS ARE PRODUCED BY A COMBINATION OF MIRROR IMAGE BIPOLAR PULSE GRADIENTS. This form of gradient pulses is effective for eliminating phase shifts generated by constant velocity.*

Flow Measurement

A variety of MR techniques for flow measurements have been proposed. In general, all MR flow measurements are classified into two major categories: the first group utilizes longitudinal magnetization (time-of-flight techniques) and the other group utilizes transverse magnetization (phase techniques). Techniques employing longitudinal magnetization detect the amplitude of MR signals. On the other hand, techniques using transverse magnetization detect spin phase changes due to flow in magnetic field gradient.

Time-of-flight techniques rely on specific temporal and spatial changes in longitudinal magnetization of specified spin population in flowing blood. Many time-of-flight techniques dependent upon signal intensity changes associated with velocity changes have been investigated. However, these approaches have not been so successful, because the signal intensity changes associated with velocity are not simple and are influenced by various factors, including velocity, acceleration, direction, or flow phase effects [4,5,26,27]. Flow phase effects are caused by the application of magnetic field gradient during the slice selective 90° and 180° pulses. Intravoxel dephasing due to velocity and concomitant phase dispersion within a voxel are significant for fast flow. Consequently, signal changes are difficult to use for velocity quantification [5]. An alternative and probably more practical approach is a bolus tracking method [28-30]. Recent development of this technique employed gradient-echo sequences [30]. A restricted region of blood is labelled or tagged by RF presaturation pulses at the right angle to the direction of flow. An initial 90° pulse tips the longitudinal magnetization into the transverse plane; a gradient pulse of large amplitude called a spoiler follows to disperse the residual transverse magnetization. Subsequent imaging sequences are applied in the direction parallel to the flow (i.e., orthogonal to the 90° presaturation pulse) (Fig. 7). When imaged with gradient-echo sequences, presaturated spins provide low signal intensity. The low signal tagged bolus is easily discriminated from the rest of blood, which is bright on gradient-echo images. Because the initial position of the presaturation is recognized on adjacent stationary tissues as a dark line, velocity is simply quantified as distance traveled divided by the time between tagging and data readout.

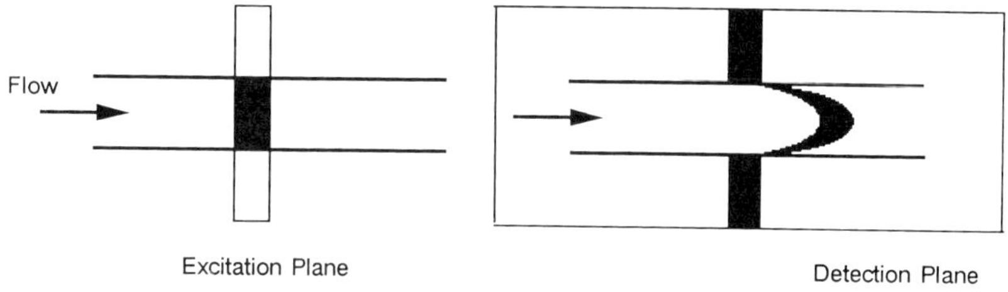

Figure 7. *DIAGRAMS SHOWING THE TIME-OF-FLIGHT FLOW MEASUREMENT TECHNIQUES. Initial excitation of spins is performed at right angle to the flow direction. The excited spins, in contrast, are detected along the flow direction.*

Phase techniques are based upon the fact that phase shifts of the MR signal is linearly proportional to the constant velocity along a magnetic field gradient. From the MR signal, two different types of information can be extracted: magnitude and phase of transverse magnetization. Standard MR anatomical images are reconstructed from the signal magnitude. However, phase information are not apparent on the standard magnitude images. Although there are various method to display the flow phase information, phase mapping methods have been proposed for clinical application.

Phase mapping methods provide phase values for each imaging voxel of phase images [11,12,25,31] (Figs. 8 and 9). On the phase image, signal intensity is set so as to be proportional to the phase and, therefore, velocity. To avoid the contamination of flow phase effects in multiple directions, phase mapping can be accomplished by

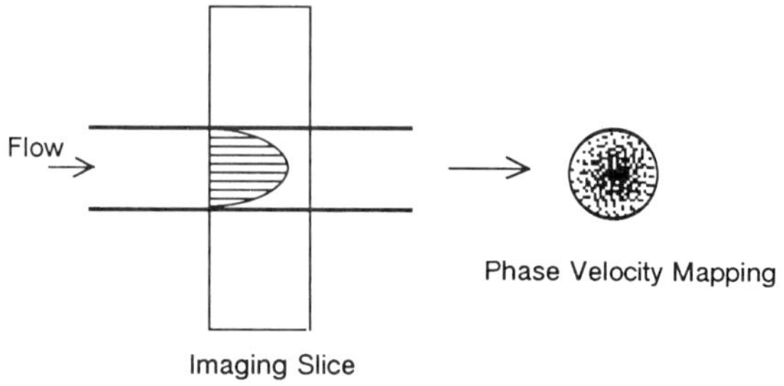

Figure 8. *DIAGRAMS SHOWING THE PHASE VELOCITY MAPPING TECHNIQUES. Signal intensity at each pixel on phase velocity maps is proportional to the velocity of flow.*

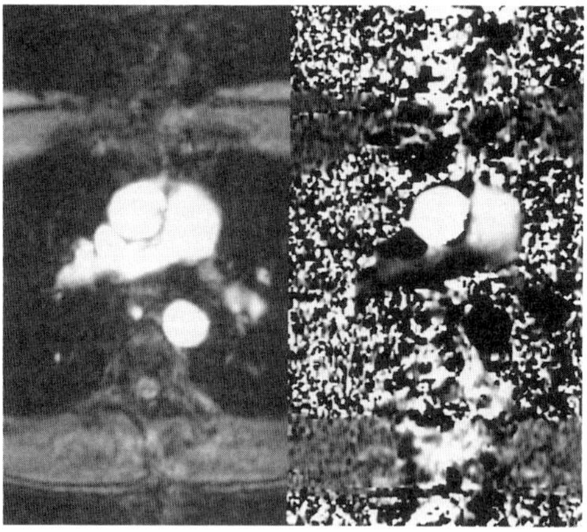

(a) (b)

Figure 9. *FROM THE MR SIGNAL, TWO TYPES OF IMAGES CAN BE RECONSTRUCTED: MAGNITUDE (a) AND PHASE IMAGES (b). Standard MR images are reconstructed from signal magnitude (a). Velocity phase mapping (b) provides pixel based velocity encoded phase data as a difference of signal intensity on images.*

subtraction of two interleaved phase data sets which have been differently encoded along only one desired direction [25]. Phase mapping can be combined with flow compensation techniques which are effective for minimizing signal loss duc to velocity dispersion in a vessel or high order terms of spin position [25]. Cinematic display of phase mapping with high temporal resolution can be attained with the use of gradient-echo sequences [25].

Fourier flow imaging is an alternative method to provide flow phase information [32,33]. In this technique, velocity is encoded by the use of bipolar gradient pulses in the same fashion as the phase mapping methods. However, the phase encoding gradients are increased in stepwise fashion similar to encoding a line location in standard MR images. Two-dimensional Fourier transformation of these phase data gives the image intensity which is the relative number of spins flowing at a particular velocity and spatial location in the image in the frequency encoding direction. Because the one dimension is used for velocity encoding, the final image has only one spatial resolution and cross sectional velocity distribution is projected on one plane. To obtain velocity distribution with two-dimensional spatial resolution, three-dimensional Fourier transformation is required, resulting in prolonged imaging time. Compared to phase mapping, Fourier flow imaging has the advantage of avoiding partial volume averaging of velocity data within a voxel. Signal from static tissue can be discriminated from flowing spins within the same voxel, and, therefore, the accuracy of measuring velocity is not reduced.

Some phase techniques produce magnitude images whose signal intensity represents the degree of flow velocity [34,35]. Flow velocity is encoded by using bipolar gradient pulses. The polarity of the bipolar pulses is inverted in alternating manner, so that the resulting phase shift for the same spin is equal but opposite for the two sets of data. After complex subtraction of these phase data sets, signal intensity of the magnitude images is proportional to the degree of phase shift and thus velocity. This technique can provide clear MR angiograms on which signal intensity represents flow velocity. The accuracy of flow measurements by this technique, however, are influenced by the assumption of a flow profile (parabolic or plug), and will be strongly influenced by the signal changes due to intra-voxel phase dispersion or inflow enhancement.

Accuracy of Flow Quantification

The requirements for accuracy of MR flow measurements are dependent upon the purpose of the study and flow conditions, such as the magnitude of flow velocity, direction of flow and the presence or absence of turbulence. Each of the several MR flow methods has its own efficacy and limitations in terms of accuracy depending upon different flow conditions. The accuracy of MR flow techniques has been compared with other independent flow measurements using flow phantom and/or *in vivo* flow studies.

Accuracy of time-of-flight techniques has been evaluated in several studies. Among these studies, bolus tracking method could correctly measure flow velocity up to 35 cm/s in a constant flow phantom [30]. Another type of bolus tracking method correctly determined high flow velocity (up to 3 m/s) [29] and slow flow (5 cm/s) [36] generated in a phantom. In vivo accuracy of the bolus tracking technique was demonstrated in the abdominal aorta [37] and portal vein [38] compared with Doppler ultrasound measurements.

A recent study reported an interesting application of the bolus tracking technique using flow profiles along flow direction [39]. The trailing edge of the tracked bolus directly reflects the flow profiles such as a parabolic contour on flow images. The shape of parabolic profile by MR was very similar to that determined by laser Doppler measurements. The fluid velocity profile of tracked bolus demonstrated the development of parabolic flow from an initially flat or plug-like profile at the entrance region of a tube. Shear stress at a vascular wall could be estimated by measuring the slope of the fluid velocity profile at the vessel wall. The MR determined shear stress agreed with theoretical values calculated from developed parabolic profiles. These capabilities may be employed in the future to examine vascular wall shear stress and its impact on vascular damage in vivo.

The accuracy of phase modulation techniques has been evaluated in several studies. Recent phantom studies in our laboratory demonstrated that velocity measurements by this technique was very accurate for the velocities over a wide range (20 - 410 cm/s) (Fig. 10). In this experiments, the velocity with critical Reynolds number (= 2500) for the transition from laminar to turbulent flow corresponds to 40 cm/sec. The results suggest that the capability to measure high flow velocity with this technique is maintained even under the occurrence of turbulence. The effect of turbulence is considered to decrease

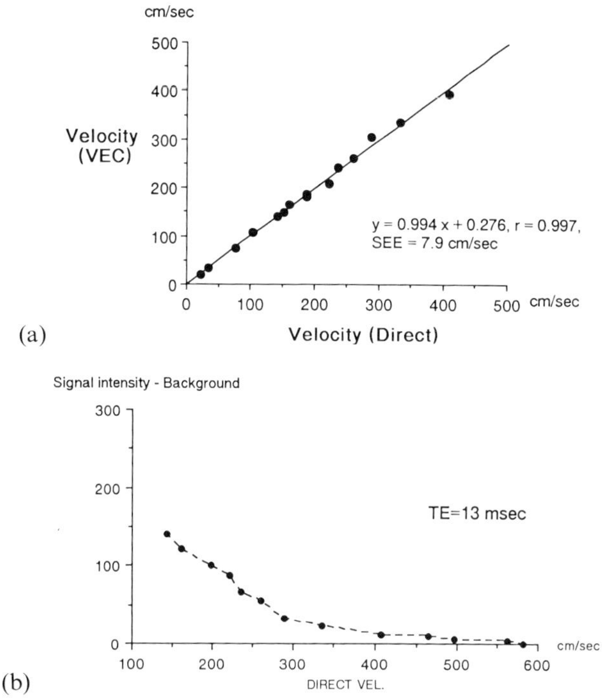

Figure 10. *(a) In constant flow phantom experiments, velocities were correctly determined by MRI in the range from 20 to 410 cm/s using a TE of 13 ms at 1.5 Tesla. With increasing velocity, signal intensity on magnitude images decreased and were completely lost at 450 cm/s (b). Above this velocity, velocity could not be measured.*

signal intensity. With increasing velocity, signal from flowing material decreased (Fig. 10). Sequences with the TE of 13 ms were not able to measure velocity above 450 cm/s because signal was completely lost at this point. The effect of signal loss can be diminished with decreasing the TE. When the TE was lowered to 7 ms, velocity could be accurately measured up to 580 cm/s (Fig. 11). In contrast, extremely slow velocity (5 mm/sec) could be correctly measured with phase techniques as well [40].

Other studies demonstrated the feasibility of the phase technique for pulsatile flow. Pulsatile flow velocity determined by the techniques was correct when compared with Doppler ultrasound measurements in the abdominal aorta [41] or pulmonary artery [42].

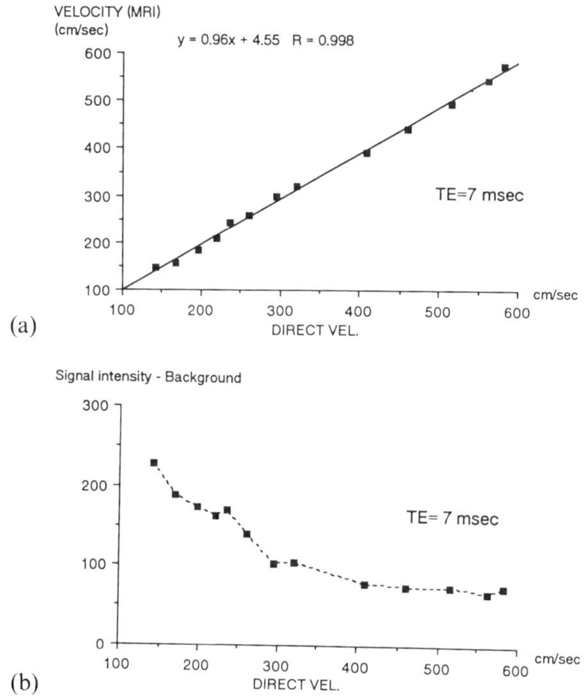

Figure 11. *(a) In constant flow phantom experiments, velocities were correctly determined by MRI up to 580 cm/sec using a TE of 7 msec at 1.5 Tesla. Although with increasing velocity signal intensity on magnitude images decreased, signal was still maintained at the highest velocity (b) and the capability of velocity measurements was maintained.*

Aortic or pulmonary flow volume by phase techniques correlated well with stroke volume determined by ventricular volumetric measurements with spin echo [43] or cine MR images [42] (Fig. 12). These results suggest that higher order derivatives of spin position associated with pulsatile flow may not have significant impacts on the accuracy of flow quantification with phase techniques under normal flow conditions.

The accuracy of phase techniques, however, is not constant depending upon the selection of methods. For velocity encoding, some methods use two alternating experiments with different gradient. Subtraction of the two experiments provides only phase velocity data along only a desired direction for velocity measurements. Other

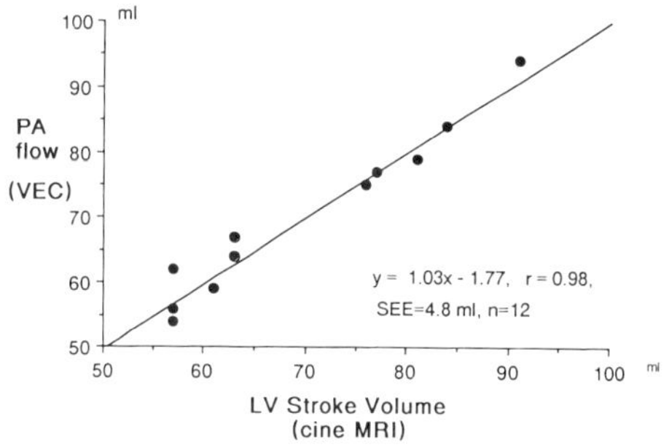

Figure 12. *LEFT VENTRICULAR STROKE VOLUMES BY MRI (VEC) CORRELATED WITH THOSE BY VOLUMETRIC ANALYSIS WITH CINE MRI.*

methods employ the same gradient as those used for conventional two dimensional Fourier transformation imaging for velocity encoding. The sequences have sensitivity to flow in both slice select and read out direction. Moreover, differently encoded phase velocity data sets were not subtracted. Therefore, the sequence is very sensitive to flow both within and perpendicular to the imaging plane. With occurrence of turbulence, velocity components transverse to the main flow direction occur. The flow in the direction of the imaging plane can add erroneous phase shift to the results [44]. Therefore, selective velocity encoding may be the critical factor for accurate velocity quantification with phase modulation techniques.

Clinical Results

MR flow quantification is still in the stage of determining feasibility, and the full application of MR to clinical flow studies has not been attained. To date, almost all non-invasive flow studies have been accomplished by the use of Doppler ultrasound. However, several reports demonstrated unique clinical capability of MR flow techniques [45-47].

Flow studies by the use of phase velocity mapping have been used in patients with intracardiac shunts [45], and coarctation of the aorta [45]. In these cases, flow velocity mapping can identify abnormal flow signal similar to Doppler colour flow mapping and more importantly can demonstrate the velocity profile in a cross-section of a vessel. Such cross sectional flow images can differentiate and quantify antegrade and retrograde flow in a vessel separately. Abnormally large amount of retrograde flow at mid to late systole in the main pulmonary artery was recognized in patients with pulmonary arterial hypertension (Fig. 13) [46]. In contrast, retrograde flow in the aorta was significantly reduced in patients with coronary artery disease compared with normal subjects [47]. Such information may be related to the severity or pathophysiology of disease process, but further studies are necessary to clarify clinical significance or rele-vance of these findings.

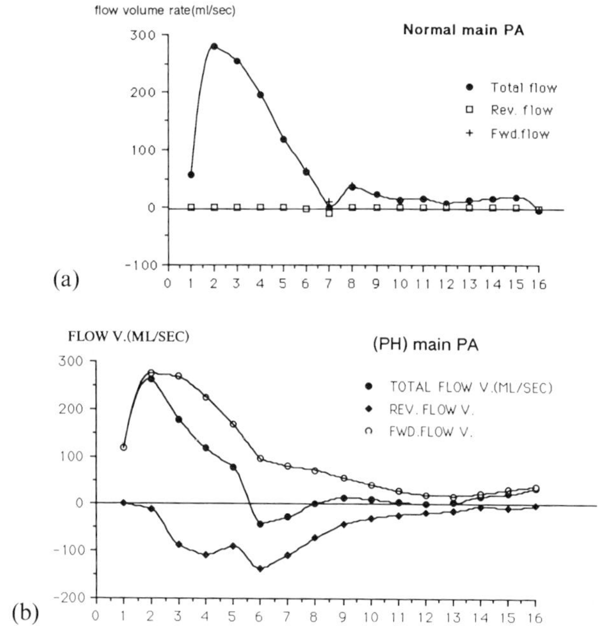

Figure 13. *PULMONARY FLOW PROFILES IN A NORMAL SUBJECT (a) AND A PATIENT WITH PRIMARY PULMONARY HYPERTENSION (b). After mid-systole, substantial amount of retrograde flow (REV. FLOW) in the patient with pulmonary hypertension was recognized, which was not present in normal subjects.*

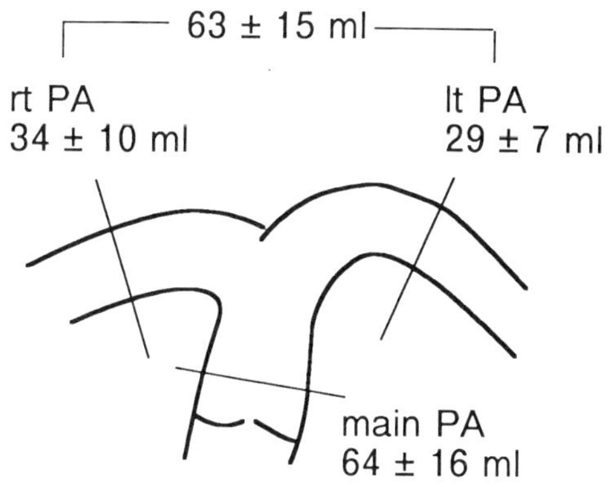

Figure 14. *BLOOD FLOW VOLUMES IN ONE CARDIAC CYCLE AT THE RIGHT AND LEFT PULMONARY ARTERIES WERE MEASURED SEPARATELY. The sum of the amount of blood flow at each artery was similar to the flow volume measured at the main pulmonary artery.*

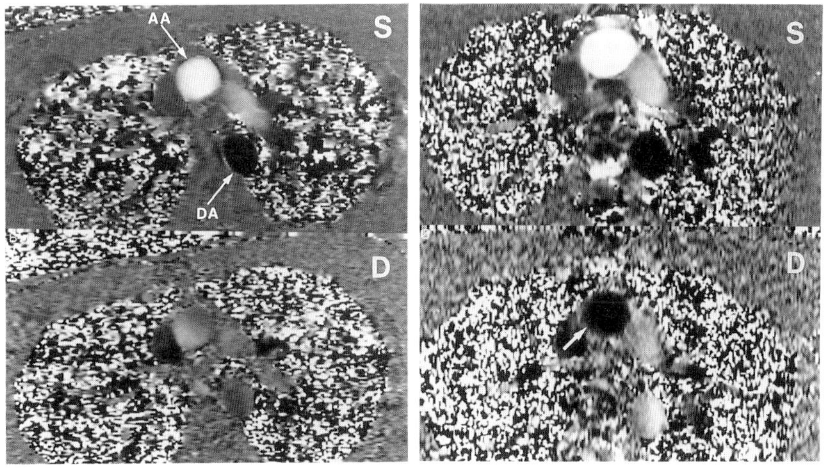

Figure 15. *PHASE IMAGES FROM A NORMAL SUBJECT (a) AND A PATIENT WITH AORTIC REGURGITATION (b). Note the reversal of coloration of signal in the ascending and descending aorta in the patients with aortic regurgitation (arrow). This indicates substantial retrograde flow in diastole. S = Systole; D = Diastole; AA = Ascending aorta; DA = Descending aorta.*

Potential advantages of velocity flow mapping over Doppler echocardiography may be demonstrated on flow studies at medium or relatively small sized vessel in the deep sites of the body. Because MR images can be acquired with a desired oblique imaging plane, the effect of obliquity between flow direction and sampling direction can bc corrected. Recent studies in our laboratory showed that blood flow at the right and left pulmonary arteries could be separately measured in normal subjects by using such an oblique imaging plane (Fig. 14). The ratio of the flow volume at each artery was similar to that

(a)

(b)

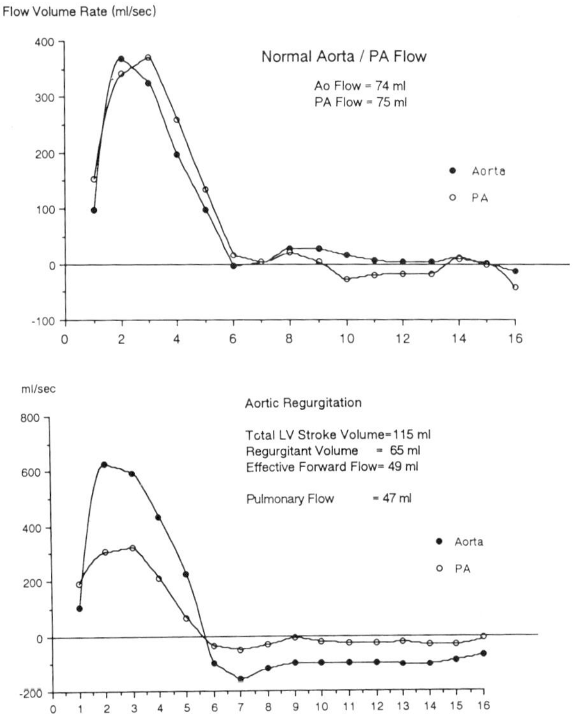

Figure 16. *AORTIC FLOW PROFILES IN A NORMAL SUBJECT (a) AND A PATIENT WITH AORTIC REGURGITATION (b). Flow with negative value implies regurgitant flow in the ascending aorta. Initial positive flow during systole was followed by regurgitant flow throughout the diastole. Subtraction of the regurgitant volume from total stroke volume determined by initial positive flow provided effective forward flow form the left ventricle. Separately measured pulmonary flow was close to the effective forward flow volume.*

reported by nuclear techniques [48]. The sum of the amount of blood flow at both arteries was close to flow volume measured at the main pulmonary artery (Fig. 14). MR flow studies of portal venous system showed that the response of increasing portal blood flow after glucose administration was depressed in patients with chronic hepatitis [36]. Similarly, abnormal reverse portal blood flow was documented in patients with portal hypertension [38]. Although the capability of MR flow measurements at small vessels may be limited by spatial resolution, various vessels which are difficult to approach by Doppler ultrasound can be approached with MR flow studies.

Another possible application of velocity flow mapping is to evaluate valvular heart disease. Because retrograde flow as well as antegrade flow in the aorta may be directly measured on flow images, time integrated retrograde flow volume over one cardiac cycle will provide regurgitant volume through an incompetent aortic valve. Our preliminary experience in the patients with aortic regurgitation showed that the amount of total stroke volume at the aorta was significantly larger than that of effective stroke volume measured at the main pulmonary artery (Figs. 15 and 16). Abnormal retrograde flow was recognized throughout diastole. Subtraction of the retrograde flow from total stroke volume provided a similar value to the effective stroke volume. Measurement of retrograde flow in the aorta may be utilized to quantify regurgitant volume directly and grade the severity of aortic regurgitation quantitatively. Similar to Doppler echocardiography, estimation of pressure gradient at stenotic valve or vessel may be accomplished by MR flow studies. To date, however, signal loss caused by severe dephasing due to turbulent flow has limited such applications of MR flow phase techniques. Decreasing the echo delay time may be helpful in minimizing signal loss and enable measurements of flow through stenotic valves.

References

1. Singer JR. Blood flow rates by nuclear magnetic resonance measurements. *Science* 1959;**130**:1652-1653.
2. Kaufman L, Crooks LE, Sheldon PE, Rowan W, Miller T. Evaluation of NMR imaging for detection and quantification of obstructions in vessels. *Invest Radiol* 1982;**17**:554-560.
3. Singer JR. Nuclear magnetic resonance blood flow measurements in the human brain. *Science* 1983;**221**:654-656.

4. Feinberg DA, Crooks L, Hoenninger J, Arakawa M, Watts J. Pulsatile blood velocity in human arteries displayed by magnctic resonance imaging. *Radiology* 1984;**153**:177-180.
5. Wehrli FW, Shimakawa A, MacFall JR, Axel L, Perman W. MR imaging of venous and arterial flow by a selective saturated-recovery spin echo (SSRSE) method. *J Comput Assist Tomogr* 1985;**9**:537-545.
6. Edelman RR, Mattle HP, Atkins DJ, Hoogewoud HM. MR angiography. *AJR* 1990;**154**:937-046.
7. Axel L. Blood flow effects in magnetic resonance imaging. *AJR* 1984;**143**:1157-1166.
8. Wehrli FW. Time-of-flight effects in MR imaging of flow. *Magn Reson Med* 1990;**14**:187- 193.
9. Crooks LE, Mills CM, Davis PL, et al. Visualization of cerebral and vascular abnormalities by MR imaging: the effects of imaging parameters on contrast. *Radiology* 1982;**144**:843-854.
10. Dumoulin CL. Flow imaging. In Budinger TF, Margulis AR (eds). *Medical magnetic resonance. A primer.* Berkely, Society of magnetic resonance in medicine, 1988.
11. van Dijk P. Direct cardiac NMR imaging of heart wall and blood flow velocity. *J Comput Assist Tomogr* 1984;**8**:429-436.
12. Bryant DJ, Payne JA, Firmin DN, Longmore DB. Measurement of flow with NMR imaging using a gradient pulse and phase difference technique. *J Comput Assist Tomogr* 1984;**8**:588-593.
13. Moran PR. A flow velocity zeugmatographic interplace for NMR imaging in humans. *Magn Reson Imaging* 1982;**1**:197-203.
14. Moran PR, Moran RA, Karstaedt K. Verification and evaluation of internal flow and motion. *Radiology* 1985;**154**:433-441.
15. von Schulthess GK. Blood flow. In Higgins CB, Hricak H (eds). *Magnetic resonance imaging of the body.* New York: Raven Press, 1987;119-143.
16. Ehman RL, McNamara MT, Brasch RC, Felmlee JP, Gray JE, Higgins CB. Influence of physiologic motion on the appearance of tissue in MR images. *Radiology* 1986;**159**:777-782.
17. Haacke EM, Patrick JL. Reducing motion artifacts in two dimensional Fourier transform imaging. *Magn Res Imag* 1986;**4**:359.
18. Edelman RR, Atkinson DJ, Silvcr MS. FRODO pulses: a new method for elimination of motion flow and wrap-around artifact. *Radiology* 1988;**166**:231-236.
19. Felmlee JP, Ehman RL. Spatial presaturation: a method for suppressing flow artifacts and improving dcpiction of vascular anatomy in MRI. *Radiology* 1987;**164**:559-564.
20. Wehrli FW. Fast-scan imaging: principles and contrast phenomenology. In Higgins CB, Hricak H (eds). *Magnetic resonance imaging of the body.* New York:Raven Press, 1987;23-38.
21. Ehman RL, Felmlee JP. Flow artifact reduction in MRI: a review of the roles of gradient moment nulling and spatial presaturation. *Magn Reson Med* 1990;**14**:293-307.
22. Laub GA, Kaiser WA. MR angiography with gradient motion rephasing. *J Comput Assist Tomogr* 1988;**12**:377-382.
23. Haacke EM, Lenz GW. Improving MR image quality in the presence of motion by using rephasing gradients. *AJR* 1987;**148**:1251-1258.
24. Pattany PM, Phillips JJ, Chiu LC, Lipcamon JD, Duerk JL, McNally JM, Mohapatra SN. Motion artifacts suppression technique (MAST) for MR imaging. *J Comput Assist Tomogr* 1987;**11**:369-377.
25. Nayler GL, Firmin DN, Longmore DB. Blood flow imaging by cine magnetic resonance. *J Comput Assist Tomogr* 1986;**10**:715-722.
26. Wehrli FW, MacFall JR, Axel L, Sutts D, Glover GH, Herfkens RJ. Approaches to in-plane and out-of-plane flow imaging. *Non-invasive Med Imaging* 1984;**1**:127-136.

27. Wehrli FW, Shimakawa A, Gullberg GT, MacFall JR. Time-of-flight MR flow imaging: selective saturation recovery with gradient refocusing. *Radiology* 1986;**160**:781-785.
28. Axel L, Shimakawa A, MacFall J. A time-of-flight method of measuring flow velocity by magnetic resonance imaging. *Magn Reson Imaging* 1986;**4**:199-205.
29. Shimizu K, Matsuda T, Sakurai T, et al. Visualization of moving fluid: quantitative analysis of blood flow velocity using MR imaging. *Radiology* 1986;**159**:195-199.
30. Edelman RR, Mattle HP, Kleefield J, Silver MS. Quantification of blood flow with dynamic MR imaging and presaturation bolus tracking. *Radiology* 1989;**171**:551-556.
31. Pettigrew RI, Dannels W. Use of standard gradients with compound oblique angulation for optimal quantitative MR flow imaging in oblique vessels. *AJR* 1987;**148**:405-409.
32. Feinberg DA, Crooks L, Sheldon P, Hoenninger III J, Watts J, Arakawa M. Magnetic resonance imaging the velocity vector components of fluid flow. *Magn Reson Med* 1985;**2**:555-566.
33. Henning J, Muri M, Brunner P, Friedburg H. Quantitative flow measurement with the fast Fourier flow technique. *Radiology* 1988;**166**:237-240.
34. Dumoulin CL, Hart HR. Magnetic resonance angiography. *Radiology* 1986;**161**:717-720.
35. Walker MF, Souza SP, Dumoulin CL. Quantitative flow measurement in phase contrast angiography. *J Comput Assist Tomogr* 1988;**12**:304-313.
36. Tamada T, Moriyasu F, Ono S, et al. Portal blood flow: measurement with MR imaging. *Radiology* 1989;**173**:639-644.
37. Matsuda T, Shimizu K, Sakurai T, et al. Measurement of aortic blood flow with MR imaging: comparative study with Doppler US. *Radiology* 1987;**162**:857-861.
38. Edelman RR, Zhao B, Liu C, Wentz K, Mattle HP, Finn JP, McArdle C. MR angiography and dynamic flow evaluation of the portal venous system. *AJR* 1989;**153**:755-760.
39. Kraft KA, Fatouros PP, Fei DY, Rittgers SE, Kishore PRS. MR imaging of model fluid velocity profiles. *Magn Reson Imaging* 1989;**7**:69-77.
40. Martin AJ, Drake JM, Lemaire C, Henkelman RM. Cerebrospinal fluid shunts: flow measurements with MR imaging. *Radiology* 1989;**173**:243-247.
41. Maier SE, Meier D, Boesiger P, Moser UT, Vieli A. Human abdominal aorta: comparative measurements of blood flow with MR imaging and multigated Doppler US. *Radiology* 1989;**171**:487-492.
42. Kondo C, Caputo GR, Semelka R, Foster E, Shimakawa A, Higgins CB. Right and left ventricular stroke volume measurements with velocity encoded cine MR: in vivo and in vitro validation. *Circulation* 1990 (submitted).
43. Firmin DN, Nayler GL, Klipstein RH, Urnderwood SR, Rees RSO, Longmore DB. In vivo validation of MR velocity imaging. *J Comput Assist Tomogr* 1987;**11**:751-756.
44. Meier D, Maier S, Bosiger P. Quantitative flow measurements on phantoms and on blood vessels with MR. *Magn Reson Med* 1988;**8**:25-34.
45. Underwood SR, Filmin DN, Klipstein RH, Rees RSO, Longmore DB. Magnetic resonance velocity mapping: clinical application of a new technique. *Br Heart J* 1987;**57**:404-412.
46. Bogren HG, Klipstein RH, Mohiaddin RH, Firmin DN, Underwood SR, Rees RSO, Longmore DB. Pulmonary artery distensibility and blood flow patterns: a magnetic resonance study of normal subjects and of patients with pulmonary arterial hypertension. *Am Heart J* 1989;**118**:990-999.
47. Bogren HG, Mohiaddin RH, Klipstein RH, Firmin DN, Underwood SR, Rees RSO, Longmore DB. The function of the aorta in ischemic heart diseasc: a magnetic resonance and angiographic study of aortic compliance and blood flow pattems. *Am Heart J* 1989;**118**:234-247.

48. Karvonen J, Ahonen A, Kari-Koskinen O, Koskinen M, Timisjarvi J, Hirvonen L. Determination of reference values for regional lung ventilation and perfusion. In Hutas I, Debreczeni LA (eds). *Advances in Physiological Sciences Vol. 10 Respiration.* Pergamon Press 1981.

Coronary interventional procedures

Udo Sechtem, Julius Michael Curtius and Hans-Wilhelm Höpp
University of Cologne, Cologne, Germany

Introduction

Since the first procedure performed by Gruentzig in 1977 [1], percutaneous transluminal balloon coronary angioplasty (PTCA) has developed into very effective treatment modality for coronary artery disease. Advances in catheter technology and increased operator experience now permit successful balloon dilatation in more than 90% of lesions [2,3] despite application of the technique to increasingly complex anatomic situations. Today, PTCA is routinely applied in many centres for distal coronary disease, stenoses in multiple vessels [4,5], bifurcation lesions [6], total occlusions [7], and stenosed bypass grafts [8,9]. In contrast to established anatomic indications, the use of PTCA is more controversial in some clinical situations. One major topic is the optimal integration of thrombolytic therapy and angioplasty in patients with acute myocardial infarction. Another recently debated issue is the application of PTCA to patients with clinical features that make bypass surgery an unacceptable form of treatment. Both questions are discussed in the first part of this chapter.

Despite the progress made over the last decade, balloon angioplasty still suffers from some limitations. Abrupt closure, often requiring emergency bypass surgery, occurs in 3 - 5% of cases even in the hands of experienced operators [2,10]. Complex stenoses such as those with calcification, eccentricity or lengths of more than 10 mm have lower success rates and higher complication rates [11]. Total occlusions are difficult to recanalize and keep patent, especially those older than 3 months [12]. Finally, restenosis occurs in about one-third of dilated segments and this rate seems resistant to all pharmacological attempts at improvement [13]. A multitude of new interventional techniques has been developed to overcome these shortcomings of balloon angioplasty. Despite the initial enthusiasm for these new tools, all of them have to be judged against the current gold standard of interventional cardiology before being accepted as clinically useful. Therefore, these procedures have to either increase the primary success rates of balloon angioplasty, eliminate or help manage complications, or reduce restenosis. Hence, the second part of this chapter will give an overview of new catheter-based treatment modalities such as stents, lasers and atherectomy devices and put their advantages and disadvantages into perspective. Finally, the potential of imaging techniques such as angioscopy and intravascular ultrasound will be discussed.

Balloon Angioplasty in Acute Myocardial Infarction

Different goals may be achieved by application of PTCA in the setting of acute myocardial infarction [14]:

1. It may be used to directly recanalize the infarct-related artery without prior thrombolytic therapy (direct PTCA).
2. During urgent angiography after thrombolytic therapy, immediate PTCA is directed towards treatment of the underlying stenoses.
3. Rescue PTCA is used for recanalization of vessels persistently occluded despite thrombolytic therapy.
4. PTCA directed at prophylaxis of recurrent ischaemia may be deferred for several days to allow for stabilization of arterial injury (deferred PTCA).
5. PTCA is termed elective if performed more than 1 week after the index event with the intention of treating angina or provocable ischaemia.

Direct PTCA

Direct PTCA may be used as an alterative to thrombolytic therapy in centres with extensive operator expertise and permanently accessible catheterization laboratories. Hartzler et al, were the first to use PTCA without prior thrombolytic therapy as the primary tool to restore coronary artery flow in patients with acute myocardial infarcts [15]. This approach has been shown to result in a high rate (94%) of successful dilatation of the infarct vessel in a follow-up report in 500 patients from this institution [16]. Their results have been confirmed in other studies of direct PTCA, where patency rates of 78 - 95%, depending on the definition of success [17], were reported [17-20]. Despite the fact that patients, who would not have fulfilled the entry criteria for thrombolytic trials, were included in this study, in-hospital mortality was only 7.2% [16]. When rigorous exclusion criteria were applied to patients (no prior bypass surgery, no cardiogenic shock, no presentation > 4 hours after onset of chest pain) mortality was only 1.8% compared to 4 - 7% in recent intravenous thrombolytic trials [21-23]. Positive long-term effects of direct angioplasty in acute myocardial infarction include a low late mortality of 2 - 5% for hospital survivors [16,18,24].

Patients presenting with haemodynamic instability can be successfully treated with direct PTCA. Haemodynamic improvement is most pronounced in patients with low ejection fractions who carry a high risk of postinfarction morbidity and mortality [16]. Immediate recanalization in cardiogenic shock reduced mortality from the traditional 80% range to 40% in small series [16,25,26], whereas previous studies with thrombolytic agents failed to demonstrate a benefit for such patients [27,23].

There are several other advantages of direct angioplasty in the treatment of acute myocardial infarction. The substantial group of patients [23] who would not receive thrombolytic therapy under contraindications (Table 1) for current thrombolytic trials could nevertheless benefit from restoration of vessel patency. The incidence of bleeding complications including intraplaque and intramyocardial haemorrhage, which are frequent (15 - 29%) in patients with combined treatment of thrombolysis and PTCA [29], is markedly reduced [16]. Intracranial haemorrhage, which occurs in 0.5 - 1.9% of patients treated with thrombolytic agents [23,28,30-32], is uncommon with direct PTCA [16].

On the other hand, there are also important drawbacks to direct angioplasty in acute myocardial infarction. It is impractical because it requires the availability of experienced operators on a 24 hour basis as well as immediately available catheterization laboratories. The time delay, which occurs, if the catheterization laboratory is not immediately available because of an ongoing procedure in another patient, often results in longer time delays in restoring coronary flow for direct PTCA compared to intravenous thrombolysis. The reocclusion rate after successful reperfusion by direct PTCA is still 15% [16] which is similar to reocclusion rates reported after thrombolytic therapy with streptokinase [33]. High grade stenoses at immediate angiography, probably caused by residual thrombus, have been shown to undergo further lysis within the next days such that approximately 15% of the infarct population have minimal lesions (< 60% diameter stenosis) at repeat catheterization [21,23]. These patients would probably not profit from urgent revascularization, which would merely consist of compression of thrombotic material and inflict additional injury to the vessel wall with potentially adverse long-term effects [34].

Table 1. *Exclusion criteria for intravenous thrombolytic therapy in acute myocardial infarction [21,42,60]*

Absolute contra-indications	Active bleeding
	Bleeding diatheses
Relative contra-indications	Age > 75 years
	Uncontrolled hypertension after treatment of pain (blood pressure > 180/110 mmHg)
	Stroke or transient ischaemic attack within 6 months
	Recent prolonged resuscitation
	Surgery within 14 days

Although it may be the treatment of choice in patients with severe left ventricular dysfunction or cardiogenic shock, where even minimal functional recovery may be of value, and in patients who have contraindications for intravenous thrombolytic therapy, PTCA as the primary and sole means of reperfusion is not realistically available for most patients with acute myocardial infarction. Furthermore, despite the excellent results from the Hartzler group [16,35,36], concern remains that additional injury inflicted by mechanical interaction upon an already unstable vessel wall might be detrimental to overall outcome as suggested by several trials of immediate PTCA after chemical thrombolysis (see below). A randomized trial addressing this question is clearly warranted.

Immediate versus Deferred PTCA

The concept of immediate angiography and PTCA is based on the observation that although intravenous thrombolysis decreases mortality in patients with acute myocardial infarction as compared to conventional treatment [23,30,37-39], the incidence of reinfarction and postinfarction angina is higher [23,31,40]. Because high grade stenoses remain in a high proportion of patients after successful thrombolysis [41], immediate removal of the obstruction by angioplasty might decrease reocclusion, improve regional blood flow, and enhance recovery of the injured myocardium. Furthermore, early visualization of the infarct-related artery affords the opportunity of identifying those patients whose artery remains occluded after thrombolysis and attempt mechanical recanalization.

Three large randomized trials [21,22,42] recently addressed the question whether immediate PTCA after thrombolysis, carried out in all patients with suitable coronary anatomy (no severe multivessel disease, no left main stenosis, no minimal lesions < 50% [21]), was a superior concept in the treatment of acute myocardial infarction as compared to the more conservative strategy of deferred PTCA (Table 2). The astonishing conclusion reached unanimously by all three studies was that coronary angiography and PTCA performed within the early hours of myocardial infarction, either during or immediately after thrombolytic therapy, offer no added benefit and may even be harmful as compared with PTCA performed with a delay of 18 hours to several days.

Mortality was lower in the groups with delayed or no PTCA (1% TAMI 1,6% TIMI IIA, 3% European Study) than in the immediate group (4%,7%,7%). Notably, the difference in mortality was lower in the TIMI IIA trial in which the delayed group underwent angiography rather early after the event. The other end point, global left ventricular function at discharge, was not significantly different between the immediate angioplasty and the other group in any of the studies. Hospital course was more complicated in the immediate PTCA group and bleeding complications were higher (19.5% vs. 7.2% in TIMI IIA). For a more detailed discussion of these studies, the reader is referred to recent reviews of this topic [14,43,44]. One-year follow-up from patients enrolled in the TAMI I trial [45] demonstrates a very low postdischarge mortality (1.9%) and combined rate of death or non-fatal myocardial infarction (6%) for the entire cohort. The group with delayed PTCA at 7 - 10 days after the infarct had more nonfatal myocardial infarctions and cardiac hospitalizations than the immediate PTCA group, but these differences were small and not statistically significant. One year follow-up from the TIMI phase II pilot study confirms the relative paucity of deaths and recurrent myocardial infarctions occurring between 6 weeks and 1 year after thrombolysis and early PTCA [46]. Long-term follow-up from TIMI II and the European study group is not yet available.

Table 2. *Therapeutic options in trials for thrombolysis and PTCA in acute myocardial infarction*

Study	Cardiac Catheterization	PTCA
TAMI [21]	Immediate	Immediate vs. 7 days
TIMI IIA [42]	Immediate vs. 18 - 48 hours	Immediate vs. 18 - 48 hours
ECSG [22]	Immediate vs. before discharge	Immediate vs. none
TIMI [23]	18 - 48 hours vs. only in patients with ischaemia	18 - 48 hours vs. only in patients with ischaemia

Adapted from ref. 43 with permission

Immediate PTCA therefore appears unnecessary or even potentially detrimental in patients during or after intravenous thrombolysis with rt-PA for acute myocardial infarction. The unexpectedly negative outcomes may be explained by the 'sick artery concept' [14], which implies that an artery with a ruptured plaque, platelet aggregation, and residual thrombus after fibrinolytic treatment is not likely to tolerate further injury inflicted by PTCA without adverse reactions. This concept also suggests that immediate PTCA is not a valid concept after thrombolysis with other agents than rt-PA. Deferral seems to be a better setting for PTCA, possibly due to some healing of the initial endothelial damage.

Deferred PTCA versus Elective PTCA

The assumption inherent in the approach of immediate or deferred angioplasty is that the frequency of recurrent ischaemic events can be reduced in patients with residual high grade stenoses, who have been shown to be at high risk for reocclusion after thrombolysis with streptokinase [41,47-50]. In contrast, recurrent ischaemic events after thrombolysis with rt-PA, which are even more frequent than after thrombolysis using streptokinase, cannot be predicted by quantitative and morphological assessment at the time of urgent angiography [51]. This inability to identify on the basis of early clinical or angiographic findings which patients might benefit from immediate or delayed revascularization provides one important rationale for a conservative approach.

Consequently, the TIMI II study [23] compared early deferred angioplasty within 18 - 48 hours to the more conservative strategy of elective catheterization and PTCA only in patients with spontaneous recurrent ischaemia during hospitalization or demonstration of ischaemia on predischarge submaximal exercise testing. In this trial, deferred prophylactic PTCA did not offer an advantage in terms of reduction in mortality (5.2% deferred vs. 4.7% elective PTCA) or nonfatal reinfarction (5.9% deferred vs. 5.4% elective PTCA) over the more conservative strategy of diagnostic and mechanical intervention only when clinically indicated. This observation has been corroborated by another randomized trial which compared late prophylactic PTCA 5 days after thrombolytic therapy to angiography and PTCA only for documented ischaemia [52]. Thus, cardiac catheterization does not seem necessary for the majority of patients treated with thrombolytic therapy for acute myocardial infarction, except for those with recurrent ischaemia or exercise-induced ischaemia. A possible exception might be for those patients with particularly high post-discharge mortality with medical therapy [53] such as those in Killip class III or IV [54], previous infarction, the elderly [33,55], and those with ST depression infarction [44].

The long-term follow-up of TIMI II and other studies has to be awaited before final conclusions can be made regarding the management of patients after thrombolytic therapy for acute myocardial infarction. The question is still whether the conservative strategy which yields similar short-term results as the early PTCA approach will produce the same excellent long-term results reported after aggressive reperfusion strategies. Postdischarge mortality and reinfarction rates (Table 3) following these aggressive reperfusion schemes are considerably lower than those reported for patients with thrombolytic therapy alone [53] or for patients from the prethrombolysis era [56,57]. In addition, rates of excellent functional status and return to work [53] suggest that costs of such strategy may in part be offset by improved outcome beyond survival benefits. A word of caution is necessary as regards the comparison with historical controls. Since the older studies were reported, significant changes have occurred in adjunctive therapy, particularly the routine use of aspirin and beta-adrenergic-blocking agents. These factors alone may have favourably altered prognosis of the relatively young and previously healthy patients included in the aggressive reperfusion studies independent of reperfusion strategy.

Rescue PTCA

Despite successful reperfusion after intravenous thrombolytic therapy in the majority of patients, recanalization will not be achieved in at least 10% - 15% of eligible patients [21,27,42,59-62]. Many studies have demonstrated that a patent infarct-related artery is a major determinant of early and late survival [63,64] and failure to achieve this goal is associated with adverse outcome [17,24,65]. Consequently, this group of patients with 'resistance' [66] to thrombolysis, might benefit from a strategy of emergency coronary angioplasty as a fallback means of achieving vessel patency.

Indeed, rescue PTCA results in significant myocardial salvage and improvement of outcome when thrombolytic therapy failed [24,65, 67,68]. The largest series of 192 patients with failed thrombolysis and coronary anatomy suitable for rescue PTCA was recently reported from the TAMI studies [69]. Successful mechanical recanalization was achieved in 88%. Compared to patients with successful chemical thrombolysis, in-hospital mortality was similar (4.6% vs. 5.9% rescue PTCA group). However, reocclusion was more frequent in the angioplasty patency group. A major impact on mortality by rescue angioplasty is suggested by the high mortality rate in patients with failed rescue angioplasty as compared to patients in whom the procedure was successful (39.1% vs. 5.9%). A strong argument for

Table 3. *Postdischarge mortality and reinfarction rates in trials using aggressive mechanical strategies in comparison with thrombolysis alone (GISSI) and prethrombolysis era figures (MPRG)*

Study	Patients included	In-hospital mortality	Postdischarge mortality at 1 year	Postdischarge myocardial infarction at 1 year	Postdischarge death or myocardial infarction
TAMI I [45]	386	7.0%	1.9%	4.0%	6.0%
TIMI IIA [46]	288	5.2% (6 wk)	3.5%	2.2%	4.5%
Stack [24]	342	11.0%	2.0%	4.0%	6.0%
Rothbaum [18]	151	8.6%	2.2%	2.9%	not reported
Holmes [68]	63	3.0%	1.6%	6.3%	not reported
O'Keefe [16]	500	7.2%	5.0%	3.0%	16.0%*
GISSI [53]	4865	10.7%	7.2%	3.6%**	not reported
MPRG [56,57]	866	not available	9.0%	9.0%	not reported

* = survival without recurrent myocardial infarction or bypass surgery
** = reinfarction rates at 6 months

early identification of thrombolysis failure and institution of rescue angioplasty comes from the fact that patients discharged from the hospital with thrombolysis patency or angioplasty patency have similar rates of mortality, non-fatal myocardial infarction, additional revascularization procedures or subsequent hospitalization, although baseline ejection fraction was lower in the angioplasty patency group. The increased reocclusion rate after rescue angioplasty, which was not observed in patients scheduled for immediate angioplasty after successful thrombolysis with rt-PA [21] may have several explanations. Apart from more extensive vessel wall damage [70] and possibly different thrombus composition [71] seen in patients refractory to chemical thrombolysis, the delay to reperfusion caused by the study design [69] could lead to more extensive myocardial necrosis and oedema inhibiting coronary flow.

The strategy of rescue angioplasty is limited by the difficulty of non-invasive assessment of the perfusion status of the infarct-related artery [72] after thrombolysis. In the TAMI trials, assessment of chest pain and ST segment changes was unreliable for prediction of perfusion or reperfusion TAMI (Table 4). Reperfusion arrhythmias were also not predictive of reperfusion status. Therefore, measures that improve the ability to detect successful lysis are urgently needed.

At present, immediate angiography remains the only reliable means of early identification of persistently occluded infarct-related arteries. However, angiography during the lytic state is fraught (13% - 47%) with bleeding complications [21,73-76] which would mainly occur in the majority of patients who would not benefit from this diagnostic procedure. Moreover, the practical problem of limited financial and manpower resources associated with direct angioplasty also applies for urgent catheterization. Holmes and Topol [43] warned before the escalation of therapeutic interventions which they called 'reperfusion momentum'. The 'oculostenotic reflex' [14] to aggressively treat stenoses demonstrated at early coronary angiography in patients with patent infarct-related arteries may lead to unwarranted concern of the treating physician resulting in overuse of angioplasty, for instance for some lesions which consist mainly of thrombus and would have undergone spontaneous lysis anyhow [21].

The excessive mortality after failed rescue angioplasty [17,25,65, 69] may have several explanations. The invasive procedure itself causes additional stress, hypotension and negative inotropic influence related to contrast agents, anaemia to bleeding and other complications. Rescue angioplasty of the right coronary artery is associated with a high rate of complications and a high mortality [77]. Thereforc, caution is advised in applying rescue PTCA to patients with uncomplicated inferior wall infarction. With so many pros and cons, only further randomized trials will be able to determine the ultimate role of rescue angioplasty in acute myocardial infarction.

Table 4. *Efficacy of simple clinical measurements to predict perfusion status of infarct-related artery after thrombolysis*

	Percentage of study group (n = 386)	Patent infarct artery in % of subgroup
Chest pain		
Unchanged	20%	60%
Improved	51%	71%
Completely resolved	29%	84%
ST elevation		
Unchanged	56%	63%
Improved	38%	84%
Return to baseline	6%	96%
Arrhythmias		
None	64%	72%
Ventricular tachycardia > 100	6%	67%
Ventricular tachycardia < 100	7%	75%
Ventricular fibrillation	8%	77%
2° atrioventricular block	3%	64%
3° atrioventricular block	5%	74%
Severe sinus bradycardia	16%	72%

Adapted from ref. 72 with permission

The observation that patients with successful rescue angioplasty have a good long-term prognosis despite a decreased ejection fraction at discharge [63] or lack of improvement of ejection fraction by the procedure [63,64] has raised the question of whether restoration of arterial patency has a beneficial effect on survival independent of myocardial salvage. Although this issue is still debated, possible mechanisms include limitation of infarct expansion [78,79] and electrical instability [80,81]. Another question, which relates to this finding but cannot be answered presently, is whether occluded arteries should be recanalized independent of ongoing ischaemia. An argument in favour of attempting to recanalize occluded arteries even 72 hours after onset of symptoms is the experience of Guerci and coworkers [82] who reported substantial improvement in ventricular function in patients with late recanalization.

Conclusions

It has become clear that for most patients treated with thrombolytic therapy for myocardial infarction, cardiac catheterization and balloon angioplasty are not necessary, except for those with recurrent ischaemia or exercise induced ischaemia. Unresolved issues include whether direct angioplasty without thrombolytic therapy, if logistically possible, is superior to thrombolytic therapy followed by a conservative revascularization strategy. Another debated issue is whether the reduction in mortality and morbidity observed after successful rescue angioplasty justifies the side effects and costs of routine immediate angiography in all patients, or at least those without improvement in chest pain or ST-segment changes which would be necessary to identify all patients with occluded infarct-related arteries after intravenous thrombolysis. Finally, more studies are needed to define the interaction of other thrombolytic agents with early mechanical intervention because most of the results discussed above relate to treatment with intravenous tissue plasminogen activator.

Balloon Angioplasty in High Risk Patients

As PTCA is still associated with a risk of acute vessel closure of 3% - 5% [83,10] and the necessity for emergency bypass surgery in approximately 3.5% [83], patients at high risk for the development of haemodynamic instability after acute vessel closure, such as those with poor left ventricular function or a target vessel supplying substantial amounts of myocardium, are usually not considered to be good candidates for PTCA. In the event of abrupt closure, these patients may not survive long enough to undergo bypass surgery. Also, balloon inflation results in ischaemia and compromise of left ventricular function that could last for a period of time after inflation and may be poorly tolerated.

Perfusion catheters

Several techniques are available for augmenting myocardial perfusion during PTCA in high risk patients. Autoperfusion techniques were developed to permit prolonged balloon inflation times to achieve a better PTCA result, or, in the event of abrupt vessel closure, to avoid the need for an extracorporal perfusion pump system [84,85]. The Stack autoperfusion balloon catheter [86,87] has sideholes proximal and distal to the balloon (Fig. 1) and provides adequate distal perfusion such that balloon inflations up to 90 minutes are tolerated without evidence of myocardial necrosis.

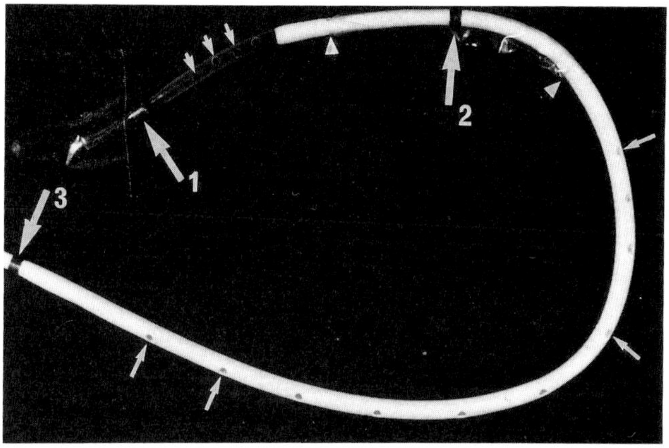

Figure 1. *STACK PERFUSION™ CORONARY DILATION CATHETER (Advanced Cardiovascular Systems, Temecula, CA). Three rings marks the tip (arrow 1), the middle of the balloon (arrow 2), and the end of proximal side holes (arrow 3). There are 10 proximal (small arrows) and four distal side holes. The proximal and distal ends of the balloon are marked by arrowheads. When the balloon is inflated, perfusion can take place through the sideholes and the central lumen of the catheter as long as aortic pressure is of sufficient magnitude.*

Another Stack catheter [88], the so called bail-out reperfusion catheter, has 36 side holes arranged in a spiral pattern over the distal 10 cm of the catheter to provide distal perfusion in the setting of abrupt vessel closure during PTCA. With repeated flushing of the catheter at short intervals thrombotic occlusion of the catheter is uncommon [89].

Despite good results with the reperfusion catheter up to 90 minutes [89], small areas of myocardial necrosis developed after 6 hour occlusions in a canine preparation, despite the use of the perfusion catheter [90]. Although the time span for which the perfusion catheter may be safely left in place has not been determined in humans, these data suggest that the use of the autoperfusion catheter does not substitute for prompt surgical standby in the case of abrupt vessel closure. Moreover, in patients with extensive intracoronary thrombosis before insertion of the reperfusion catheter, maintenance of adequate flow may be impossible despite successful placement of catheter [38]. Another current problem is the stiffness of the distal portion of the catheter and the rather large profile which make it difficult to position the catheter across high grade stenoses or through tortuous proximal vessels.

However, in haemodynamically stable patients without extensive intracoronary thrombosis, the autoperfusion catheter with or without balloon seems to be useful as an adjunctive modality in patients who fail PTCA and are awaiting emergency coronary bypass surgery [90]. Time can be bought for the surgeon, especially in patients where prolonged exposure of the heart can be expected, such as in previous thoracotomy or chest radiation, or to permit preparation of the internal mammary artery. The use of the autoperfusion catheter is problematic in patients with severe haemodynamic compromise where this passive form of arterial perfusion is most likely ineffective due to the low coronary flow. Combination of aortic balloon counterpulsation or cardiopulmonary bypass support with the autoperfusion catheter may be a solution under these circumstances.

Intra-aortic Balloon Counter Pulsation

Several interventions have been proposed to support the circulation during the procedure and make PTCA a safe undertaking even in these high-risk patients. Prophylactic intra-aortic balloon pumping was the first technique proposed [91]. The experience of several groups in high risk patients with ejection fractions of less than 25% suggests that even multivessel dilatation can be successfully performed with improved ischaemic tolerance [92,93]. The main complication is vascular injury associated with percutaneous placement of the balloon requiring surgical intervention.

Cardiopulmonary Bypass Support

The idea of using prophylactic cardiopulmonary bypass in these patients developed after the initial success of PTCA performed in the operating theatre on cardiopulmonary bypass [94]. This technique, termed 'supported angioplasty', was introduced by Vogel and coworkers [95], who initially placed the cannulas using local cut-down. The insertion technique employed more recently consists of percutaneous placement of a 20 Fr arterial cannula in the iliac artery after angiographic evaluation of iliofemoral anatomy and another 20 Fr multihole venous cannula at the junction of the inferior vena cava and the right atrium [96]. A portable cardiopulmonary support system (CR Bard) using a centrifugal, non-occlusive pump, a polypropylene hollow fibre membrane oxygenator and a water-based heat exchanger actively aspirates blood from the right atrium and thus provides flow rates of 2 to 6 l/min. Cardiopulmonary support is initiated before instrumentation of the coronaries and adjusted to provide adequate blood pressure and peripheral perfusion during balloon inflation and to reduce diastolic pulmonary artery pressure below approximately 5 mmHg [96]. The technique was reported to be useful in a group of 100 high risk patients [95] who tolerated balloon inflation times of up to 10 minutes [96] without evidence of myocardial injury.

Complications at the femoral insertion site with blood loss requiring transfusion initially occurred in almost half the patients [95,96]. With further experience and increasing use of 'standby support' [95] by inserting smaller cannulas which may then be rapidly exchanged and bypass instituted in case of haemodynamic collapse [97], morbidity has considerably declined to less than 20% [98]. The mortality of 3 - 4% associated with the procedure in this group of patients which is mainly related to late vessel closure, has remained constant [98]. Long term follow-up revealed excellent relief of symptoms in 87% of patients surviving for more than 1 year (82%) [96].

Although maintenance of mentation and peripheral perfusion are well preserved on cardiopulmonary support, myocardial ischaemia [99] and possibly myocardial infarction, may occur during PTCA because direct myocardial perfusion is not provided by the device. Hence, a difficult situation can be envisaged in which termination of bypass after PTCA will not be feasible in a conscious patient because of left ventricular dysfunction. Other groups studying patients who fulfilled entry criteria for the National Registry for elective high risk cardiopulmonary bypass supported by PTCA but underwent the procedure without bypass support, reported similar clinical and angiographic success rates with significantly lower mortality and morbidity [100]. Therefore, the clinical role of supported PTCA has still to be demonstrated in a randomized trial and should presently be restricted to the few centres developing the technique.

Other systemic support approaches include transaortic valve turbine pumping [101,102] and percutaneous left ventricular assist devices [103]. Experience with both techniques is still at the experimental level. The transaortic haemopump device cannot yet be inserted percutaneously and left atrial-left femoral bypass requires transseptal puncture with its associated risks.

Coronary Sinus Retroperfusion

Myocardial salvage during ischaemic conditions can be achieved by retrograde perfusion of the myocardium through the coronary sinus [104]. Both passive and active retrograde perfusion using pressure-controlled synchronized intermittent occlusion of the coronary sinus and synchronized retroperfusion of arterial blood respectively, have been shown to reduce infarct size after LAD occlusion in a canine model [105]. The best results were achieved, however, by combining both techniques [105].

The technique of retroperfusion during PTCA requires placement of a catheter with a gas-inflated balloon within the distal great cardiac vein. The synchronized pump is timed to the electrocardiogram and is R-wave triggered. The coronary sinus balloon is inflated by an electropneumatic inflation device. Arterial blood from the opposite femoral artery is pumped into the coronary sinus during diastolic balloon occlusion [105,106]. Initial results from a randomized multi-centre trial evaluating the safety and efficacy of synchronized retroperfusion during angioplasty of the left anterior descending branch (LAD) demonstrated that there were slight reductions in the occurrence of chest pain and slight increases in the time to onset of pain [106]. ST-segment changes occurred slightly less often and were slightly less pronounced in retroperfusion-treated inflations than in untreated control inflations. Although synchronized retroperfusion seems to have promise for improving or delaying the ischaemic response during LAD angioplasty, it is clear that the technique is not effective in all patients and that the ischaemic response is not totally abolished. Importantly, only one case report exists on PTCA and retroperfusion in high risk patients [107] and patients with cardiogenic shock were excluded from the multicentre trial.

Comparison of perfusion techniques do not yet exist in humans. However, animal data demonstrate that catheter autoperfusion leads to a substantially greater degree of myocardial salvage (70% vs. 34% of area at risk) than coronary sinus retroperfusion in identical canine experimental preparations [90,108].

Conclusions

PTCA seems to be relatively safe even in high risk patients and requires intra-aortic balloon pumping or cardiopulmonary bypass support, the apparently most effective technique of circulatory support, only in a minority of patients. The intra-aortic balloon pump has to be used prophylactically or therapeutically in less than 10% of patients with an ejection fraction < 40% [92]. Hence, unprotected PTCA works without an excess of complications even in high risk patients. On the other hand, it has to be remembered that even prophylactic use of the balloon pump cannot guarantee good results or replace good judgement, technique and careful patient selection. Careful review of patients considered for supported coronary angioplasty by surgical colleagues is essential for optimal selection of surgical revascularization or catheter revascularization and surgical standby. If the prophylactic use of support devices is considered to be necessary, stand-by support seems most appropriate, because both devices may be inserted within a few minutes in the case of haemodynamic instability. The autoperfusion catheter, although somewhat difficult to handle in its present design, improves distal coronary perfusion and may offer additional benefit in the case of acute vessel occlusion.

Intracoronary Stents

Acute occlusion of a coronary artery during PTCA is a significant limitation of the procedure, despite improvements in equipment and increased experience of operators. Acute occlusion is usually caused by dissection [109] with secondary thrombosis. Spasm as the sole cause of occlusion is rare and accounts for less than 5% of acute occlusions [110]. After application of intracoronary vasodilators, treatment in haemodynamically stable patients consists of repeat balloon inflations [111] and, if this measure cannot permanently reopen the artery, long inflations with low inflation pressure and a slightly oversized balloon [112] or a perfusion balloon catheter [113] (see above) may be helpful. Although repeat PTCA is successful in between 50% and 85% [11,111,114-118], a significant minority of 10% [118] to 55% [11] of patients has to undergo emergency bypass grafting and Q-wave infarcts develop in up to 56% [111,119] of these patients.

Restenosis is another important problem associated with PTCA. The incidence of restenosis remains between 25% and 35% [13] and does not seem to be improved by a wide variety of medical interventions. Restenosis can be viewed as a response to localized injury with accumulation of platelets immediately following angioplasty and resulting production of growth factors, which cause proliferation of smooth muscle cells [120]. Coronary morphological and procedural factors for an increased risk of restenosis are listed in Table 5. Aortocoronary venous grafts are especially prone to restenosis with rates above 50%, mainly at the proximal anastomosis and proximal graft shaft [121].

Stents were originally introduced for prevention of restenosis in peripheral arteries [122]. In the coronary arteries, several stent designs (Table 6) have been used to tack up the dissecting membrane and seal off the subintimal space in patients with abrupt coronary occlusion after PTCA and to prevent restenosis after PTCA in native coronary vessels and within aortocoronary bypass grafts. Several authors [123-125] recently reviewed coronary stent designs and initial experimental and clinical results.

Stent design has to permit rapid, precise, and safe deployment of the device into the often tortuous and dissected coronary vessels. Therefore, flexibility, tractability and profile of the stent are important. On the other hand, the stent has to maintain a relatively stable, non-flexing surface on which endothelial cells and neointima can grow most efficiently. Biocompatibility is of great concern, i.e. thrombogenicity and the potential to stimulate neointimal proliferation. Thrombogenicity, which is inherent to all metal surfaces, seems to be least pronounced with stainless steel and may further be reduced by polymer coating [126,127].

Table 5. *Morphological and procedural risk factors for development of restenosis*

Morphological	Total occlusions Lesion severity LAD lesions Proximal lesions Bifurcation lesions Length > 10 - 15 mm Calcified lesions Eccentric lesions Diffusely diseased vessels Saphenous vein grafts
Procedural	Severity of residual stenosis Absence of localized intimal tear Large dissection

Reproduced from ref. 13 with permission

Table 6. *Characteristics of coronary stents currently available for human investigation*

	Composition	Deployment	Length (mm)
Wallstent	0.08 mm stainless steel filaments	PTCA balloon/ self-expanding	15 to 23
Palmaz design	0.015 mm stainless steel filaments	PTCA balloon-expandable	15
Gianturco design	0.015 mm stainless steel filaments	PTCA balloon-expandable	20

Reproduced from ref. 124 with permission

Medinvent Wallstent

The selfexpandable Medinvent stent (Fig. 2) is flexible along its long axis and fully expanded has a diameter of between 2.5 and 6 mm. A stent diameter 0.5 mm larger than the reference diameter of the stenosed vessel is recommended [128]. The stent can be positioned within the coronary arteries through standard 8F or 9F guiding catheters.

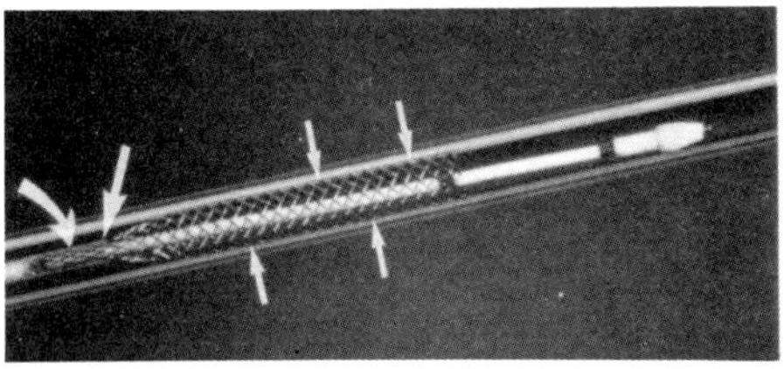

Figure 2. *THE SELF-EXPANDING MEDINVENT WALLSTENT DURING DEPLOYMENT. After retainment of the membrane (arrow on tip of membrane), the compressed stent (curved arrow) is liberated and exerts pressure against the vessel wall (small arrows). With permission from U. Sigwart, 1990. The self-expanding mesh stent. In: Topol EJ, (ed). Textbook of interventional cardiology, p 609. Philadelphia: W. B. Saunders.*

The thicker filaments of the wallstent increasing its thrombogenicity may be one reason for a rather high number of early stent occlusions [128-130]. However, the anticoagulation regimen, which nowadays consists of pretreatment with aspirin (325 mg) and dipyridamole (20 mg/day) to be continued for 6 months and additional anticoagulation with warfarin for 3 months for all stent types clinically used today, evolved throughout this early series and was initially handled less stringently [123].

When used for tacking down the dissection flap in patients with acute occlusions during PTCA, the wallstent was successful in all 25 attempted cases [131,132]. Complications consisted of mural thrombosis immediately after implantation requiring local thrombolytic treatment, side branch occlusion possibly caused by embolization of material during the repeated balloon inflations, and late occlusion requiring repeated balloon angioplasty or resulting in myocardial infarction.

In aortocoronary bypass grafts, implantation of the wallstent after successful PTCA or even before PTCA was attempted in grafts of poor quality and brittle appearance and was technically successful in all grafts [131,133]. The restenosis rate of 38% in the small series of patients reported up to [133] now is, however, similar to the high restenosis rate observed after balloon angioplasty alone.

Recent data illustrate the effect of Medinvent stent placement for prevention of restenosis [128,134]. Fibro-intimal hyperplasia lead to marked diffuse narrowing of stented arterial segments at 7 months of follow-up [128]. Using a stenosis diameter of > 50% as the definition for restenosis, restenosis was found in 14% of patients with open stents. However, stent occlusions occurred in 25% of those with angiographic follow-up [128]. Therefore, this stent type does not improve restenosis rates and is fraught with a high rate of acute and subacute occlusions.

Gianturco Stent

The coil stent (Fig. 3) has a flexible structure and the necessary cold deforming structural properties for balloon expandability and structural integrity [125]. Unlike the Medinvent and Palmaz-Schatz stents, this stent does not shorten when expanded. Up to now, the stent has mainly been used at a single centre and data are scarce. Treatment of acute vessel closure after PTCA has been satisfactorily accomplished in a small number of patients [135], but restenosis has occurred in a significant percentage of patients [136]. Therefore, further development of this stent will include a change of material from stainless steel to tantalum and the bonding of pharmacological agents such as anticoagulants or specific antimitotic agents to decrease the incidence of thrombosis and restenosis.

Palmaz Stent

Of all stent types, this rigid stent, originally described by Palmaz in 1985 [137], has been most extensively used clinically. Initially, its construction (Fig. 4) confined its use to straight proximal segments of the coronary arteries. More recently, a modified version (Fig. 4) consisting of two shorter rigid segments (7 mm each) joined by a flexible bridge (1 mm) has improved the implantability of the device, although difficulties in placement still exist [138]. A new sheathed F5 delivery system [139] seems to reduce problems such as proximal deployment and embolization, which occurred in approximately 5%

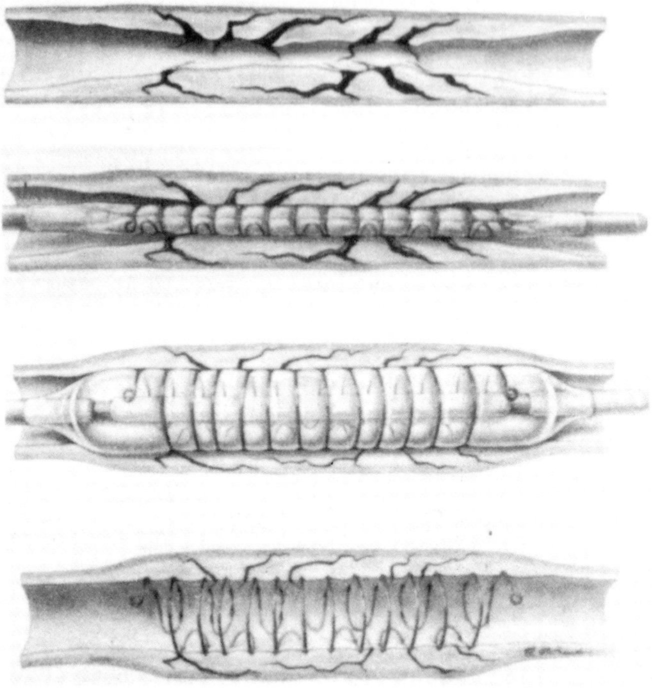

Figure 3. *DIAGRAMMATIC REPRESENTATION OF COIL STENT BEING BALLOON-DILATED IN DISSECTED CORONARY ARTERY. Top: several cracks are visible within the intima and media after previous balloon angioplasty. The three panels below show positioning of another balloon mounted with the stent, inflation and final result after withdrawal of the catheter. With permission from G.S. Roubin et al. Intracoronary stenting during percutaneous transluminal coronary angioplasty. Circulation, 1990:81(suppl. IV):92-100.*

of attempted placements and were mainly due to snagging of the stent on the diseased proximal vessel anatomy.

The Palmaz stent has now been used in several hundred patients. A large series from Toulouse reported a success rate of 93.1% in 160 patients who had stents implanted for acute closure (Fig. 5) or restenosis after previous angioplasty [140]. Apart from unsuccessful stent delivery in five of their patients, six patients suffered from major complications such as abrupt closure (n = 5) occurring up to 6 days after stent placement and dissection of the right coronary artery ostium (n = 1). In another series of 37 patients with right coronary

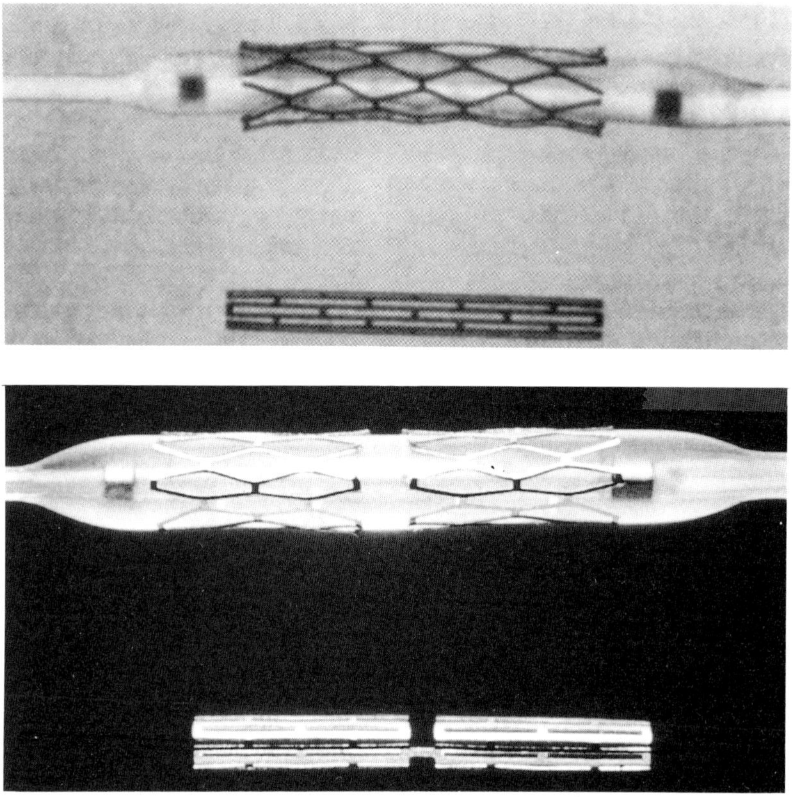

(a)

(b)

Figure 4. *(a) ORIGINAL BALLOON EXPANDABLE PALMAZ STENT (Johnson & Johnson, New Brunswick, New Jersey). (Reprinted with permission from RA Schatz: A view of vascular stents. Circulation 1989;79:445-457). (b): Recent modification to increase flexibility. A small metal bridge links two shorter stent components.*

artery stenoses believed to have a poor short- or long-term prognosis with balloon angioplasty because of prior restenosis or adverse lesion morphology, attempted stent placement was successful in 35 (95%) [141]. Successfully dilated stenoses showed further reduction of stenosis diameter after stenting.

Although acute thrombosis did not occur in this series [141], one patient developed subacute closure of the vessel after self-discontinuation of warfarin. Subacute stent thrombosis within 10 days remains an important problem with stent implantation and may lead to angina, acute myocardial infarction, and death. Subacute thrombotic events

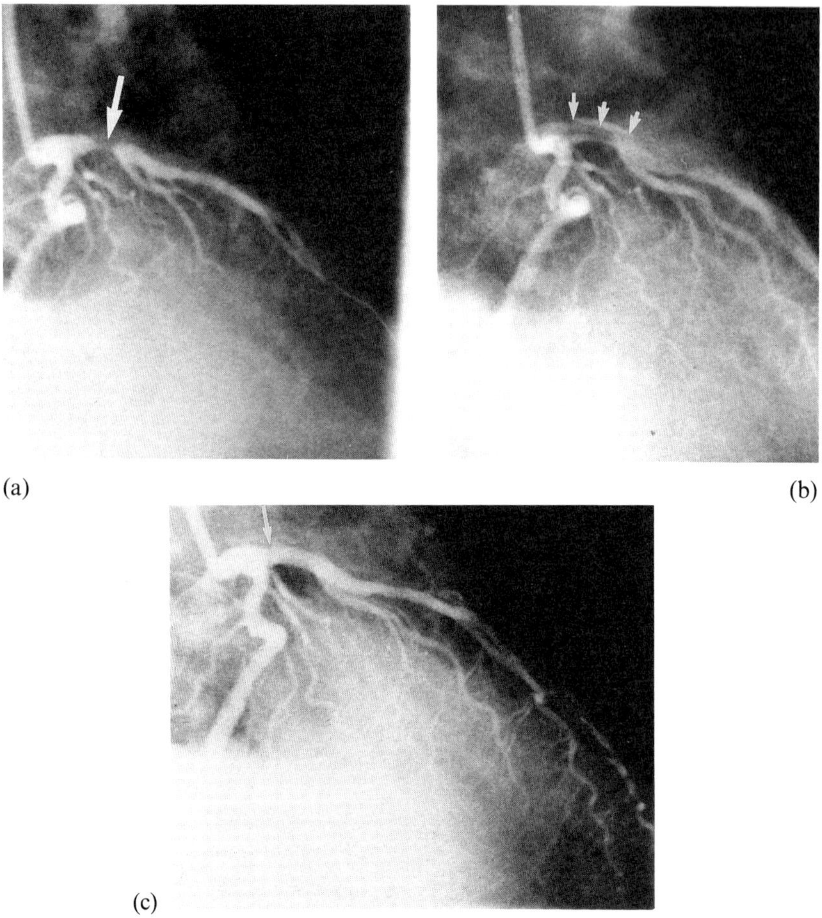

(a) (b) (c)

Figure 5. *(a) Tight LAD stenosis (arrow) before PTCA. (b) After PTCA, a flow limiting dissecting membrane (small arrows) extends into the left main coronary artery. (c) Emergency stenting with a Schatz-Palmaz stent results in a smooth contour of the proximal LAD. A small irregularity is seen at the proximal end of the stent (arrow).*

occurred in 12% of patients not treated with warfarin and 5% of patients fully anticoagulated using the scheme described above [142].

Restenosis rates including reocclusion at 2 - 6 months after placement of Palmaz stents are similar to those observed after simple balloon angioplasty [141,143-145], although a high percentage of patients with prior restenosis were included in the cohort and suboptimal anticoagulation therapy was used in the initial patients.

However, figures for the entire cohorts have to be split into patients with multiple stents and those who received only a single stent. Placement of multiple stents results in increased surface density of metal at the point of overlap and leads to a high risk of restenosis with rates ranging from 57% - 67% [141,146]. In contrast, restenosis rate is only 15% to 17% for single stents [141,146]. Stenting does not seem to delay the temporal course of the restenosis process and progression of restenosis does not occur beyond 6 months following stenting [141,147]. Restenoses can be redilated with a high success rate [141,144] although bypass grafting is frequently used for patient management.

Other Stent Designs

Poor radiopacity of current stent designs, due to the thin stainless steel filaments used to reduce thrombogenicity, currently limits precise positioning and may lead to stent embolization because slippage off the stent may initially go unnoticed. Two types of tantalum stents (Medtronic Wiktor and Cordis Corp.) appear to have improved visibility and good biocompatibility in animal [148] and initial human implantation [149]. However, full anticoagulation for at least 3 months is mandatory because subacute thrombosis occurred in 24% of patients with a less stringent anticoagulation regimen [150].

Nitilol, a thermal memory alloy, is an attractive material for stents because of its ability to re-expand to a predesigned shape at body temperature. This stent has not yet been used in the coronary arteries clinically. Stents made of L-polylactide which are bioabsorbable within 8 months have recently undergone first animal studies. The authors concluded that this stent design was worth further investigation due to good deployability, endothelialization and stent patency [151].

Conclusions

The present role of stents as an adjunct to balloon angioplasty has not yet been fully elucidated. Although it seems clear that acute vessel closure can be successfully managed by stent implantation, the device has shown disappointing overall results in the prevention of restenosis. This may be due to stretching medial smooth muscle cells, stimulating mural thrombosis, or attracting increased numbers of macrophages and monocytes to the stented vessel wall [125]. However, in patients with single stents, there may be trend towards lower restenosis rates. Stents are unique in their capability to serve as a source for locally applied pharmaceuticals designed to prevent restenoses. However, before this vision of the future becomes realistic, the control mechanisms governing the process of restenosis must first be fully understood. Further follow-up is necessary to resolve the question of whether stents will maintain long-term patency after emergency stenting for acute closure. Unless this can be demonstrated, use of a bail-out catheter and emergency bypass grafting may be a safer way of avoiding the sequelae of vessel closure during PTCA.

Laser Angioplasty

The use of laser energy to dissolve coronary atherosclerotic plaque was initially described by Lee and coworkers [152] in 1981. Since then, laser technology has made much progress and several systems are now used in the coronary arteries of living humans.

Laser angioplasty has been expected to improve disappointing conventional PTCA results in three clinical circumstances. Firstly, success rates in the treatment of chronic total occlusions remain in the order of only 50% - 70% [153-155], because it is often impossible with conventional balloon angioplasty to cross the occluded segment with the guide-wire or with the balloon catheter itself after successful guide-wire advancement. Laser angioplasty might be more successful by vaporizing the occluding organized thrombus. Secondly, lasers are expected to debulk lesions by the same mechanism, which might prevent restenosis or at least reduce the high restenosis rates observed after poor primary PTCA results with substantial residual plaque [156]. Thirdly, dilatation of long, diffusely narrowed segments with balloon angioplasty is not optimal and associated with increased complication rates [109].

Technical Considerations

Types of Lasers

Continuous wave lasers were initially used to achieve improved results in the recanalization of occluded peripheral arteries. These lasers remove atherosclerotic plaque [152,157] and other tissue by conversion of solid matter to gas. Laser energy is converted to heat, which rapidly vaporizes water within tissue and leaves a central zone of vaporization surrounded by a zone of charring. Neodymium (Nd):YAG, argon ion, and carbon-dioxide lasers operate by this photothermal mechanism. However, ablation of calcified plaque is not possible due to absence of water.

As the ragged surface created by continuous wave lasers leads to thrombosis and long lasting laser action results in diffusion of thermal energy which may destroy vessel walls and cause perforation, continuous wave lasers were pulsed with pulse durations that limited thermal diffusion by restricting the transfer of thermal energy to adjacent tissue. However, pulse duration in the nanosecond range requires enormous peak energies of visible and infrared light to be delivered through optical fibres in order to achieve tissue ablation with reduced thermal effects.

The excimer laser emits ultraviolet light of shorter wave length at 308 nm for xenon chloride gas and at 351 nm for xenon fluoride gas. Both lasers are currently undergoing clinical evaluation in the coronary arteries but most results were acquired using the 308 nm laser. Because heat can be dissipated between pulses, tissue ablation occurs with minimal thermal effects [158]. The virtual absence of thermal conduction leads to regular, precise incision margins at the cost, however, that vaporization is concentrated to an area corresponding to the diameter of the optical fibre. The high energy delivered at the tip of the fibre can even be used to ablate dense calcifications [159]. Although a photochemical mechanism with direct breakage of molecular bonds has been proposed [160], mechanical tearing due to gas trapped under the fibre and small thermal damage zones were found by others when the fibre is in direct contact with the tissue during ablation [161].

Catheter Design

Catheters have to guide the photoenergy to the appropriate anatomical location. To achieve this in the coronary arteries, a fair amount of flexibility is required. Unfortunately, fibre optics are quite stiff and very small diameters are necessary to give them some flexibility. Therefore, coronary catheters for excimer lasers are made of fibre bundles using fibre diameters in the order of 100 - 200 μm [160,162] which accommodate a coronary guide-wire in a central lumen. Because the angiographic success depends on the size of the laser catheter [163], larger catheters with diameters of 2 mm and more are required for successful 'laser only' angioplasty without additional widening of the initial channel by balloon angioplasty. However, catheter diameters are limited by the fact that at ratios close to 1 between vessel lumen and catheter size, any lumen eccentricity or tortuosity will result in lateral deviation of the ablative front surface with a high risk of perforation [164].

The small channels [165], the high rate of perforation [166], difficulties in directing to the target, and the extensive thermal damage at the tip of the bare fibres [167] were the reasons for the development of catheters capped with tapered, metallic tips, so called 'hot tip' catheters, which are heated with laser energy from argon or Neodymium (Nd):YAG generators [168]. Although successfully applied in the peripheral arteries with a very low perforation rate by some groups [169], others reported distal embolization in 33% of patients with peripheral angioplasty using 'hot tip' lasers. Material harvested by atherectomy catheter showed gross charring with thermal injury [170].

Another thermal laser catheter uses a balloon to align the optical fibre coaxially to the vessel. The fibre has an optical lens at its tip and derives its energy from an argon source [171]. This catheter has theoretical advantages over catheters guided by a central wire in total occlusions. However, the initial success rate for recanalizing chronic total coronary occlusions (59%) was similar to the results of standard balloon angioplasty [171].

Litvack et al, described their experience with an alternative heat source for the 'hot tip' catheter [160]. They used much cheaper radiofrequency energy to heat the tip to 130°C similar to the temperature achieved by laser generators. The device was used with a success rate similar to that reported using lasered 'hot tip' catheters.

Clinical use of Thermal Devices

Thermal 'hot tip' devices have been used with limited success in the coronary arteries. Cumberland et al, [172] reported myocardial infarction within 24 hours of the procedure in three of their four patients which was attributed to thrombus formation or vasospasm. Crea et al, [173] performed percutaneous, intra-operative recanalization of high-grade LAD stenoses in six patients. Perforation occurred in one patient and luminal obstruction was not relieved in two others due to the small size of the catheter used. Another problem was the limited flexibility of the catheter.

Laser-thermal catheters coaxially guided over a central guide-wire using quick short bursts of laser energy were recently reported to successfully recanalize chronic total occlusions [174]. Due to thermal energy being confined to a small thermal band around the probe and short bursts of thermal energy being used, the authors claim a diminished tendency for vasospasm and thermal damage to the vessel wall. However, the authors commented that the use of conventional balloon dilatation might also have resulted in a successful procedure. The concern about thrombosis, spasm, and perforation within the small and tortuous coronary arteries is heightened by a report from Rosenthal, who observed side branch occlusions and thermal damage in the coronaries with poor outcome following use of a thermal laser [175]. Animal experiments by Gal and coworkers [176] demonstrated a high tendency for spasm in the peripheral arteries when subjected to an argon laser in contrast to pulsed lasers which did not induce spasm.

With the 'hot tip' laser, basically all authors conclude that probe modification will be necessary for safety and better handling. It seems therefore that 'hot tip' angioplasty of the coronary arteries is still an investigational procedure and it is not clear whether improvements with regard to safety as well as to acute and long-term efficacy in the coronaries will be achievable.

Clinical use of the Excimer Laser

Since its clinical introduction in the late 1980s, the excimer laser has become increasingly popular and is now the most extensively used laser device in the coronaries. Initial applications in coronary arteries [177] and aortocoronary vein grafts [178] demonstrated the feasibility of safely performing percutaneous excimer laser coronary angioplasty. Excimer laser treatment was not associated with chest pain or burning sensations [179].

The Excimer Laser Coronary Angioplasty Registry has recently reported on the first 685 patients treated with the device [180]. The spectrum of lesions treated was similar to that of standard balloon angioplasty; 9% were total occlusions and 12% vein grafts. Laser success defined as a $\geq$ 20% reduction of stenosis or creation of a lumen near the catheter diameter, was achieved in 83%. Procedural success, defined as a final stenosis diameter $<$ 50% including additional conventional balloon angioplasty, was 93%. However, laser-only procedures resulted in procedural success in only 43% for the entire group and 56% with the 2.0 mm catheter. These success rates were achieved with a spectrum and a rate of complications similar to those seen with balloon angioplasty (acute occlusion 5.2%, perforation 1.0%, major dissection 13%, myocardial infarction 0.4%, CABG 2.2%, death 0.2%). Despite claims that pulsed lasers would not induce spasm, this complication was seen in 8.5% of patients [181] whereas Karsch and coworkers, using slightly different catheters, saw spasm in eight of their first 15 patients [179]. Ironically, conventional balloon angioplasty was successfully used in the majority of patients with occlusion after failed laser angioplasty [181,182]. The good news was certainly that lesion length was no problem for the excimer laser and stenoses longer than 20 mm still showed a procedural success of 92%. Angiographic analysis in a subgroup of patients showed that the complexity of a lesion including moderate to heavy calcifications did not result in an adverse outcome after excimer laser angioplasty [183]. Therefore, complex lesions, especially long and diffusely sclerotic lesions, may become a potential laser application.

The crucial question of whether excimer laser angioplasty will improve success rates in chronic total occlusions was addressed by Werner and coworkers [184] and Trautwein and coworkers [185]. In their combined series, the occlusion could be crossed with the guidewire in 50 of the 58 lesions, and was then successfully treated with the laser in 47. Additional balloon angioplasty had to be performed in 33/50 lesions with a residual stenosis > 50%. Restenosis rate was 50% in 48 patients with repeat angiograms [185,186]. These studies could not demonstrate any additional benefit derived from excimer laser angioplasty as compared to balloon PTCA. With respect to the rather disappointing long-term results, the higher costs, especially in the majority of patients who required additional balloon angioplasty, do not appear to be justified.

The restenosis rates after laser angioplasty of stenotic lesions are also not any better than those of conventional balloon angioplasty. In their initial 107 patients with 6 month follow-up angiograms, Haase and coworkers [187] found a restenosis rate of 43%. The rate of restenosis was even 56% in patients with more extensive vessel damage produced by the combined use of laser and balloon angioplasty (n = 50) whereas patients after excimer laser angioplasty only (n = 57) showed a rate of 32%. In the small group of 35 patients with follow-up angiography reported from Göttingen, Germany, 12 (34%) had restenosis [186].

Fluorescence Guided Lasers

It is clear that the use of a guide-wire, although increasing the safety of laser catheters, abolishes one of the theoretical advantages of the device - the ability to reopen occlusions without the need to first cross them with a wire. One way of improving safety without the need for a guide-wire would be to know what lies ahead and adjust laser firing accordingly. This concept has been followed by Leon and Geschwind and coworkers who used spectroscopic atheroma detection to discriminate between atheromatous and normal tissue and guide the use of laser energy during recanalization of peripheral arteries. Although spectroscopic identification of normal tissue resulted in appropriate interruption of laser firing and laser perforation occurred in only two of 55 patients, mechanical vessel perforation was frequent [188].

The same group [189] found fluorescence-guided laser coronary angioplasty using a pulsed dye or Holmium:YAG laser to be fraught with major complications in 7/12 patients. Shock wave effects and poor ablation efficiency associated with the laser generators and not inefficient fluorescence guidance were felt to be responsible for this unacceptable frequency of complications. Further work in the coronaries seems justifiable only after major design refinements of the laser system.

Laser Balloon Angioplasty

The concept of thermal vascular welding using Nd:YAG and other laser sources has led to the development of laser balloon angioplasty which is now clinically tested for its ability to seal acute dissections and reduce the incidence of restenosis. In addition to a conventional PTCA balloon, this special catheter is fitted with a tip inside the balloon which diffuses thermal laser energy in a cylindrical pattern and heats the surrounding tissue through the balloon walls. In an animal model, application of both pressure and thermal energy in the setting of obstructing dissections has been shown to result in readaptation and fusion of intimal flaps with the vessel wall [190]. Absorption of laser radiation by thrombotic material is expected to result in rapid dissecation of thrombus [191], and a reduction in elastic recoil and vasoconstrictive potential by destruction of smooth muscle cells is hoped to reduce restenosis rate.

A multicentre trial using the Spears balloon laser angioplasty catheter after conventional PTCA has demonstrated in 232 patients that vessel diameter could be acutely increased further after suboptimal PTCA. Six month follow-up data showed similar results in the laser and the conventional balloon groups [192]. Formal restenosis rates were not reported from this trial. Laser balloon angioplasty was found to be effective in restoring blood flow and avoiding emergency bypass operations in 72/85 patients with abrupt closure following PTCA [193]. However, it is not clear whether alternative conventional bail-out strategies would not have resulted in a similarly high success rate.

Follow-up angiography from one centre in the trial revealed restenoses in 8/15 (53%) patients and atherectomy specimens showed neointimal proliferation typical of post-PTCA patients [194]. Similarly high restenosis rates were reported from another subgroup of 48 patients. Restenoses seemed to increase in frequency in proportion to the amount of laser energy used [195].

Conclusions

Over the past several years, laser angioplasty for coronary artery disease has undergone considerable development. Although useful in femoral artery occlusions, thermal lasers with and without metal caps do not seem to be suitable tools within the coronaries because of perforation, spasm and thrombosis. Laser balloon angioplasty does not seem to provide advantages over conventional balloon techniques. Excimer laser angioplasty was received with much enthusiasm and large numbers of patients with a multitude of lesion characteristics have already undergone this procedure. Recent results indicate that this laser may possibly expand the applications of angioplasty to patients with complex disease such as long and irregular or calcified stenoses. Further development of catheter devices is mandatory, however, before any of these techniques can be recommended for routine clinical use.

The two major goals of laser angioplasty, recanalization of total occlusions and reduction of restenosis rate will probably remain elusive. Total occlusion is extremely difficult to tackle with lasers because the advantage of the laser - the ability to vaporize organized thrombus and other tissue - is, at the same time, its Achilles heel, as this ability may also result in vessel perforation. Better guidance of the laser catheter tip by a central lumen guide-wire, on the other hand, requires passage of the guide-wire through the occlusion before laser energy can be applied. Precisely this necessity, however, is the major shortcoming of conventional PTCA in the treatment of total occlusions.

Atherectomy

Directional Coronary Atherectomy

The Simpson atherotome is the most extensively studied device that works by actual removal of atherosclerotic plaque. It was suggested that this mechanism would result in less residual stenosis as compared to balloon angioplasty and reduce the incidence of dissection. Consequently, a higher primary angiographic success rate with a lower rate of complications was expected. In addition, the smoother surface allegedly left by the device should avoid elastic recoil, thrombus formation and turbulence within the diseased arterial segment which in combination with the removal of atheroma, should reduce the restenosis rate [196].

The over-the-wire coronary atherectomy catheter designed for controlled excision and retrieval of tissue features a distal non-flexible cylinder which contains the collection chamber, a window, a cup-shaped high-speed rotating cutter driven by a small hand-held motor, and a small balloon. Once the bulky and stiff catheter is positioned within the stenosis, the balloon is inflated at low pressure to stabilize the housing chamber and press the window against the plaque, protruding parts of which are then cut through the window by pushing the rotating cutter forward [197]. Atheromatous material can be retrieved from the collecting chamber after removal of the catheter (Fig. 6).

Dotter effects certainly contribute to the overall impact of the device on the lesion because the catheter is relatively large and bulky and cannot get rid of tissue in front of it like a front-firing laser catheter. Although removal of tissue is probably most important, an additional balloon angioplasty effect must be assumed because only 34% of the tissue forming a stenotic lesion is actually removed from the vessel [198]. Actually, less than half the increase in final lumen

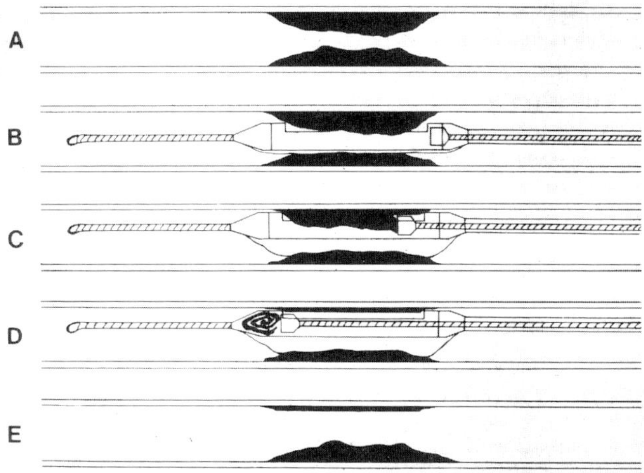

Figure 6. *ATHERECTOMY PROCEDURE. (a): Lesion before atherectomy; (b): Catheter in position across lesion; (c): Balloon support inflated; (d): Cutter advanced and specimen trapped in housing; (e): Balloon deflated and catheter removed. With permission from J.B. Simpson et al. Transluminal atherectomy for occlusive peripheral vascular disease. Am J Cardiol 1988;61:96G-101G.*

diameter can be explained by the rather low amount of excised tissue [199].

The latest update of results from the multicentre study of the US Directional Coronary Atherectomy Investigator Group in 958 patients showed a success rate of 85% in a variety of common coronary lesions [200]. In an additional 7%, lesions were successfully treated by balloon angioplasty. Success rates were lower in diffuse (79%) [201] and calcified lesions (69%) [202].

Complications rates in these 958 patients were similar to those after balloon angioplasty [203]: occlusion of a major vessel occurred in 3.7%, side branch occlusion in 3.6%, distal embolization in 1.9%, spasm in 2.5%, and perforation 0.7%. Emergency bypass surgery was required in 4.0% and emergency balloon angioplasty in 2.0%. Enzymatic myocardial infarction occurred in 5.0%, Q-wave infarcts in 0.8%, and 0.5% of patients died. Complications were more often seen in atherectomy of the right coronary artery, in lesions with diffuse narrowing > 20mm, calcification [202], excentricity, and de novo lesions [203]. These data certainly do not support earlier claims that this procedure was safer than PTCA.

Follow-up data are available from the first 62 patients undergoing atherectomy and repeat catheterization at Sequoia Hospital [204]. Restenosis was present in 38% in 56 native lesions, and in 55% of 20 vein graft lesions. Subgroup analysis showed that restenosis rate was lower in de novo lesions (24%) than in those with previous restenosis (44%) [205]. Long lesions also had a higher rate of restenosis (63%) [201]. Safian and coworkers reported a 30% 6-month lesion restenosis rate which was also lower in patients undergoing primary rather than secondary atherectomy performed for postangioplasty restenosis (20% vs. 40%) [206].

Facing similar complication rates and restenosis rates as in PTCA, it is difficult to define indications for directional atherectomy in the treatment of coronary artery lesions. Although initial results suggested ostial and RCA stenoses to be especially favourable for the procedure, the higher restenosis rates in the former and the higher rate of complications in the latter refute these expectations. Other lesion attributes which are unfavourable for PTCA such as calcification, eccentricity, and length > 20 mm do not seem to show improved short- and long-term results after directional atherectomy. In vein grafts, restenosis rate is high [207] irrespective of the interventional technique applied. Atherectomy may possibly be used as the primary tool with a good success rate (92%) in lesions with ulceration, dissection, or intimal flaps [208]. It is not yet clear whether this technique will be helpful in the treatment of PTCA induced dissections [208-210]. At least in extensive dissections, there is a danger of vessel perforation. Interestingly, conventional balloon angioplasty may be used effectively to manage vessel occlusion resulting from atherectomy [210].

Directional atherectomy is the first technique which permits retrieval of biopsy specimens from human vessels. Excised endovascular tissue provides a unique opportunity of exploring the biochemical and genetic basis of restenosis. Research on restenosis may importantly benefit from such material because observations from animal models of atherosclerosis have only limited applicability to human disease. In de novo lesions without previous mechanical interaction, removed tissue has the well known appearance of atherosclerosis. In restenotic segments, histology shows three components:

1. Fibrocellular tissue.
2. Typical atherosclerotic morphology.

3. Organizing thrombus which suggests that thrombus may be an important underlying factor in restenosis [211].

The number of specimens containing parts of the media and adventitia varies depending on the population studied. In the initial 100 Sequoia patients, adventitia was seen in only 1% and media in 3% [197]. In a smaller series, other investigators found media tissue in 64% and adventitia in 23% [212]. However, short- or long-term outcome did not depend on the presence or absence of these layers [213]. Excellent primary results or vessel ectasia after atherectomy suggest a high likelihood of excision of normal vessel wall [214,215], although vessel perforations are infrequent. Nevertheless, striving for the perfect angiographic result in an attempt to achieve lower restenosis rates seems potentially dangerous.

In conclusion, directional coronary atherectomy appears to be yet another mechanical device which will probably not fulfil its initial promise. Although further modifications of the device may facilitate crossing of tortuous proximal vessels and tight lesions, major complications are not likely to be reduced to a level significantly lower than in balloon angioplasty. Restenosis rates are at least as high as after balloon angioplasty and seem to be caused by the same biological reaction to the triad of Dotter, balloon and cutter injury of the vessel wall. At least for the present, atherectomy cannot be recommended for most complex lesions which are difficult to dilate with a balloon. Nevertheless, further research is warranted to possibly define subgroups of patients who might benefit from this approach. Finally, atherectomy will definitely have a role in future efforts to clarify the complex process of restenosis formation.

Other Atherectomy Devices

The Auth Rotablator was designed to grind obstructive atheroma into fine particles. The abrasive tip of the over-the-wire catheter is coated with minute diamond particles (Fig. 7) and rotates at 150 000 r.p.m. Macroscopically visible debris were not encountered in animal experiments and the average size of the particles was < 5μm [216]. The device is effective in increasing the luminal diameter of stenosed coronary artery segments [217], leaving a smooth surface. However, embolization of atheromatous particles was the likely reason for the development of transient atrioventricular block in six of 27 patients studied by Bertrand and coworkers [218]. Other complications

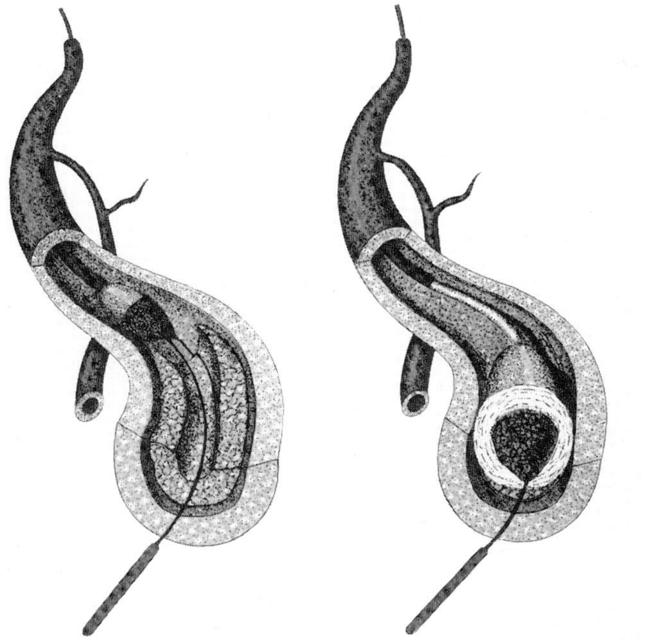

Figure 7. *Left: the conically shaped tip of the Rotablator™ is advanced over the guide-wire into the stenosis. Right: the rotating tip abrases the atheroma and minute debris are washed into the distal coronary arterial bed. With permission from R. Erbel et al. Hochfrequenz Rotationsatherektomie bei koronarer Herzkrankheit. DMW 1989;114:487-495.*

included spasm distal to the stenosis, thrombotic occlusion and acute myocardial infarction. Limitations of the technique include that the size of the burr cannot be increased beyond the internal diameter of the guiding catheter. Obviously, small burrs cannot create optimal angiographic results in larger vessels and additional balloon angioplasty is necessary in a high proportion of patients [217,219]. On the other hand, larger burrs produce larger particles and the danger of embolization and vessel perforation increases. Despite the favourable initial results for the device, its impact on future treatment strategies will be limited by the high rate of restenosis [220]. However, it is conceivable that distal lesions in smaller arteries might be successfully treated with the rotablator.

Extraction atherectomy is another newly developed technique to remove atheromatous material from the coronary arteries. The over-the-wire catheter carries a conical front cutting tip which is rotated at 750 r.p.m. under control of the operator (Fig. 8). Suction is simultaneously applied through the openings of the cutting windows and plaque fragments are collected in a reservoir at the rear of the control piece [221]. Initial clinical results from 155 lesions [222] showed primary success rates of 93% with 5% emergency bypass operations. Restenosis rates depended on baseline pathology and varied between 29% in the right coronary artery and 52% in the LAD.

Experience with these two devices is limited but these preliminary results suggest that short- and long-term success rates will not be superior to the Simpson atherectomy catheter.

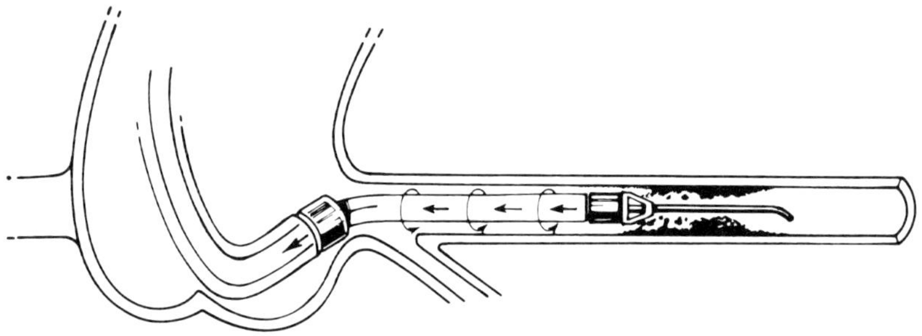

Figure 8. *TRANSLUMINAL EXTRACTION CATHETER CUTTING THROUGH ATHEROMATOUS LESION. The fragmented material is simultaneously aspirated into a collecting chamber at the end of the control device. Reprinted with permission from R. S. Stack et al. Extraction atherectomy. In: Topol E J, (ed). Textbook of interventional cardiology, pp 590-602. Philadelphia: W. B. Saunders.*

New Imaging Modalities to Assess the Effects of Intervention

Angioscopy

The examination of blood vessels using miniature fibrescopes has provided new perspectives in the pathophysiology of coronary artery disease and has shed new light on the relation between the endothelial surface and certain clinical syndromes such as unstable angina and myocardial infarction.

Light is transmitted into the coronary tree via a bundle of very thin glass fibres which have an outer diameter as small as 0.3 mm. At its tip, a wide angle lens focuses the reflected light, which comes from a xenon-based light source, into the centrally located imaging fibres. Light is transmitted through an outer ring of larger illumination fibres. The viewing angle of the lens is important for orientation within the vessel and 90° wide angle lenses are recommended for better image quality [223]. To improve imaging technology at the viewer's end of the angioscope, high resolution cameras have been developed and image processing has been refined.

Because blood between the lens and the target completely obscures the view of the inner surface of the vessel, a blood-free field of view is mandatory. This goal may be achieved using a high pressure irrigation pump which delivers sufficient fluid at pressures in excess of systolic blood pressure through a subselective guiding catheter to provide a clear field of view. Because guiding catheter and endoscope lead to some obstruction of blood flow, pressurized irrigation is usually sufficient to provide good antegrad vision. However, ST changes usually follow the injection of a larger amount of 37°C warm saline or Ringer solution similar to those seen after contrast injection and some patients may experience slight chest compression. The tip of the endoscope is quite rigid and laceration of the vessel wall may occur. Hence, more recent endoscopes are designed to be advanced over a guide-wire. A problem, which is often encountered with non-steerable angioscopes, is repeated positioning of the tip of the catheter against a vessel wall which precludes the acquisition of diagnostic images. To overcome this limitation, steerable angioscopes have been developed at the price of a larger diameter and less space for the central channels. Alternatively, a balloon mounted angioscope may be used to coaxially align the viewing system to the coronary artery and obstruct the inflow of blood with low inflation pressures for short intervals [224]. A combination of steerability, distal balloon and/or irrigation channel is desirable for maximum image quality.

Forrester and coworkers concluded from their experience with coronary angioscopy that each clinical coronary syndrome has a distinct endothelial cause and corresponding findings at angioscopy [225]. Coronary lesions in patients with chronic stable angina are composed of smooth, yellow-white atheroma and normal and diseased vessel walls can be easily distinguished. Ulcerated atheroma is distinctly unusual in patients with stable angina. In contrast, the majority of patients with crescendo angina exhibit plaque ulceration. Surrounding subintimal haemorrhage and strands of fibrin may be seen around these arterial ulcers. A high proportion of patients with angina at rest have subocclusive thrombi which may be adherent to the arterial wall despite treatment with heparin [226]. All patients with acute myocardial infarction studied by Mizuno and coworkers harboured thrombotic material within the coronary artery [227]. In patients with recent myocardial infarction, ulcerated surfaces are commonly seen [227].

Angioscopic appearances of the vessel wall following PTCA include relatively smooth surfaces which may show subintimal haemorrhage or small intimal tears [228], ruptured plaque covered with thrombotic material, larger irregular intimal tears and large flaps created by circumferential dissection [223,224]. After thermal laser or radiofrequency angioplasty, the stenotic segment may look brownish with exfoliated endothelial flaps [224,228]. Some of these alterations cannot be detected angiographically.

In the absence of integrated angioscopic systems with optimized design of fibre-optics, lenses, flushing provisions and imaging hard- and software, the clinical role of angioscopy is difficult to define. However, several potential clinical applications have emerged during early clinical trials. In patients with failed PTCA, angioscopy may be more sensitive in the detection of obstructive intimal flaps and thrombus than angiography [223]. This may have potential therapeutic consequences because extensive thrombosis is preferentially approached with intracoronary thrombolysis and/or a bail-out reperfusion catheter, whereas large intimal flaps can be successfully treated with repeat PTCA. Another potential clinical role for angioscopy may be after thrombolytic therapy for acute myocardial infarction, where it is important to distinguish between a minimal lesion associated with a large thrombus and a high grade stenosis as the underlying lesion to previous total occlusion. This distinction is very difficult to make angiographically [14]. Continued thrombolytic therapy would be beneficial in the former instance, whereas PTCA would be indicated in the latter. Finally, intra-operative angioscopy of anastomoses after peripheral vascular surgery may result in correction of several unsuspected technical errors [229]. As angiography is not usually carried out during bypass operations, angioscopy may expand the surgeon's armamentarium to detect intimal flaps within or plaque distal to the anastomosis.

Present percutaneous coronary angioscopy systems are not sufficiently developed to proclaim their routine use and reports on the use of this technique in patients are scarce. Examinations have been mostly restricted to the straight proximal coronary segments. Complications such as the creation of obstructive intimal flaps may occur if the angioscope is extensively manipulated to reach the lesion of interest. Due to difficulties in obtaining a clear field-of-view, the procedure still takes several minutes to be completed [224]. Furthermore, quantitation of stenoses cannot be reliably performed because the distance of the object from the lens must be known and the angioscope has to be directed coaxially to the long axis of the vessel. Although it has been used to direct interventional devices such as thermal lasers [165] or atherectomy catheters in order to avoid vessel perforation, key information on the composition and thickness of the vessel wall is not provided by the technique.

In conclusion, angioscopy, although being a very attractive imaging device, is still significantly limited by technical factors. Clinically useful information may be obtained during certain interventions such as after failed PTCA or after thrombolytic therapy. In these circumstances, it may serve as an adjunct to angiography.

Intracoronary Ultrasonic Imaging

As mentioned above, angioscopic information is limited to the intima and intraluminal structures but does not delineate the extent and distribution of atheroma along the vessel wall. In contrast, ultrasonic images display the vessel from inside similar to pathological cross-sections (Fig. 9).

Ultrasonic endovascular imaging is expected to be used as an adjunct to angiography which does not provide optimal information about coronary anatomy. Although the longitudinal silhouette of the vessel lumen is clearly displayed by angiography, the cross-sectional distribution of atherosclerosis is difficult to judge. Diffuse disease may be underestimated, because the structure of the diseased vessel wall itself is not visualized [230]. During and after interventions in the coronary arteries, better information about the composition of atheroma, integrity of the intimal surface, presence or absence of ulcerations, dissection, intimal flap, and thrombus would be advantageous. The availability of a wide selection of interventional tech-

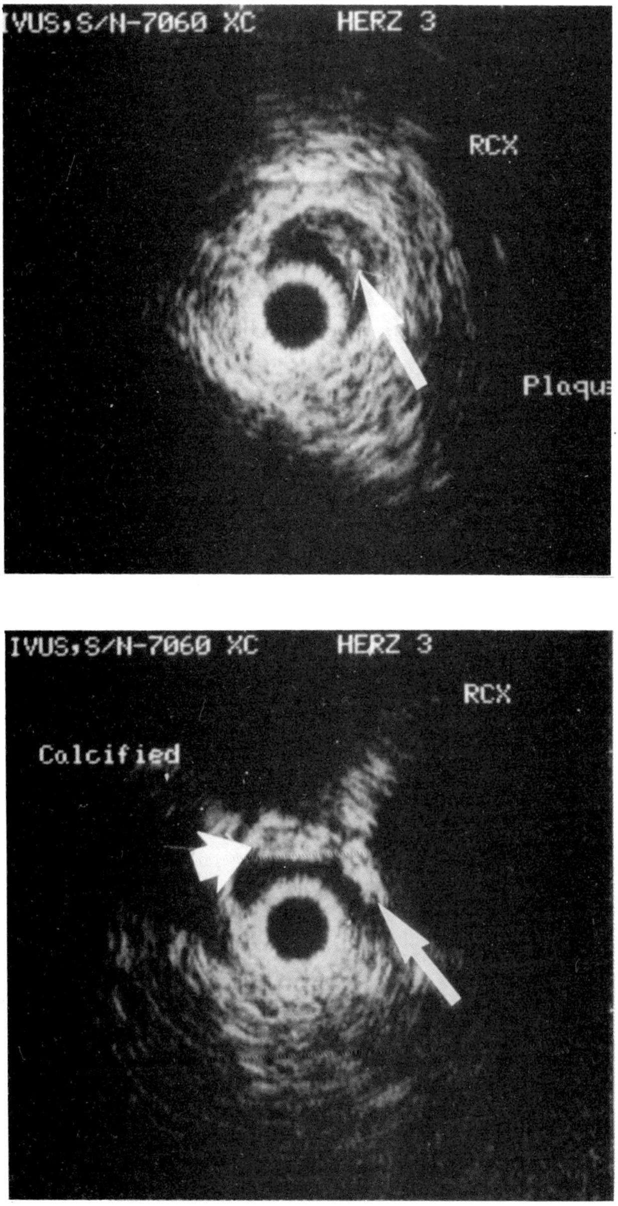

(a)

(b)

Figure 9. *IN VITRO INTRACORONARY ULTRASOUND IMAGE FROM PRESSURE PERFUSED HUMAN HEART. (a) A soft, histologically fibrous plaque (arrow) protrudes into the lumen. (b) Calcified plaques (arrows) have higher signal intensity and cause a characteristic distal shadowing.*

niques makes better criteria for the selection of the appropriate interventional technique for each individual lesion highly desirable.

Since the first real-time, catheter based ultrasound system was developed by Bom and coworkers more than 20 years ago [231], miniaturization of transducers has resulted in catheters which are small enough to be introduced into the coronary arteries. Three basic catheter designs are now commercially available: an electronically switched phased array system, which has 32 acoustic elements positioned around the tip and contains a microchip that controls firing of the elements in order to reduce the number of electric wires running through the full length of the catheter [232,233] and two mechanical systems. The rotating element system contains a single transducer which is mounted in an slight forward angle with respect to the main axis and is driven at about 900 r.p.m. by a motor drive unit and a cable running through the catheter [234]. The pulsed ultrasound waves traverse the fluid filled catheter tip and the acoustically transparent catheter wall before reaching the vessel wall at the same angle under which the acoustic element is mounted (Fig.10). This angle leads to some distortion of true vessel dimensions which are measured perpendicular to its long axis. In contrast, the other mechanical design features a beam plane perpendicular to the vessel wall. This effect is achieved by a rotating mirror, which reflects the acoustic waves emitted by the stationary transducer in the desired manner. Another advantage of this design is the ability to image an artery with a diameter as small as the catheter shaft without a ring-down artefact [235] (Fig. 9).

The main technical problem with the phased array system is the low resolution due to difficulties to mount more elements on the catheter tip. Mechanical systems suffer from image artefacts because the rotating element at the tip does not identically follow the rotation of the motor due to limited torsional rigidity of the shaft. Flexibility of the catheter which is required to adjust to the bends in the coronary arteries demands low flexural rigidity which is opposed to the need for high torsional rigidity. Other image artefacts in the moving coronaries result from the rather slow rotation of the shaft which as of now precludes perfect real-time imaging. The development of smaller catheters with diameters below the currently available 1.6 mm are mandatory to image stenotic coronary segments. However, smaller transducer elements also require higher centre frequencies to maintain image quality and ring-down artefacts become more of a

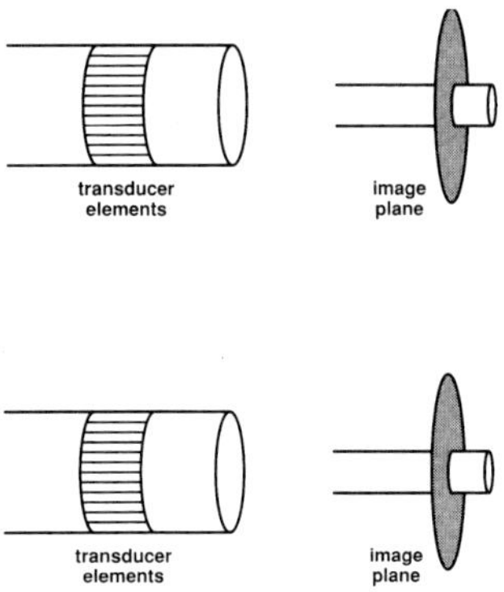

(b)

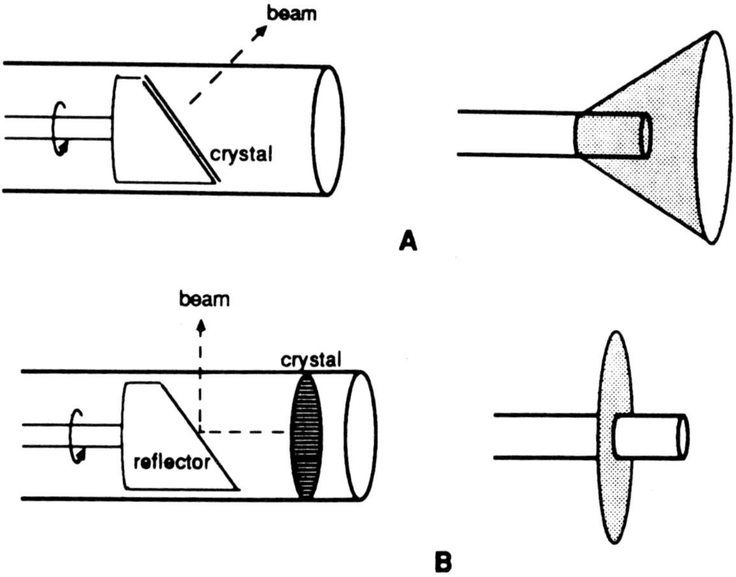

Figure 10. *SCHEMATIC ILLUSTRATIONS OF ULTRASOUND TECHNOLOGY. (a) Multiple-element electronically switched catheter transducer. Sequential firing of the radially arranged transducer elements causes a beam sweep perpendicular to the catheter. (b) Upper panel (A): Mechanical transducer design in which transducer crystal is directly rotated. The crystal is mounted at a slight angle relative to catheter axis which results in a cone shaped ultrasonic beam. Lower panel (B): Another mechanical design in which the crystal is mounted in the tip of the catheter facing backward. The rotating reflector produces a scan plane perpendicular to the long axis of the catheter. Importantly, the longer beam path allows the ring-down artefact to be dissipated within the catheter. With permission from P. Yock et al. J Am Soc Echo 1989;2:296-304.*

problem with reduced vessel size.

The ultrasonic display of an artery depends on whether an elastic or muscular type of artery is imaged. Images of elastic arteries such as the aorta or the pulmonary trunk show a media which is as echogenic as the surrounding intima and adventitia [236] and can thus not be distinguished from these layers. In contrast, muscular arteries such as the coronary arteries present a typical three-layered wall provided the resolution of the system is sufficient and the media is of sufficient thickness. Microdissection studies revealed that this three-layered pattern is caused by the intima - internal elastic lamina (inner ring), media (middle echolucent ring) and external elastic lamina - adventitia (outer ring) [237].

Localized atheroma protrudes into the vessel lumen and is easily identified by the alteration of the normally round lumen. Four types of plaque components can to a limited extent be characterized by ultrasound in atherosclerotic lesions. Hypoechoic lesions reflect a significant deposition of lipid, whereas soft echoes are indicative of fibromuscular tissue such as commonly found in restenosis after PTCA [233]. Bright echoes are characteristic of collagen-rich fibrous tissues and bright echoes with shadowing behind the lesion represent calcified atheroma [236]. Distinction of thrombus from atheroma seems to be possible with similar accuracy as with angioscopy [239], although thrombus age cannot be determined. However, tissue characterization and identification cannot be easily accomplished from the observation of the intensity of the reflected ultrasound, which is importantly influenced by the imaging parameters of the machine. Therefore, more detailed analysis of the interaction of the unprocessed radiofrequency signals with components of the vessel wall will be necessary [240].

Several recent in vitro and in vivo studies have demonstrated that luminal areas and diameters of arteries before and after balloon angioplasty measured from ultrasound images correlate well ($r > 0.9$) with those obtained from histopathological sections [241,242] and angiographic measurements [233]. Measurements of wall thickness correlated less close with histopathology ($r = 0.79$) [243], possibly due to eccentric catheter location, angulation relative to the arterial wall or altered transmission of ultrasound through tissues of differing acoustic impedance [244]. Nevertheless, ultrasound measurements are sensitive enough to demonstrate thinning of the media at locations with significant atherosclerosis [245].

Following PTCA, ultrasound imaging can be safely performed [246] and demonstrates the presence of tears in the atheroma as well as dissections between media and the plaque in most patients [247]. In addition, ultrasound imaging may show a large residual atheroma following balloon angioplasty which may be one explanation for the high incidence of restenosis [247].

A catheter combining ultrasound imaging and mechanical atherectomy was employed by Yock and coworkers in an effort to achieve more aggressive plaque debulking without causing vessel perforation [248]. Ultrasound images could be used to direct the housing towards accumulations of atheroma and away from more normal segments. Another exciting development is the development of combined intracoronary ultrasound imaging and angioplasty catheters [249]. With such a catheter, immediate analysis of the effects of balloon angioplasty on the vessel wall may become possible. Future combination of Doppler ultrasound and imaging capabilities into one catheter would possibly provide information about the haemodynamic consequences of a stenosis by allowing calculation of absolute flow rates.

Comparison of intravascular ultrasound and fibre-optic angioscopy, performed in peripheral arteries after interventional procedures, revealed the superior nature of angioscopy in evaluating suture lines, valves and side branches of venous grafts, and intraluminal lesions such as thrombi and dissections [250,251]. In contrast, ultrasound was superior for assessment of the depth and tissue character of lesions as well as of intraluminal dimensions. Hence, the technique appeared helpful in choosing between atherectomy and angioplasty, and in evaluating the success of the procedures [250,251]. Classifications of endoluminal findings by angioscopy and intravascular ultrasound correlated well with histological distinction between stable and disrupted atheroma [252].

In conclusion, intravascular ultrasound, which is still in the developmental stages, may become useful in performing interventional procedures because of the unique information provided about alterations of the vessel wall itself. Although angioscopy has advantages for the visualization of intraluminal pathology, the comparative ease of performance of ultrasound imaging, and the possibility of having balloon catheters with ultrasound imaging capabilities may become important considerations for future clinical use. Both techniques will not replace angiography with its superior overview of the vascular tree but could be used for detailed analyses of individual sites complementary to angiography. Potentially, both techniques provide additional information to the angioplasty operator which may guide therapeutic decisions, for instance, in cases of acute occlusion. However, only extensive clinical studies will be able to demonstrate whether the new imaging techniques will indeed improve patient care.

Final Remarks

Over the past decade, PTCA has developed into a highly effective treatment modality for increasingly complex anatomic and clinical situations in patients with coronary artery disease. In patients with acute myocardial infarction and cardiogenic shock or haemodynamic deterioration due to failure of thrombolytic therapy, coronary angiography and PTCA should be performed as early as possible. However, routine angiography and PTCA is not necessary in all patients and may be omitted without compromising clinical outcome, unless a patient shows spontaneous myocardial ischaemia or has a pathological predischarge limited stress test. In patients at high risk for coronary bypass surgery such as those with poor left ventricular function or debilitating diseases, PTCA can be safely performed, although support devices such as the intra-aortic balloon pump or cardiopulmonary bypass may be necessary in some instances.

Despite the improved success of PTCA, stents, lasers, and atherectomy devices have been developed to;

1. Further improve primary success rates.
2. Eliminate or help manage complications.
3. Reduce restenosis.

Unfortunately, at their present stage of development, primary success rates of all new techniques are, at best, the same as for conventional balloon angioplasty. Today, the most common reason for PTCA failure is the inability to cross a lesion with either guide-wire or balloon catheter due to the presence of total chronic occlusion, severe proximal tortuosity, or complex lesion characteristics. Current multifibre laser catheters and atherectomy devices have high profiles and relatively inflexible shafts, making these devices unpractical in exactly the same type of lesion which is difficult to dilate by balloon angioplasty. Moreover, all coronary excimer lasers and atherectomy devices under investigation require guide-wire support for safe coaxial advancement which in turn will preclude significantly improved success rates for chronic total occlusion in the near future. Its inability to dilate certain rigid lesions is the only, (albeit uncommon), shortcoming of PTCA, which might be overcome by the new devices.

Management of acute complications may be facilitated by autoperfusion (balloon) catheters and probably balloon-expandable stents, whereas hot balloon catheters, whether heated by laser or high-frequency energy sources, do not seem to provide significant advantages. However, situations which cannot be managed by repeated and prolonged dilatations are infrequent.

The final rationale to replace the time honoured balloon angioplasty by new interventional devices would be the demonstration of a reduction in restenosis rates. Unfortunately, initial data indicate that none of the newer systems reduces the intimal hyperplastic response to arterial manipulation. In a recent editorial [253], Block considered the development of mechanical interventions that attempt to overcome the response to injury caused by intravascular therapeutic interventions as 'probably futile'. The injury caused by all endoluminal devices sets in motion a complex biological response of the vessel wall which is, as yet, poorly understood. The end result in a third of patients will be restenosis, despite or possibly even because of mechanical interaction with coronary atheroma. However, with the development of all new devices still in the early stages, a final judgment cannot be made and further improvements in their performance can be anticipated.

Angioscopy, under optimal circumstances, provides clear and easily interpretable images, but is more complicated to perform than intravascular ultrasound, which has the additional advantage of affording a look beyond the endothelial surface of the vessel. However, both imaging techniques will only have a major clinical impact if the information provided can indeed be used to guide and improve coronary intervention.

References

1. Gruentzig AR, Myler RK, Hannah EH, Turina, MI. Coronary transluminal angioplasty. *Circulation* 1977;**56(Suppl. III)**:III-84.

2. Detre K, Holubkov R, Kelsey S, Cowley M, Kent K, Williams D, Myler R, Faxon D, Holmes DJr, Bourassa M, Block P, Gosselin A, Bentivoglio L, Leatherman L, Dorros G, King SB, Galichia J, Al-Bassam M, Leon M, Robertson T, Passamani E. the and Co-Investigators of the NHLBI's Percutaneous Transluminal Coronary Angioplasty Registry. Percutaneous transluminal coronary angioplasty in 1985-1986 and 1977-1981. The National Heart, Lung and Blood Institute Registry. *N Engl J Med* 1988;**318**:265-270.
3. Tuzcu EM, Simpfendorfer C, Dorosti K, Franco I, Hollman J, Badwhar K, Whitlow P. Changing patterns in percutaneous transluminal coronary angioplasty. *Am Heart J* 1989;**117**:1374-1377.
4. Myler RK, Cote G, Topol EJ, Stertzer SH, Fishman-Rosen J, Murphy MC. Multiple vessel angioplasty: definition, classification and results. *J Am Coll Cardiol*;**7**:237A-241A.
5. Gaul G, Hollman J, Simpfendorfer C, Franco I. Acute occlusion in multiple lesion coronary angioplasty: frequency and management. *J Am Coll Cardiol* 1989;**13**:283-288.
6. O'Keefe JH, Holmes DR, Reeder GS, Bresnahan DR. A new approach for dilation of bifurcation stenoses: the dual probe technique. *Mayo Clin Proc* 1989;**64**:277-281.
7. Stone GW, Rutherford BD, McConahay DR, Johnson WL, Giorgi LV, Ligon RW, Hartzler G.O. Procedural outcome of angioplasty for total coronary artery occlusion: an analysis of 971 lesions in 905 patients. *J Am Coll Cardiol* 1990;**15**:849-856.
8. Reed DC, Beller GA, Nygaard TW, Tedesco C, Watson DD, Burwell LR. The clinical efficacy and scintigraphic evaluation of post-coronary bypass patients undergoing percutaneous transluminal coronary angioplasty for recurrent angina. *Am Heart J* 1989;**117**:60-65.
9. Cote G, Myler RK, Stertzer SH, Clark DA, Fishman-Rosen J, Murphy M, Shaw RE. Percutaneous transluminal angioplasty of stenotic coronary artery bypass grafts: 5 years' experience. *J Am Coll Cardiol* 1987;**9**:8-17.
10. Ellis SG, Roubin GS, King SB, Douglas JS, Shaw RE, Stertzer SH, Myler RK. In hospital cardiac mortality after acute closure after coronary angioplasty: analysis of risk factors from 8,207 procedures. *J Am Coll Cardiol* 1988;**11**:211-216.
11. Ellis SG, Roubin GS, King SB, Douglas JS, Weintraub WS, Thomas RG, Cox WR. Angiographic and clinical predictors of acute closure after native vessel coronary angioplasty *Circulation* 1988;**77**:372-379.
12. DiSciascio G, Vetrovec GW, Cowley MJ, Wolfgang TC. Early and late outcome of percutaneous transluminal coronary angioplasty of subacute and chronic total occlusions versus conventional stenoses. *Am Heart J* 1986;**111**:833-839.
13. Fanelli C, Aronoff R. Restenosis following coronary angioplasty. *Am Heart J* 1990;**119**:357-368
14. Topol EJ. Mechanical interventions for acute myocardial infarction. In Topol EJ (ed). *Textbook of interventional cardiology.* (Philadelphia: W B. Saunders), 1990;269-299.
15. Hartzler GO, Rutherford BD, McCohanay DR, Johnson WL, McCallister BD, Gura GM, Conn RC, Crockett JE. Percutaneous transluminal coronary angioplasty with and without prior thrombolytic therapy for treatment of acute myocardial infarction. *Am Heart J* 1983;**106**:965-973.
16. O'Keefe JH, Rutherford BD, McConahay DR, Ligon RW, Johnson Wl, Giorgi LV, Crockett JE, McCallister BD, Conn RD, Gura GM, Good TH, Steinhaus DM, Bateman TM, Shimshak TM, Hartzler GO. Early and late results of coronary angioplasty without antacedent thrombolytic therapy for acute myocardial infarction. *Am J Cardiol* 1989;**64**:1221-1230.

17. Flaker GC, Webel RR, Meinhardt S, Anderson S, Santolin C, Artis A, Krol R. Emergency angioplasty in acute anterior myocardial infarction. *Am Heart J* 1989;**118:**1154-1160.
18. Rothbaum DA, Linnemeier TJ, Landin RJ, Steinmetz EF, Hillis JS, Hallam CC, Noble RJ, See MR. Emergency percutaneous transluminal coronary angioplasty in acute myocardial infarction: a 3-year experience. *J Am Coll Cardiol* 1987;**10:**264-272.
19. Marco J, Caster L, Szatmary LJ, Fahjadet J. Emergency percutaneous transluminal coronary angioplasty without thrombolysis as initial therapy in acute myocardial infarction. *Int J Cardiol* 1987;**15:**55-63.
20. O'Neill W, Timmis GC, Bourdillon PD, Lai P, Ganghadarhan V, Walton J, Ramos R, Laufer N, Gordon S, Schork A, Pitt B. A prospective randomized clinical trial of intracoronary streptokinase versus coronary angioplasty for acute myocardial infarction. *N Engl J Med* 1986;**314:**812-818.
21. Topol EJ, Califf RM, George BS, Kereiakes DJ, Abbottsmith CW, Candela RJ, Lee KL, Pitt B, Stack RS, O'Neill WW, and the Thrombolysis and Angioplasty in Myocardial Infarction Study Group. A randomized trial of immediate versus elective angioplasty after intravenous tissue plasminogen activator in acute myocardial infarction. *N Engl J Med* 1987;**317**:581-588.
22. Simoons ML, Arnold ME, Betriu A, de Bono DP, Col J, Dougherty FC, von Essen R, Lambertz H, Lubsen J, Meier B. Thrombolysis with rt-PA in acute myocardial infarction: no beneficial effect of immediate PTCA. *Lancet* 1988;**I:**197-203.
23. The TIMI Study Group. Comparison of invasive and conservative strategies after treatment with intravenous tissue plasminogen activator in acute myocardial infarction. *N Engl J Med* 1989;**320**:618-627.
24. Stack RS, Califf RM, Hinohara T, Phillips HR, Pryor DB, Simonton CA, Carlson EB, Morris KG, Behar VS, Kong Y, Peter RH, Hlaiky MA, O'Connor CM, Mark DB. Survival and cardiac event rates in the first year after emergency coronary angioplasty for acute myocardial infarction. *J Am Coll Cardiol* 1988;**11:**1141-1149.
25. Ellis SG, O'Neill WW, Bates ER, Walton JA, Nabel EH, Werns SW, Topol EJ. Implications for patient triage from survival and left ventricular functional recovery analyses in 500 consecutive patients treated with coronary angioplasty for acute myocardial infarction. *J Am Coll Cardiol* 1989;**13:**1251-1259.
26. Lee L, Bates ER, Pitt B, Walton JA, Laufer N, O'Neill WW. Percutaneous transluminal coronary angioplasty improves survival in acute myocardial infarction complicated by cardiogenic shock. *Circulation* 1988;**78:**1345-1351.
27. Topol EJ. Coronary angioplasty for acute myocardial infarction. *Ann Intern Med* 1988;**109:**970-980.
28. Gruppo Italiano per lo Studio della Streptochinasi nell'Infarto Miocardio (GISSI). Effectiveness of intravenous thrombolytic treatment in acute myocardial infarction. *Lancet* 1986;**I:**397-401.
29. Cairns JA, Collins R, Fuster V, Passamani ER. Coronary thrombolysis. *Chest* 1989;**95:**73S-87S.
30. Wilcox RG, von der Lippe G, Olsson CG, Jensen G, Skene AM, Hampton JR. Trial of tissue plasminogen activator for mortality reduction in acute myocardial infarction. *Lancet* 1988;**II:**525-530.
31. The I.S.A.M. Study Group. A prospective trial of intravenous streptokinase in acute myocardial infarction (I.S.A.M.). *N Engl J Med* 1986;**314:**1465-1471.
32. O'Connor CM. Califf RM, Massey EW, Mark DB, Kereiakes DJ, Candela RJ, Abbottsmith C, George B, Stack RS, Aronson L, Mantell S, Topol EJ. Stroke and acute myocardial infarction in the thrombolytic era: Clinical correlates and long-term prognosis. *J Am Coll Cardiol* 1990;**16:**533-540.

33. Chesebro JH, Knatterud G, Roberts R, Borer J, Cohen LS, Dalen J, Dodge HT, Frands CK, Hillis D, Ludbrook P. Thrombolysis in Myocardial Infarction (TIMI) trial. Phase I: a comparison between intravenous tissue plasminogen activator and intravenous streptokinase. Clinical findings through hospital discharge. *Circulation* 1987;**76:**142-154.
34. Ischinger T, Gruentzig AR, Hollman J, King SB, Douglas J, Meier B, Bradford J, Tankersley R. Should coronary arteries with less than 60% diameter stenosis be treated by angioplasty? *Circulation* 1983;**68:**148-154.
35. Kahn JK, Rutherford BD, McConahay DR, Johnson WL, Giorgi LV, Shimshak TM, Ligon R, Hertzler GO. Results of primary angioplasty for acute myocardial infarction in patients with multivessel coronary artery disease. *J Am Coll Cardiol* 1990;**16:**1089-1096.
36. Stone GW, Rutherford BD, McConahay DR, Johnson WL, Giorgi LV, Ligon RW, Hertzler GO. Direct coronary angioplasty in acute myocardial infarction: Outcome in patients with single vessel disease. *J Am Coll Cardiol* 1990;**15:**534-543.
37. Van de Werf F, Arnold AER, and the European Cooperative Study Group for Recombinant Tissue-Type Plasminogen Activator (rt-PA). Intravenous tissue plasminogen activator and size of infarct, left ventricular function, and survival in acute myocardial infarction. *Br Med J* 1988;**297:**1374-1379.
38. ISIS-2 Collaborative Group. Randomized trial of intravenous streptokinase, oral aspirin, both, or neither among 17,187 cases of suspected acute myocardial infarction: ISIS-2. *Lancet* 1988;**I:**349-360.
39. The AIMS Trial Study Group. Effect of intravenous APSAC on mortality after acute myocardial infarction. *Lancet* 1988;**I:**545-549.
40. Simoons ML, Serruys PW, Brand M, Bär F, De Zwaan C, Res J, Verheigt FWA, Krauss XH, Remme WJ, Vermeer F, Lubsen J. Improved survival after early thrombolysis in acute myocardial infarction: a randomized trial by the Interuniversity Cardiology Institute in the Netherlands. *Lancet* 1985;**II:**578-582.
41. Harrison DG, Ferguson DW, Collins SM, Skorton DJ, Ericksen EE, Kioschos JM, Marcus ML, White CW. Rethrombosis after reperfusion with streptokinase: importance of geometry of residual lesions. *Circulation* 1984;**69:**991-999.
42. The TIMI Research Group. Immediate versus delayed catheterization and angioplasty following thrombolytic therapy for acute myocardial infarction: TIMI IIA results. *JAMA* 1988;**260:**2849-2858.
43. Holmes DR, Topol EJ. Reperfusion momentum: Lessons from the randomized trials of immediate coronary angioplasty for myocardial infarction. *J Am Coll Cardiol* 1989;**14:**1572-1578.
44. Ellis SG. Interventions in acute myocardial infarction. *Circulation* 1989;**81(suppl. IV):**43-50.
45. Califf RM, Topol EJ, George BS, Kereiakes DJ, Aronson LG, Lee KL, Martin L, Candela R, Abbotsmith C, O'Neill WW, Pryor DB, Stack RS,and the TAMI study group. One-year outcome after therapy with tissue plasminogen activator: Report from the thrombolysis and angioplasty in myocardial infarction trial. *Am Heart J* 1990;**119:**777-785.
46. Chaitman BR, Thompson BW, Kern MJ, Vandormael MG, Cohen MR, Ruocco NA, Solomon RE, Braunwald E, for the TIMI Investigators. Tissue plasminogen activator followed by transluminal angioplasty: One-year TIMI phase II pilot results. *Am Heart J* 1990;**119:**213-221.
47. Gold HK, Leinbach RC, Palacios IF, Yasuda T, Block PC, Buckley MJ, Akins CW, Daggett WM, Austen WG. Coronary reocclusion after selective administration of streptokinase. *Circulation* 1983;**68(Suppl. IV):**50-54.

48. Serruys PW, Wijns W, Van den Brand M, Ribeiro V, Fioretti P, Simoons ML, Kooijman CJ, Reiber JHC, Hugenholtz PG. Is transluminal coronary angioplasty mandatory after successful thrombolysis? Qantitative coronary angiographic study. *Br Heart J* 1983;**50:**257-265.
49. Gash AK, Spann JF, Sherry S, Belver AD, Carabello BA, McDonough MT, Mann RH, McCann WD, Gault JH, Gentzler RD, Kent RL. Factors influencing reocclusion after coronary thrombolysis for acute myocardial infarction. *Am J Cardiol* 1986;**57:**175-177.
50. Badger RS, Brown BG, Kennedy JW, Mathey D, Gallery CA, Bolson EL, Dodge HT. Usefulness of recanalization to luminal diameter of 0.6 mm or more with intracoronary streptokinase during acute myocardial infarction in predicting 'normal' perfusion status, continued arterial patency and survival at 1 year. *Am J Cardiol* 1987;**59:**519-522.
51. Ellis SG, Topol EJ, George BS, Kereiakes DJ, Debowey D, Sigmon KN, Pickel A, Lee KL, Califf RM. Recurrent ischaemia without warning. Analysis of risk factors for in-hospital ischaemic events following successful thrombolysis with intravenous tissue plasminogen activator. *Circulation* 1989;**80:**1159-1165.
52. Barbash GI, Roth A, Hod H, Modan M, Miller HI, Rath S, Zahav JH, Keren G, Motro M, Shachar A, Basan S, Agranat O, Rabinowitz B, Laniado S, Kaplinsky E. Randomized controlled trial of late in-hospital angiography and angioplasty versus conservative management after treatment with recombinant tissue-type plasminogen activator in acute myocardial infarction. *Am J Cardiol* 1990;**66:**538-545.
53. Gruppo Italiano per lo Studio della Streptochinasi nell'Infarto Miocardio (GISSI). Long-term effects of intravenous thrombolysis in acute myocardial infarction: final report from the GISSI Study. *Lancet* 1987;**II:**871-874.
54. Vema E, Repetto S, Boscarini M, Ghezzi I, Binaghi G. Emergency coronary angioplasty in patients with severe left ventricular dysfunction or cardiogenic shock after acute myocardial infarction. *Eur Heart J* 1989;**10:**958-966.
55. Holland KJ, O'Neill WW, Bates ER, Pitt B, Topol EJ. Emergency percutaneous transluminal coronary angioplasty during acute myocardial infarction for patients more than 70 years of age. *Am J Cardiol* 1989;**63:**399-403.
56. The Multicenter Post-infarction Research Group. Risk stratification after survival after myocardial infarction. *N Engl J Med* 1983;**309:**331-336.
57. Dwyer Jr EM, McMaster P, Greenberg H, and the Multicenter Postinfarction research Group. Nonfatal cardiac events and recurrent infarction in the year after acute myocardial infarction. *J Am Coll Cardiol* 1984;**4:**695-702.
58. Califf RM, Topol EJ, George BS, Kereiakes DJ, Aronson LG, Lee KL, Martin L, Candela R, Abbottsmith C, O'Neill WW, Pryor DB, Stack RS, and the TAMI study group. One-year outcome after therapy with tissue plasminogen activator: Report the Thrombolysis and Angioplasty in Myocardial Infarction trial. *Am Heart J* 1990;**119:**777-785.
59. Van de Werf F, Arnold AER, and the European Cooperative Study Group for Recombinant Tissue-Type Plasminogen Activator (rt-PA). Intravenous tissue plasminogen activator and size of infarct, left ventricular function, and survival in acute myocardial infarction. *Br Med J* 1988;**297:**1374-1379.
60. Verstraete M, Bory M, Brower RW, Collen D, de Bono DP, Erbel R, Huhmann W, Lennane RJ, Mathey D, Michels HR, Schartl M, Uebis R, Bernard R, Lubsen J, Meyer J, Rutsch W, Schmidt W, von Essen R. Randomized trial of intravenous recombinant tissue-type plasminogen activator versus intravenous streptokinase in acute myocardial infarction. *Lancet* 1985;**I:**842-847.
61. Neuhaus KL, Feuerer W, Jeeb-Tebbe S, Niedere W, Vogt A, Tebbe U. Improved thrombolysis with a modified dose regimen of recombinant tissue-type plasminogen activator. *J Am Coll Cardiol* 1989;**14:**1566-1569.

62. Smalling RW, Schumacher R, Morris D, Harder K, Fuentes F, Valentine RP, Battey LL, Merhige M, Pitts DE, Lieberman HA, Nishikawa A, Adyanthaya A, Hopkins A, Grossbard E. Improved infarct-related arterial patency after high dose, weight-adjusted, rapid infusion of tissue-type plasminogen activator in myocardial infarction: Results of a multicenter randomized trial of two dosage regimens. *J Am Coll Cardiol* 1990;**15:**915-921.
63. Stadius ML, Davis K, Maynard C, Ritchie JL, Kennedy JW. Risk stratification for one-year survival based on characteristics identified in the early hours of acute myocardial infarction: The western Washington intracoronary streptokinase trial. *Circulation* 1986;**74:**703-711.
64. Dalen JE, Gore JM, Braunwald E, Borer J, Goldberg RJ, Passamani ER, Forman S, Knatterud D, and the TIMI Investigators. Six- and twelve-months follow-up of the phase I Thrombolysis in Myocardial Infarction (TIMI) trial. *Am J Cardiol* 1988;**62:**179-185.
65. Califf RM, Topol EJ, George BS, Boswick JM, Lee KL, Stump D, Dillion J, Abbottsmith C, Candela RJ, Kereiakes DJ, O'Neill W, Stack RS, and the TAMI Study Group. Characteristics and outcome of patients in whom reperfusion with intravenous tissue-type plasminogen activator fails: Results of the Thrombolysis and Angioplasty in Myocardial Infarction (TAMI) I Trial. *Circulation* 1988;**77:**1090-1099.
66. Topol EJ. Ultra-thrombolysis. *J Am Coll Cardiol* 1990;**15:**922-924.
67. Fung AY, Lai P, Topol EJ, Bates ER, Bourdillon PDV, Walton JA, Mancini GBJ, Kryski T, Pitt B, O'Neill WW. Value of percutaneous transluminal coronary angioplasty after unsuccessful intravenous streptokinase therapy in acute myocardial infarction. *Am J Cardiol* 1986;**58:**686-691.
68. Holmes DR, Gersh BJ, Bailey KR, Reeder GS, Bresnahan JF, Bresnahan DR, Vlietstra RE, Emergency 'rescue' percutaneous transluminal coronary angioplasty after failed thrombolysis with streptokinase. *Circulation* 1990;**81(suppl. IV):**51-56.
69. Abbottsmith CW, Topol EJ, George BS, Stack RS, Kereiakes DJ, Candela RJ, Anderson LC, Harrelson-Woodlief SL, Califf RM. Fate of patients with acute myocardial infarction with patency of the infarct-related vessel achieved with successful thrombolysis versus rescue angioplasty. *J Am Coll Cardiol* 1990;**16:**770-778.
70. Richardson SG, Callen D, Morton P, Murtagh JG, Scott ME, O'Keefe DB. Pathological changes after intravenous streptokinase treatment in eight patients with acute myocardial infarction. *Br Heart J* 1989;**61:**390-395.
71. Jang IK, Gold HK, Ziskind AA, Fallon JT, Holt RE, Leinbach RC, May JW, Collen D. Different sensitivity of erythrocyte-rich and platelet-rich arterial thrombi to lysis with recombinant tissue-type plasminogen activator. A possible explanation for resistance to coronary thrombolysis. *Circulation* 1989;**79:**920-928.
72. Califf RM, O'Neill W, Stack RS, Aronson L, Mark DB, Mantell S, George BS, Candela RJ, Kereiakes DJ, Abbottsmith C, Topol EJ, and the TAMI study group Failure of simple clinical measurements to predict perfusion status after intravenous thrombolysis. *Ann Intern Med* 1988;**108:**658-662.
73. Kennedy JW, Ritchie JL, Davis KB, Fritz JK. Western Washington randomized trial of intracoronary streptokinase in acute myocardial infarction. *N Engl J Med* 1983;**309:**1477-1482.
74. Rentrop KP, Feit F, Blanke H, Stecy P, Schneider R, Rey M, Horowitz S, Goldman M, Karsch K, Meilman H, Cohen M, Siegel S, Sanger J, Slater J, Gorlin R, Fox A, Fagerstrom R, Calhoun, WF. Effects of intracoronary streptokinase and intracoronary nitroglycerin infusion on coronary angiographic patterns and mortality in patients with acute myocardial infarction. *N Engl J Med* 1984;**311:**1457-1463.

75. Williams DO, Borer J, Braunwald E, Chesebro JH, Cohen LS, Dalen J, Dodge HT, Francis CK, Knatterud G, Ludbrook P, Markeis JE, Mueller H, Desvigne-Nickens P, Passamani ER, Powers ER, Rao AK, Roberts R, Ross A, Ryan TJ, Sobel BE, Winniford M, Zaret B, and Co-Investigators. Intravenous recombinant tissue-type plasminogen activator in patients with acute myocardial infarction: a report from the NHLBI thrombolysis in myocardial infarction trial. *Circulation* 1986;**73:**338-346.
76. The TIMI Study Group. The Thrombolysis in Myocardial Infarction (TIMI) trial. *N Engl J Med* 1985;**312:**932-936.
77. Gacioch GM, Topol EJ. Sudden paradoxical clinical deterioration during angioplasty of the occluded right coronary artery in acute myocardial infarction. *J Am Coll Cardiol* 1989;**14:**1202- 1209.
78. Hochman JS, Choo H. Limitation of myocardial infarct expansion by reperfusion independent of myocardial salvage. *Circulation* 1987;**75:**299-306.
79. Warren SE, Royal HD, Markis JE, Grossman W, McKay RG. Time course of left ventricular dilatation after myocardial infarction: Influence of infarct-related artery and success of coronary thrombolysis. *J Am Coll Cardiol* 1988;**11:**12-19.
80. Sager PT, Perlmutter RA, Rosenfeld LE, McPherson CA, Wackers FJ, Batsford WP. Electrophysiologic effects of thrombolytic therapy in patients with a transmural anterior myocardial infarction complicated by left ventricular aneurysm formation. *J Am Coll Cardiol* 1988;**12:**19-24.
81. Kersschot IE, Brugada P, Ramentol M, Zehender M, Waldecker B, Stevenson WG, Geibel A, De Zwaan C, Wellens H. Effects of early reperfusion in acute myocardial infarction on arrhythmias induced by electrical stimulation: a prospective, randomized study. *J Am Coll Cardiol* 1986;**7:**1234-1242.
82. Guerci AD, Gerstenblith G, Brinker JA, Chandra NC, Gottlieb SO, Bahr RD, Weiss JL, Shapiro EP, Flaherty JT, Bush DE, Chew PH, Gottlieb SH, Halperin HR, Ouyang P, Walford GD, Bell WR, Fatterpaker AK, Llewellyn M, Topol EJ, Healey B, Siu CO, Becker LC, Weisfeldt ML. A randomized trial of intravenous tissue plasminogen activator for acute myocardial infarction with subsequent randomization to elective coronary angioplasty. *N Engl J Med* 1987;**317:**1613-1618.
83. Detre K, Holubkov R, Kelsey S, Cowley M, Kent K, Williams D, Myler R, Faxon D, Holmes DJr, Bourassa M, Block P, Gosselin A, Bentivoglio L, Leathemman L, Dorros G, King SB, Galichia J, Al-Bassam M, Leon M, Robertson T, Passamani E, and the Co-Investigators of the NHLBI's Percutaneous Transluminal Coronary Angioplasty Registry. Percutaneous transluminal coronary angioplasty in 1985-1986 and 1977-1981. The National Heart, Lung, and Blood Institute Registry. *N Engl J Med* 1988;**318:**265-270.
84. Anderson HV, Leimgruber PP, Roubin GS, Nelson DI, Gruentzig AR. Distal coronary artery perfusion during percutaneous transluminal coronary angioplasty. *Am Heart J* 1985;**110**;720-726
85. McDonald FM, Fuchs M, Kreuzer J, Hopp HW, Arnold HG, Heyman L, Hirche HJ, Hombach V. Hemodynamic and anti-arrhythmic protective effects of intracoronary perfusion during percutaneous transluminal coronary angioplasty. *Eur Heart J* 1985;**6:**284-293.
86. Quigley PJ, Hinohara T, Phillips HR, Peter RH, Behar VS, Kong Y, Simonton CA, Perez JA, Stack RS. Myocardial protection during coronary angioplasty with an autoperfusion balloon catheter in humans. *Circulation* 1988;**78:**1128-1134.
87. Turi ZG, Rezkella S, Campbell CA, Kloner RA. Amelioration of ischaemia during angioplasty of the left anterior descending coronary artery with an autoperfusion catheter. *Am J Cardiol* 1988;**62:**513-517.

88. Hinohara T, Simpson JB, Phillips HR, Stack RS. Transluminal intracoronary reperfusion catheter: A device to maintain coronary perfusion between failed coronary angioplasty and emergency coronary bypass surgery. *J Am Coll Cardiol* 1988;**11**:977-982.
89. Christensen CW, Lassar TA, Daley LC, Rieder MA, Schmidt DH. Regional myocardial blood flow with a reperfusion catheter and an autoperfusion balloon catheter during total coronary occlusion. *Am Heart J* 1990;**119**:242-248.
90. Zalewski A, Berry C, Kosman ZK, Shi Y, Goldberg S. Myocardial protection with autoperfusion during prolonged coronary artery occlusion. *Am Heart J* 1990;1 19:41-46.
91. Alcan KE, Sterzer SH, Walsh JE, DePasquale NP, Bruno MS. The role of intra-aortic balloon counterpulsation in patients undergoing percutaneous transluminal coronary angioplasty. *Am Heart J* 1983;**105**:527-530.
92. Kahn JK, Rutherford BD, McConahay DR, Johnson WL, Giorgi LV, Hartzler GO. Supported 'high risk' coronary angioplasty using intra-aortic balloon pump counterpulsation. *J Am Coll Cardiol* 1990;**15**:1151-1155.
93. Koolen JJ, Cisser CA, Piek JJ, David GK, Dunning AJ. Improved ischaemic tolerance during coronary angioplasty of high-risk patients by intra aortic balloon pumping. *Circulation* 1990;**82(Suppl. III)**:III-680
94. Jones EL, King SB. Intraoperative balloon catheter dilatation in the treatment of coronary artery disease. *Am Heart J* 1984:**107**:836-837.
95. Vogel R, Tommaso C, Gundry S. Initial experience with angioplasty and aortic valvuloplasty using elective semipercutaneous cardiopulmonary support. *Am J Cardiol* 1988;**62**:811-813.
96. Shawl FA, Domanski MJ, Punja S, Hernandez TJ. Percutaneous cardiopulmonary bypass support in high-risk patients undergoing percutaneous transluminal coronary angioplasty. *Am J Cardiol* 1989;**64**:1258-1263.
97. Teirstein PS, Vogel RA, Dorros G, Stertzer SE, Vandormael MG, Smith SC, Overlie PA. Prophylactic vs standby cardiopulmonary support for high risk PTCA. *Circulation* 1990;**82(Suppl. III)**:III-680.
98. Vogel RA, Shawl FA, for the registry participants. Report of the National Registry. of Elective Supported Angioplasty: Comparison of the 1988 and 1989 results. *Circulation* 1990;**82(suppl. III)**:III-653
99. Geannopoulos C, Peters T, Leya F, Euler D, Wallock M, Orlow S, Johnson S, Scanlon P. Does percutaneous cardiopulmonary support protect the heart from ischaemic dysfunction during coronary occlusion? *J Am Coll Cardiol* 1990;**15**:43A.
100. Herz I, Fried G, Feld H, Schulhoff N, Hollander G, Greengart A, Gelbfish J, Lichstein E, Frankel R, Sacchi T, Shani J. High risk PTCA without cardiopulmonary bypass support. *Circulation* 1990;**82(Suppl. III)**:III-654.
101. Smalling RW, Cassidy DB, Merhige M, Felli PR, Wise GM, Barrett RL. Improved hemodynamic and left ventricular unloading during acute ischaemia using the hemopump left ventricular assist device compared to intraaortic balloon counter pulsation. *J Am Coll Cardiol* 1989;**13**:160A.
102. Lincoff AM, Popma JJ, Bates ER, Deeb GM, Bolling SF, Meagher JS, Kelly AM, Wampler RK, Nicklas JM. Successful coronary angioplasty in two patients with cardiogenic shock using the Nimbus Hemopump support device. *Am Heart J* 1990;**120**:970-972.
103. Shani J, Hollander G, Nathan I, Greengart A, Toporoff B, Jacobowitz I, Glassman E, Cunningham J, Lichstein E. Percutaneous left atrial-left femoral bypass with a pulsatilc pump: initial human experience in cardiogenic shock. *J Am Coll Cardiol* 1989;**13**:53A.

104. Meerbaum S, Lang TW, Osher JV, Hashirnoto K, Lewis GW, Feldstein C, Corday E. Diastolic retroperfusiorl of acutely ischaemic myocardium. *Am J Cardiol* 1976;**37:**588-598.
105. Jacobs AK, Simon P, Hogfeldt V, Faxon DP, Owen A, Ryan TJ. Increase in myocardial salvage by combining coronary sinus occlusion and retroperfusion. *J Am Coll Cardiol* 1989;**13:**53A.
106. Jacobs AK, Faxon DP. Retroperfusion and PTCA. In Topol EJ (ed). *Textbook of interventional cardiology.* (Philadelphia: WB. Saunders), 1989:477-495.
107. Hajduczki I, Kar S, Areeda J, Ryden L, Corday S, Haendchen R, Corday E. Reversal of chronic regional myocardial dysfunction (hibemating mtocardium) by synchronized diastolic coronary venous retroperfusion during coronary angioplasty. *J Am Coll Cardiol* 1990;**15:**238-242.
108. Zalewski A, Goldberg S, Slysh S, Maroko PR. Myocardial protection via coronary sinus interventions: superior effects of arterialization compared with intermittent occlusion. *Circulation* 1985;**71:**1215-1223.
109. King SB. Prediction of acute closure in percutaneous transluminal coronary angioplasty. *Circulation* 1990;**81(Suppl. IV):**5-8.
110. Hollman J, Gruetzig AR, Douglas JSJr, King SB, Ischinger T, Meier B. Acute. occlusion after percutaneous transluminal coronary angioplasty - a new approach. *Circulation* 1983;**68:**725-732.
111. Detre KM, Holmes DRJr, Holubkov R, Cowley MJ, Bourassa MG, Faxon DP, Dorros GR, Bentivoglio LG, Kent KM, Myler RK and coinvestigators of the National Heart, Lung, and Blood Insitute's Percutaneous Transluminal Coronary Angioplasty Registry. Incidence and consequences of periprocedurall occlusion. The 1985-1986 National Heart, Lung, and Blood Insitute Percutaneous Transluminal Coronary Angioplasty Registry. *Circulation* 1990;**82:**739-750.
112. Palazzo AM, Gustafson GM, Santilli E, Kemp HG. Unusually long inflation times during percutaneous transluminal coronary angioplasty. *Cathet Cardiovasc Diagn* 1988;**14:**154-158.
113. Hodes Zl, Rothbaum DA, Linnemeier TJ, Landin RJ, Ball MW, Giebel RA. Use of the ACS Stack perfusion dilatation catheter in PTCA to avoid coronary artery bypass surgery. *J Am Coll Cardiol* 1989;**13:**155A.
114. Simpfendorfer C, Belardi J, Bellamy G, Galan K, Franco I, Hollman J. Frequency, management, and follow-up of patients with acute coronary occlusions after percutaneous transluminal coronary angioplasty. *Am J Cardiol* 1987;**59:**267-269.
115. Buccino KR, Btenner AS, Browne KF. Awte reocclusion during percutaneous transluminal coronary angioplasty: Immediate and long-term outcome. *Cathet Cardiovasc Diagn* 1989;**17:**75-79.
116. Ischinger T, Gruentzig AR, Meier B, Galan K. Coronary dissection and total coronary occlusion associated with percutaneous transluminal coronary angioplasty: Significance of initial angiographic morphology of coronary stenoses. *Circulation* 1986;**74:**1371-1378.
117. Steffenino G, Meier B, Finci L, Velebit V, von Gegesser L, Faidutti B, Rutishauser W. Acute complications of elective coronary angioplasty: A review of 500 consecutive procedures. *Br Heart J* 1988;**59:**151-158.
118. Kulick DL, Rahimtoola SH. Acute coronary occlusion after percutaneous transluminal coronary angioplasty. *Circulation* 1990;**82:**1039-1043.
119. Tebbe U, Ruschewski W, Knake W, Herse B, Figulla HR, Klein HH, Wiegand V, Dalichau H, Kreuzer H. Will emergency coronary artery bypass grafling after failed elective percutaneous transluminal coronary angioplasty prevent myocardial infarction? *Thorac Cardiovasc Surgeon* 1989;**37:**308-312.

120. Ross R. The pathogenesis of atherosclerosis - an update. *N Engl J Med* 1986;**314:**488-500.
121. Dorros G, Johnson WD, Tector AJ, Schmahl TM, Kalush SL, Janke L. Percutaneous transluminal coronary angioplasty in patients with prior coronary artery bypass grafting. *J Thorac Cardiovasc Surg* 1984;**87:**17-26.
122. Dotter CT. Transluminally placed coilspring endarterial tube grafts: long-tern patency in canine popliteal artery. *Invest Radiol* 1969;**4:**329-332.
123. Schatz RA. A view of vascular stents. *Circulation* 1989;**79:**445-457.
124. Ellis SG, Topol EJ. Intracoronary stents: Will they fulfill their promise as an adjunct to angioplasty? *J Am Coll Cardiol* 1989;**13:**1425-1430.
125. Roubin GS, King SB, Douglas JS, Lembo NJ, Robinson KA. Intracoronary stenting during percutaneous transluminal coronary angioplasty. *Circulation* 1990;**81(Suppl. IV):**92-100.
126. Van der Giessen WJ, Strauss BH, Van Beusekom HMM, Van Loon H, Van Woerkens LJ. Self-expandable mesh stents: an experimental study comparing polymer coated and uncoated wallstent stents in the coronary circulation of dogs. *Circulation* 1990;**82(Suppl. III):**542
127. Bailey SR, Guy DM, Garcia OJ, Paige S, Palmaz JC, Miller DD. Polymer coating. of Palmaz-Schatz stent attenuates vascular spasm after stent placement. *Circulation* 1990;**82(Suppl. III):**III-541.
128. Serruys PW, Strauss BH, Beatt KJ, Bertrand ME, Puel J, Rickards AF, Meier B, Goy JJ, Vogt P, Kappenberger L, Sigwart U. Angiographic follow-up after placement of a self-expanding coronary-artery stent. *N Engl J Med* 1991;**324:**13-17.
129. Puel J, Juilliere Y, Bertrand ME, Rickards AF, Sigwart U, Serruys PW. Early and late assessment of stenosis geometry after coronary arterial stenting. *Am J Cardiol* 1988;**61:**546-553.
130. Bertrand ME, Rickards AF, Serruys PW. Coronary stenting implantation for primary and secondary prevention of restenosis after PTCA: resuHs of a pilot multicenter trial (1986/87) (CASIS Trial). *Eur Heart J* 1988;**9(Suppl. 1):**55.
131. Sigwart U. The self-expanding mesh stent. In Topol EJ (ed). *Textbook of interventional cardiology.* (Philadelphia: WB. Saunders), 1990;605-622.
132. Sigwart U, Urban P, Golf S, Kaufmann U, Imbert C, Fischer A, Kappenberger L. Emergency stenting for acute occlusion after coronary balloon angioplasty. *Circulation* 1988;**78:**1121-1127.
133. Urban P, Sigwart U, Golf S, Kaufmann U, Sadeghi H, Kappenberger L. Intravascular stenting for stenosis of aortocoronary venous bypass grafts. *J Am Coll Cardiol* 1989;**13:**1085-1091.
134. Strauss BH, De Scheerder IK, Beatt KJ, Tijssen J, Serruys PW. Angiographic predictors of restenosis in the coronary wallstent. *Circulation* 1990;**82(Suppl. III):**III-540.
135. Roubin GS, Douglas JS, Lembo NJ, Black AJ, King SB. Intracoronary stenting for acute closure following percutaneous transluminal coronary angioplasty (PTCA). *Circulation* 1988;**78(Suppl. II):**II-407
136. Roubin GS, Robinson KA. The Gianturco-Roubin stent. In Topol EJ (ed). *Textbook of interventional cardiology.* (Philadelphia: WB. Saunders), 1990;633-646.
137. Palmaz JC, Sibbitt RR, Reuter SR, Tio FO, Rice WJ. Expandable intraluminal graft: Preliminary study. *Radiology* 1985;**156:**73-79.
138. Baim DS, Schatz R, Cleman M, Curry C. Predictors of unsuccessful placement of the Schatz-Palmaz coronary stent. *Circulation* 1989;**80(Suppl. II):**II-174.
139. Baim DS, Bailey S, Curry C, Walker C, Schatz RA. Improved success and safety of Palmaz-Schatz coronary stenting with a new delivery system. *Circulation* 1990;**82:(Suppl. III):**56-57.

140. Fajadet JC, Marco J, Caasagneau BG, Laurent JP, Flores YM, Robert GP. Balloon expandable intracoronary stents: analysis of complications in a consecutive series of 160 patients. *Circulation* 1990;**82(Suppl. III)**:III-539.

141. Levine MJ, Leonard BM, Burke JA, Nash ID, Safian RD, Diver DJ, Baim DS. Clinical and angiographic results of balloon-expandable intracoronary stents in right coronary artery stenoses. *J Am Coll Cardiol* 1990;**16**:332-339.

142. Leon MB, Almagor Y, Erbel R, Teirstein PS, Perez J, Schatz RA. Subacute thrombotic events after coronary stent placement: Clinical spectrum and predictive factors. *Circulation* 1989;**80(Suppl. II)**:174.

143. Schatz RA, Leon MB, Baim DS, Ellis SG, Erbel R, Hirshfeld JW, Goldberg S. Balloon expandable intracoronary stents: Initial results of a multicenter study. *Circulation* 1989;**80(Suppl. II)**:174.

144. Levine MJ, Clemen MW, Schatz RA, Buchbinder M, Erberl R, Baim DS. Management of restenosis following Palmaz-Schatz intracoronary stenting: Multicenter results. *Circulation* 1990;**82(Suppl. III)**:657.

145. Marco J, Fajadet JC, Cassagneau BG, Robert GP. Balloon expandable intracoronary stents: Immediate and meanterm results in a sereis of 160 consecutive patients. *Circulation* 1990;**82(Suppl. III)**:658.

146. Schatz RA, Goldberg S, Leon MB, Fish D, Hirshfeld JW, Walker CM. Coronary stenting following 'suboptimal' coronary angioplasty results. *Circulation* 1990;**82(Suppl. III)**:540.

147. Savage M, Fischman D, Ellis S, Leon M, Cleman M, Teirstein P, Walker C, Hirshfeld J, Schatz R, Goldberg S. Does late progression of restenosis occur beyond six months following coronary artery stenting? *Circulation* 1990;**82(Suppl. III)**:540.

148. Gammon RS, Chapman GD, Baumann RP, Muhlestein JB, Overman AB, Desper JS, MacGregor DC, deCoriolos PE, Stack RS. The Cordis balloon- expandable stent: Implantation features and long-term follow-up in an animal model. *Circulation* 1990;**82(Suppl. III)**:541.

149. Buchwald A, Unterberg C, Werner GS, Voth E, Kreuzer H, Wiegand V. Akut- und Langzeitergebnisse nach Implantation des neuen Wiktor-Stents bei akutem Koronarverschluß nach PTCA. *Z Kardiol* 1990;**79**:837-842.

150. Bertrand M, Kober G, Scheerder Y, Uebis R, Wiegand V. Initial multi-center human clinical experience with the Medtronic Wiktor coronary stent. *Circulation* 1990;**82(Suppl. III)**:541.

151. Chapman GD, Gammon RS, Bauman RP, Howell S, Clark H, Mikat EM, Palmos L, Buller CE, Stack RS. A bioabsorbable stent: Initial experimental results. *Circulation* 1990;**82(Suppl. III)**:72.

152. Lee G, Ikeda RM, Kozina J, Mason DT. Laser-dissolution of coronary atherosclerotic obstruction. *Am Heart J* 1981;**102**:1074-1075.

153. Kereiakes DJ, Selmon MR, McAuley BJ, McAuley DB, Sheehan DJ, Simpson JB. Angioplasty in total coronary artery occlusion: Experience in 76 consecutive patients. *J Am Coll Cardiol* 1985;**6**:526-533.

154. Safian RD, McCabe CH, Sipperly ME, McKay RG, Baim DS. Initial success and long-term follow-up of percutaneous transluminal coronary angioplasty in chronic total occlusions versus conventional stenoses. *Am J Cardiol* 1988;**61**:23G-28G.

155. LaVeau PJ, Remetz MS, Cabin HS, Hennecken JF, McConnell SH, Rosen RE, Cleman MW. Predictors of success in percutaneous transluminal coronary angioplasty of chronic total occlusions. *Am J Cardiol* 1989;**64**:1264-1269.

156. Leimgruber PP, Roubin GS, Hollman J, Cotsonis GA, Meier B, Douglas JS, King SB, Gruentzig AR. Restenosis after successful coronary angioplasty in patients with single vessel disease. *Circulation* 1986;**73**:710-717.

157. Abela GS, Normann S, Cohen D, Feldmann RE, Geiser EA, Conti CR. Effects of carbon dioxide, Nd:YAG and argon-laser radiation on coronary atheromatous plaques. *Am J Cardiol* 1982;**50:**1199-1205.
158. Litvack F, Grundfest WS, Goldenberg T, Laudenslager J, Forrester J. Excimer laser angioplasty. In Topol EJ (ed). *Textbook of interventional cardiology.* (Philadelphia WB. Saunders), 1990;269-299.
159. Grundfest WS, Litvack F, Goldenberg T, Shemman T, Morgenstren L, Carroll R, Fishbein M, Forrester J, Margitan J, McDermid S, Pacala TJ, Rider DM, Laudenslager JB. Pulsed ultraviolet lasers and the potential for safe laser angioplasty. *Am J Surg* 1985;**150:**220-226.
160. Litvack F, Grundfest WS, Segalowitz J, Papaioanniou T, Goldenberg T, Laudenslager J, Hestrin L, Forrester JS, Eigler NA, Cook S. Interventional cardiovascular therapy by laser and thermal angioplasty. *Circulation* 1990;**81(Suppl. IV):**109-116.
161. Sprangers RL, Gijsbers GH, van Gemert MJ. Observation of thermal and mechanical damage by excimer laser ablation. *Circulation* 1990;**82(Suppl. III):**495.
162. Karsch K, Haase KK, Mauser M, Voelker W. Initial angiographic results in ablation of atherosclerotic plaque by percutaneous coronary excimer coronary angioplasty without subsequent balloon dilatation. *Am J Cardiol* 1989;**64:**1253-1257.
163. Torre SR, Sanborn TA, Sharma SK, Cohen M, Ambrose JA. Percutaneous coronary excimer laser angioplasty: Quantitative angiographic analysis demonstrates improved angioplasty results with larger laser catheters. *Circulation* 1990;**82(Suppl III):**671.
164. Margolis JR, Litvack F, Krauthamer D, Trautwein R, Goldenberg T, Grundfest W. Exceimer laser coronary angioplasty: American multicenter experience. *Hertz* 1990;**15:**223- 232.
165. Abela GS, Seeger JM, Barbieri E, Franzini D, Fenech A, Pepine CJ, Conti CR. Laser angioplasty with angioscopic guidance in humans. *J Am Coll Cardiol* 1986;**8:**182-194.
166. Crea F, Fenech A, Smith W, Conti CR, Abela GS. Laser recanalization of acutely thrombosed coronary arteries in live dogs: Early results. *J Am Coll Cardiol* 1985;**6:**1052-1060.
167. Welch AJ, Bradley AB, Torres JH, Motamedi M, Ghidoni JJ, Pearce JA, Hussein H, O'Rourke RA. Laser probe ablation of nommal and atherosclerotic human aorta in vitro: a tirst thermographic and histologic analysis. *Circulation* 1987;**76:**1353-1363.
168. Sanborn DA, Faxon DP, Haudenschild CC, Ryan TJ. Experimental angioplasty: Circumferential distributionof laser thermal energy with a laser probe. *J Am Coll Cardiol* 1985;**5:**934-939.
169. Cumberland DC, Sanbom TA, Tayler DI, Welsh CL, Guben JK, Moore DJ, Greenfield AJ, Ryan TJ. Percutaneous laser thermal angioplasty: initial clinical results with a laser probe in total peripheral artery occlusion. *Lancet* 1986;**I:**1457-1459.
170. Katzen BT, Kaplan JO, Schwarten DM, van Breda A. Complications of 'hot tip' laser assisted angioplasty. *Circulation* 1988;**78(Suppl. II):**417.
171. Mast G, Plokker T, Ernst S, Bal E, Tjon M, Gin J, Ascoop C. Argon-laser angioplasty for chronic total coronary occlusions: first European experience. *Circulation* 1990;**82(Suppl. III):**677.
172. Cumberland DC, Oakley GDG, Smith GH, Tayler DI, Starkey IR, Fleming JS, Goiti JJ, Davis J. Percutaneous laser-assisted coronary angioplasty. *Lancet* 1986;**II:**214.
173. Crea F, Davies G, McKenna WJ, Pashazadeh M, Keogh B, Kidner P, Taylor KM, Maseri A. Laser recanalization of coronary arteries by metal-capped optical fibers: early clinical experience in patients with stable angina pectoris. *Br Heart J* 1988;**59:**168-174.
174. Chan MC, Lee G, Guo JX, Mao JM, Chen FR, Yan WD, Xie DY, Rink DL, Argenal AJ, Mason DT. Percutaneous coronary laser angioplasty using quick short bursts of laser thermal energy for chronic total occlusions. *Am J Cardiol* 1989:**64:**940-942.

175. Rosenthal E, Montarello JK, Palmer T, Curry PVL. Coronary artery thermal damage during percutaneous 'hot tip' laser-assistes angioplasty. *Am J Cardiol* 1989;**64:**116-120.
176. Gal D, Steg PG, Rongione AJ, DeJesus ST, Clarke RH, Isner JM. Vascular spasm complicates continuous wave but not pulsed laser irradiation. *Am Heart J* 1989;**118:**934-941.
177. Litvack F, Grundfest W, Eigler N, Tsoi D, Goldenberg T, Laudenslager J, Forrester J. Percutaneous excimer laser coronary angioplasty. *Lancet* 1989;**II:**102-103.
178. Litvack F, Grundfest W, Goldenberg T, Laudenslager J, Forrester J. Percutaneous excimer laser angioplasty in aortocoronary saphenous vein grafts. *J Am Coll Cardiol* 1989;**14:**803-808.
179. Karsch KR, Haase KK, Mauser M, Voelker W. Initial angiographic results in ablation of atherosclerotic plaque by percutaneous coronary excimer laser angioplasty without subsequent balloon dilatation. *Am J Cardiol* 1989;**64:**1253-1257.
180. Litvack F, Margolis J, Rothbaum D, Kent K, Breshnahan J, Untereker W, Cummins F, Forrester J and the ELCA Ivestigators. Excimer laser coronary angioplasty - acute results of the first 685 consecutive patients. *Circulation* 1990;**82(Suppl. III):**677.
181. Bresnahan DR, Bresnahan JF, Reeder GS, Holmes DR, Bell MR. Excimer laser coronary angioplasty: Single center experience in patients with anatomy suitable for coronary balloon angioplasty. *Circulation* 1990;**82(Suppl. III):**672.
182. Karsch KR, Haase KK, Voelker W, Baumbach A, Mauser M, Seipel L. Percutaneous coronary excimer laser angioplasty in patients with stable and unstable angina pectoris. Acute results and incidence of restenosis during 6-month follow-up. *Circulation* 1990;**81:**1849-1859.
183. Ghazzal ZMB, Hearn JA, Goldenberg T, Eigler N, Kent KM, King SB. Outcome predictors after excimer laser: Detailed multicenter angiographic analysis. *Circulation* 1990;**82(Suppl. III):**670.
184. Werner GS, Buchwald A, Unterberg C, Voth E, Kreuzer H, Wiegand V. Recanalization of chronic coronary occlusion by excimer-laser angioplasty. *J Am Coll Cardiol* 1990;**15:**245A.
185. Trautwein R, Margolis J, Krauthamer D, Garcia J, Martin J. Excimer laser coronary angioplasty for chronic total occlusions. *Circulation* 1990;**82(Suppl. III):**678.
186. Buchwald A, Werner GS, Unterberg C, Wiegand V. Restenosis after excimer laser angioplasty of coronary stenoses and chronic total occlusions. *Circulation* 1990;**82(Suppl. III):**313.
187. Haase KK, Mauser M, Baumbach A, Voelker W, Karsch KR. Restenosis after excimer laser coronary atherectomy. *Circulation* 1990;**82(Suppl. III):**672.
188. Leon MB, Geschwind HJ, Selzer PM, Bonner RF. Fluorescence-guided laser angioplasty. In Topol EJ (ed). *Textbook of interventional cardiology.* (Philadelphia: WB. Saunders), 1990;713-723.
189. Leon MB, Keren G, Bartorelli AL, Almagor Y, Douek P, Hansch EC, Neville R,. Bonner RF. Fluorescence-guided laser coronary angioplasty: A clinical status report. *Circulation* 1990;**82(Suppl. III):**496.
190. Jenkins RD, Sinclair IN, McCall PE, Schoen FJ, Spears JR. Thermal sealing of arterial dissections and perforations in atherosclerotic rabbits with laser balloon angioplasty. *Lasers Life Sci* 1989;**3:**13-30.
191. Spears RJ. The potential role of laser Balloon angioplasty as an adjunct to PTCA. In Topol EJ (ed). *Textbook of interventional cardiology.* (Philadelphia: WB. Saunders), 1990:673-681.

192. Reyes VP, Plokker HWT, Leatherman LL, Dear WE, Sinclair IN, Douglas JS, King SB, Safian RD, Jenkins RD, Rickards A, Sigwart U, Pichard A, Morice MC, Spears RJ, and the LBA Study Group. Laser balloon angioplasty effectively treats unsuccessful PTCA. *Circulation* 1990;**82(Suppl. III)**:71

193. Safian RD, Reis GJ, Jenkins RD, King SB, Douglas JS, Plokker HWT, Rickards A, Ferguson JJ, Leatherman LL, Dear WE, Sinclair IN, Reyes VP, Sigwart U, Dorros G, Morice MC, Spears RJ. Failed PTCA: Salvage by laser balloon angioplasty. *Circulation* 1990;**82(Suppl. III)**:673.

194. Reis GJ, Pomerantz RM, Jenkins RD, Kuntz RE, Baim DS, Safian RD. Laser balloon angioplasty: clinical, angiographic, and histologic results. *Circulation* 1990;**82(Suppl. III)**:672.

195. Mast G, Plokker T, Bal E, Ernst S, Gin MTJ, Ascoop C. Laser balloon angioplasty does not reduce restenosis rate in type A and B coronary lesions. *Circulation* 1990;**82(Suppl. III)**:313.

196. Hinohara T, Selmon MR, Robertson GC, Braden L, Simpson JS. Directional atherectomy. New approaches for treatment of obstructive coronary and peripheral vascular disease. *Circulation* 1990;**81(Suppl. IV)**:79-91.

197. Robertson GC, Hinohara T, Selmon MR, Johnson DE, Simpson JB. Directional coronary atherectomy. In Topol EJ (ed). *Textbook of interventional cardiology.* (Philadelphia: WB. Saunders), 1990:563-579.

198. Rowe MH, Robertson GC, Simpson JB, Selmon MR, Vetter JW, Braden LJ, Hinohara T. Amount of tissue remover by directional atherectomy. *Circulation* 1990;**82(Suppl. III)**:312.

199. Penny WF, Schmidt DA, Safian RD, Baim DS. Quantitation of tissue removal and luminal improvement following coronary atherectomy. *Circulation* 1990;**82(Suppl. III)**:623.

200. US Directional Coronary Atherectomy Investigator Group. Directional coronary atherectomy: Multicenter experience. *Circulation* 1990;**82(Suppl. III)**:71.

201. Robertson GC, Selmon MR, Hinohara T, Rowe MH, Leggett JH, Braden LJ, Simpson JB. The effect of lesion length on outcome of directional coronary atherectomy. *Circulation* 1990;**82(Suppl. III)**:623.

202. Ellis SG, DeCesare NB, Popma JJ, Ghazzal ZMB, Pinkerton CA, Kereiakes DJ, Holmes DR, Topol EJ. Quantitative core lab analysis of directional coronary atherectomy (DCA) results: relation to lesion morphology and operator experience. *Circulation* 1990;**82(Suppl. III)**:311.

203. US Directional Coronary Atherectomy Investigator Group. Complications of directional coronary atherectomy in a multicenter experience. *Circulation* 1990;**82(Suppl. III)**;311.

204. Simpson JB, Robertson GC, Selmon MR, Sipperly ME, Braden LJ, Hinohara T. Restenosis following successful directional coronary atherectomy. *Circulation* 1989;**80(Suppl. III)**:582.

205. Hinohara T, Rowe MH, Robertson GC, Selmon MR, Leggett JH, Braden LJ, Simpson JB. Comparison of outcome of directional coronary atherectomy in de novo lesions and restenosed ledions. *Circulation* 1990;**82(Suppl. III)**:624.

206. Safian RD, Gelbfish JS, Erny RE, Schnin SJ, Schmidt DA, Baim DS. Coronary atherectomy. Clinical, angiographic, and histological findings and observations regarding potential mechanisms. *Circulation* 1990;**82**:69-79.

207. Kaufmann UP, Garratt KN, Vlietstra RE, Holmes DR. Transluminal atherectomy of saphenous vein aortocoronary bypass grafts. *Am J Cardiol* 1990;**65**:1430-1433.

208. Robertson GC, Rowe MH, Selmon MR, Hinohara T, Vetter JW, Braden LJ, Simpson JB. Directional coronary atherectomy for lesions with complex morphology. *Circulation* 1990;**82(Suppl. III)**:312.

209. Whitlow PL, Robertson GC, Rowe MH, Douglas JS, Cowley MJ, Kereiakes DJ, Smucker ML, Hartzler GO, Hinohara T. Directional coronary atherectomy for failed percutaneous transluminal coronary angioplasty. *Circulation* 1990;**82(Suppl. III)**:1
210. Bell MR, Kaufman UP, Vlietstra RE, Holmes DR. Combined percutaneous coronary atherectomy and coronary angioplasty: Experience in 19 consecutive patients. *J Am Coll Cardiol* 1990;**15**:1146-1150.
211. Dick RJ, Haudenschild CC, Popma JJ, Yakubov SJ, Topol EJ. Insights from quantitative histological analysis of excisional atherectomy specimens. *Circulation* 1990;**82(Suppl. III)**:311.
212. Emy RE, Gelbfish JS, Safian RD, Diver DJ, Baim DS. Does tissue removal explain all atherectomy improvement? *Circulation* 1989;**80(Suppl. II)**:582.
213. Safian RD, Gelbfish JS, Erny RE, Schnitt S, Baim DS. Histologic findings of coronary atherectomy. *Circulation* 1989;**80(Suppl II)**:583.
214. Dick RJ, Kunkel JF, Debowey DL. Does ectasia following directed coronary atherectomy predict the histological depth of excision? *Circulation* 1990;**82(Suppl. III)**:623.
215. Selmon MR, Robertson GC, Simpson JB, Rowe MH, Johnson DE, Leggett JH, Hinohara T. Retrieval of media and adventitia by directional coronary atherectomy and angiographic correlation. *Circulation* 1990;**82(Suppl. III)**:624.
216. Ahn SS, Auth DC, Marcus DR, Moore WS. Removal of focal atheromatous. lesions by angioscopically guided high speed rotary atherectomy. *J Vasc Surg* 1988;**7**:292-299.
217. Buchbinder M, O'Neill W, Warth D, Zacca N, Dietz U, Bertrand ME, Fourrier JL, Leon MB. Percutaneous coronary rotational ablation using the rotablator: results of a multicenter study. *Circulation* 1990;**82(Suppl. III)**:309.
218. Bertrand ME, Fourrier JL, Auth DC, Lablanche JM, Gommeaux AF. Percutaneous coronary rotational angioplasty. In Topol EJ (ed). *Textbook of interventional cardiology*. (Philadelphia: WB. Saunders), 1990:580-589.
219. Fourrier JL, Bertrand ME, Authl DC, Lablanche JM, Gommeaux A, Brunetaud JM. Percutaneous coronary rotationai angioplasty in humans: preliminary report. *J Am Coll Cardiol* 1989;**14**:1278-1282.
220. Niazi KA, Brodsky M, Friedman HZ, Gangadharan V, Choksi N, O'Neill WW. Restenosis after successful mechanical rotary atherectomy with the Auth rotablator. *J Am Coll Cardiol* 1990;**15**:57A.
221. Stack RS, Quigley PJ, Sketch MH, Newman GE, Phillips HR. Extraction atherectomy. In Topol EJ (ed). *Textbook of interventional cardiology*. (Philadelphia: WB. Saunders), 1990:590-602.
222. Sketch MH, O'Neill WW, Tcheng JE, Walker C, Galichia JP, Sawchak S, Cress S, Phillips HR, Stack RS. Early and late outcome following coronary transluminal. extraction-endarterectomy: A multicenter experience. *Circulation* 1990;**82(Suppl. III)**:310.
223. Grundfest W, Litvack F, Segalowitz J, Goldenberg T, Forrester JS. Angioscopy: Technical details and clinical applications. In Topol EJ (ed). *Textbook of interventional cardiology*. (Philadelphia: WB. Saunders), 1990:799-815.
224. Uchida Y, Hasegawa K, Kawamura K, Shibuya I. Angioscopic observation of the coronary luminal changes introduced by percutaneous transluminal coronary angioplasty. *Am Heart J* 1989;**117**:769-776.
225. Forrester JS, Litvack F, Grundfest W, Hickey A. A perspective of coronary artery disease seen through the arteries of living man. *Circulation* 1987;**75**:505-513.
226. Sherman CT, Litvack J, Grundfest WS, Lee M, Hickey A, Chaux A, Kass R, Blanche C, Matloff J, Morgenstern L, Ganz W, Swan HJC, Forrester JC. Coronary angioscopy in patients with unstable angina pectoris. *N Engl J Med* 1986;**315**:913-919.

227. Mizuno K, Miyamoto A, Satomura K, Shibuya T, Okamoto Y, Seguchi H, Isojima K, Kurita A, Arai T, Nakamura H. Angioscopic endothelial macropathology in patients with acute coronary syndromes. *J Am Coll Cardiol* 1989;**13:**14A.
228. Höher M, Hombach V, HOpp HW, Eggeling T, Kochs M, Amold G, Hannekum A, Hügel W. Diagnostische Bedeutung der Angioskopie bei Patienten mit koronarer Herzkrankheit. *Z Kardiol* 1988;**77:**152-159.
229. Grundfest WS, Litvack F, Glick D, Segalowitz J, Treiman R, Cohen L, Foran R, Levin P, Cossman D, Carroll R, Spigelman A, Forrester JS. Intraoperative decisions based on angioscopy in peripheral vascular surgery. *Circulation* 1988;**78(Suppl. I):**13-17.
230. Nissen SE, Gurley JC, Grines CL, Booth DC, Fischer C, DeMaria AN. Coronary atherosclerosis is frequently present at angiographically normal sites: evidence from intravascular ultrasound in man. *Circulation* 1990;**82(Suppl III):**459.
231. Bom N, Lancee CT, vanEgmond FC. An ultrasonic intracardiac scanner. *Ultrasonics* 1972;**10:**72-76.
232. Hodgson JMcB, Graham SP, Savakus AD, Dame SG, Stephens DN, Dhillon PS, Brands D, Sheehan H, Eberle MJ. Clinical percutaneous imaging of coronary anatomy using an over-the-wire ultrasound catheter system. *Int J Cardiac Imaging* 1989;**4:**187-193.
233. Nissen SE, Grines CL, Gurley JC, Sublett K, Haynie D, Diaz C, Booth DC, DeMaria AN. Application of a new phased-array ultrasound irnaging catheter in the assessment of vascular dimensions. *Circulation* 1990;**81:**660-666.
234. Pandian NG, Weintraub A, Kreis A, Schwartz SL, Konstam MA, Salem DN. Intracardiac, intravascular, two-dimensional, high frequency ultrasound imaging of pulmonary artery and its branches in humans and animals. *Circulation* 1990;**81:**2007-2012.
235. Yock PG, Linker DT, White NW, Rowe MH, Selmon MR, Robertson GC, Hinohara T, Simpson JB: Clinical applications of intravascular ultrasound imaging in atherectomy. *Int J Cardiac Imaging* 1989;**4:**117-125.
236. Gussenhoven WJ, Essed CE, Frietman P, Mastik F, Lance C, Slager C, Serruys P, Gerritsen P, Pieterman H, Bom N. Intravascular echographic assessment of vessel wall characteristics: A correlation with histology. *Int J Cardiac Imaging* 1989;**4:**105-116.
237. Siegel RJ, Fishbein MC, Chae JS, Potkin B, Berlin M, Helfant RH. Origin of the three-layered appearance of human arteries by ultrasound: Microdissection with ultrasonic and histologic correlation. *J Am Coll Cardiol* 1990;**15:**17A.
238. Davison CJ, Sheikh KH, Kisslo K, Gurbel PA, Tenaglia A, Sketch MH, Kisslo J. Intracoronary ultrasound evaluation of interventional procedures. *Circulation* 1990;**82 (Suppl. III):**440.
239. Weintraub A, Schwartz S, Pandian N. How reliable are intravascular ultrasound and fiberoptic angioscopy in the assessment of the presence and duration of intraarterial thrombosis in atheromatous vessels with complex plaques. *J Am Coll Cardiol* 1990;**15:**17A.
240. Fitzgerald PJ, Cogburn MA, Law WK, Hargrave VK, McKenzie JR, Belef WM, Yock PG. Determination of arterial wall components using intravascular ultrasound backscatter analysis. *Circulation* 1990;**82 (Suppl. III):**441.
241. Nishimura RA, Edwards WD, Warnes CA, Reeder GS, Holmes DR, Tajik AJ, Yock PG. Intravascular ultrasound imaging: In vitro validation and pathologic correlation. *J Am Coll Cardiol* 1990;**16:**145-154.
242. Tobis JM, Mallery JA, Gessert J, Griffith J, Mahon D, Bessen M, Moriuchi M, McLeay L, McRaej M, Henry WL. Intravaswlar ultrasound cross-sectional arterial imaging before and afler balloon angioplasty in Vitro. *Circulation* 1989;**80:**873-882.

243. Pandian N, Kreis A, Brockway B. Further validation of catheter-based intravascular ultrasound imaging in the detailed assessment of arterial size, shape, and wall thickness. *J Am Coll Cardiol* 1990;**15:**57A.
244. Chae JS, Potkin B, Helfant R, Siegel RJ. Potential limitations ot intravascular ultrasound imaging. *J Am Coll Cardiol* 1990;**15:**28A.
245. Gussenhoven E, Pijl A, Frietman P, Gerritsen P, Essed C, Roelandt J, Rijsterborgh H, Lancee C, van Egmond F, Bom N. Thinning of the media in atherosclerosis: an in vitro/in vivo intravascular echocardioaraphic study. *Circulation* 1990;**82 (Suppl. III):**458.
246. Werner GS, Sold G, Buchwald A, Kreuzer H, Wiegand V. Intravaskuläre Sonographie der Koronargefässe nach perkutaner transluminaler Angioplastie. *Dtsch Med Wschr* 1991;**116:**81-86.
247. Tobis JM, Mahon D, Lehmann K, Moriuchi M, Hoyne J, Henry WL. Intracoronary ultrasound imaging after balloon angioplasty. *Circulation* 1990;**82(Suppl. III)**:676
248. Yock PG, Fitzgerald PJ, Jang YT, McKenzie J, Belef M, Starksen N, White NW, Linker DT, Simpson JB. Initial trials of a combined ultrasound imaging/mechanical atherectomy catheter. *J Am Coll Cardiol* 1990;**15**:105A.
249. Hodgson JM, Cacchione JG, Berry J, Savakus A, Eberle M. Combined intracoronary ultrasound imaging and angioplasty catheter: initial in-vivo studies. *Circulation* 1990;**82(Suppl. III)**:676.
250. Siegel RJ, Chae JS, Forrester JS, Ruiz CE. Angiography, angioscopy, and ultrasound imaging before and after percutaneous balloon angioplasty. *Am Heart J* 1990;**120:**1086-1090.
251. St Goar FG, Ginsberg R, Mehigan JT, Alderman EL, Popp RL. Intravascular ultrasound evaluation of interventional procedures: Comparison with fiberoptic angioscopy. *J Am Coll Cardiol* 1990;**15**:254A.
252. Siegel RJ, Fishbein MC, Chae JS, HeHant RJ, Hickey A, Forrester, JS. Comparative studies of angioscopy and ultrasound for the evaluation of arterial disease. *Echocardiography* 1990;**7:**495-502.
253. Block, PC. Coronary-artery stents and other endoluminal devices. *N Engl J Med* 1991;**324:**52-53,

Keyword Index

I

J

K

L